Punish and critique

Over the past twenty-five years, a range of critical – that is, Marxist, poststructuralist and, less frequently, feminist – perspectives has been brought to bear on the subject of punishment and, in particular, on the question of imprisonment in Western capitalist societies. Considered together, these critical views constitute a formidable challenge to traditional ways of conceptualising punishment. Yet, for all the advances made, the new critical perspectives remain deeply flawed in a significant, but as yet barely acknowledged, way – with very few exceptions they are profoundly masculinist. *Punish and Critique* begins the task of exploring what a theoretically-informed feminist analysis of penality might look like and, in the process, uncovers a series of disjunctions in the recent critical analyses – for example, disjunctions between 'social histories' of prison regimes imposed on men and feminist histories of the imprisonment of women. Most crucially, the book unveils a radical disengagement between two current critical theoretical projects: masculinist studies of the emergence of punishment regimes in the context of the state's power to punish, and feminist studies, which map the differential impact of disciplinary power on lived female bodies.

In *Punish and Critique* Adrian Howe argues that a more fully social understanding of punishment must be informed by feminist research on women's imprisonment and by poststructuralist studies of the disciplining of women's bodies.

Punish and Critique will be invaluable reading to all students, lecturers and professionals in criminology, women's studies and sociology as well as to those working in prisons and the probation service.

Adrian Howe is Lecturer in Legal Studies at La Trobe University, Australia.

SOCIOLOGY OF LAW AND CRIME

Editors: Maureen Cain, *University of the West Indies*
Carol Smart, *University of Leeds*

This new series presents the latest critical and international scholarship in sociology, legal theory, and criminology. Books in the series will integrate the sociology of law and the sociology of crime, extending beyond both disciplines to analyse the distribution of power. Realist, critical, and postmodern approaches will be central to the series, while the major substantive themes will be gender, class, and race as they affect and, in turn, are shaped by legal relations. Throughout, the series will present fresh theoretical interpretations based on the latest empirical research. Books for early publication in the series deal with such controversial issues as child custody, criminal and penal policy, and alternative legal theory.

Titles in this series include:

Child custody and the politics of gender
Carol Smart and Selma Sevenhuijsen (eds)

Feminism and the power of the law
Carol Smart

Offending women
Anne Worrall

Femininity in dissent
Alison Young

Jurisprudence as ideology
Valerie Kerruish

The mythology of modern law
Peter Fitzpatrick

Interrogating incest
Vikki Bell

Punish and critique

Towards a feminist analysis of penality

Adrian Howe

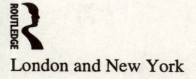

London and New York

First published 1994
by Routledge
11 New Fetter Lane, London EC4P 4EE

Simultaneously published in the USA and Canada
by Routledge
29 West 35th Street, New York, NY 10001

Typeset in Times by LaserScript, Mitcham, Surrey
Printed and bound in Great Britain by
Mackays of Chatham PLC, Chatham, Kent

British Library Cataloguing in Publication Data
A catalogue record for this book is available from the British Library

Library of Congress Cataloging in Publication Data
Howe, Adrian.
  Punish and critique: towards a feminist analysis of penality/
  Adrian Howe.
  p. cm. – (Sociology of law and crime)
  Includes bibliographical references and index.
  1. Punishment – Philosophy. 2. Imprisonment – Philosophy.
  3. Feminist theory. 4. Women prisoners. I. Title. II. Series.
  HV8693.H69   1994
  364.6 – dc20   93-36845
                                                            CIP

ISBN 0–415–05190–8 (hbk)
ISBN 0–415–05191–6 (pbk)

To the memory of my mother, Tony Howe

Contents

Series editor's preface

Maureen Cain and I have awaited the publication of this book for some time. It was Maureen who first discussed the fledgling project with Adrian Howe, but I eagerly took over as the editor designated to work with Adrian when logistics changed at an early stage in the book's development. It is a book which has been well worth waiting for.

Punish and Critique is a conversation. In saying this I mean to invoke a number of things. First, Adrian converses with her readers, adopting a style which immediately involves one in her project and which regularly foregrounds her presence as 'author'. This has the effect of making the original exercise of writing and the subsequent exercise of reading feel like a joint project. One feels as if one is on a voyage of discovery with the author rather than a passive recipient of her wisdom.

Second, *Punish and Critique* is a conversation with the ideas of other authors. There is criticism here, but none of the 'search and destroy' strategies which often accompany academic exegeses of competing analysis. And finally, it is a conversation with feminist policies which seeks to affirm the continuing possibility of such a politics under postmodern conditions.

The main contribution of this book, of course, lies in its ability to force our thinking about penalty into a confrontation with the idea of gender and with gendering practices of the late twentieth century. Adrian refers to the study of prisons and punishment as having been an 'impenetrable masculine fortress'; a site of knowledge production impervious to the tides of feminism washing over the rest of criminology and sociology. But she does not seek merely to insert women into this fortress, she aims to shift the ground of the debate altogether. Her main achievement is to argue for a blurring of the boundaries between policing and punishment; to take seriously Foucault's idea of the carceral archipelago and to look beyond the prison to find penality. If we assume that penality is only a feature of the prison, she shows that we cannot begin to appreciate the significance of gender. And, when she uses the term gender, she emphatically does not mean women. It is her argument that we need to consider fully the 'gendered characteristics of disciplinary procedures'. We are therefore talking of the construction of masculinities as well as femininities.

It is not, of course, unusual for feminists to argue that we must go beyond the additive approach to the inclusion of gender into frameworks originally conceptualised without an inkling of the existence of women, let alone gender relations. But Adrian goes far beyond this demand and starts to construct an alternative gendered vision of what she calls the punishment continuum. This should not worry the reader who is only at the foothills of feminist thought. A major strength of Adrian's conversational style is that she takes us through conventional thinking in penology and gradually builds her case for a postmodern penal politics. She is therefore able to achieve two goals. The first is to meet the needs of students who will wish to understand what is being critiqued before it is subjected to scrutiny, the second is to produce a text which satisfies readers who are already immersed in theoretical debate about how to advance feminist thinking in this field. This is a rare achievement.

Punish and Critique was, as Adrian points out, originally intended as a feminist equivalent to *The New Criminology* but in the field of penology/penality. Its original aim was to provide a text which would allow students to think beyond the existing paradigmatic framework of the field. The field of prisons and punishment has been remarkably difficult to recast and those of us who teach in the area have almost despaired of finding a text which does the theoretical work necessary to allow for a paradigmatic shift. Inasmuch as *The New Criminology* achieved this for criminology, *Punish and Critique* does follow in its tradition but, unlike *The New Criminology*, it provides more grounding in new modes of conceptualisation.

Punish and Critique is not a finished project – it is better to think of it as an ongoing conversation which calls for further debate and elaboration. It has, however, opened what was a closed door for theorising about gender. Adrian invites feminists to focus more on penality, and penologists/criminologists to take a theoretical leap forward to meet feminist theory where it currently resides (rather than on the laboured terrain of feminist empiricism). As David Garland has argued, we still need to strive for a more fully social theory of punishment, but as Adrian would suggest, we can hardly do this if we theorise the social as ungendered. Adrian Howe gives us the means to resolve this impasse and both Maureen Cain and I hope that students and teachers alike will be able to take advantage of this transgressive text.

Carol Smart
May 1994

Acknowledgements

The writing of this book was supported by a Fulbright Postdoctoral Fellow-ship to the United States in 1988. In connection with this award, I would like to thank Martha Fineman for organising a fellowship at the Law School, University of Wisconsin (Madison), and the Anthropology Depart-ment of John Jay College, New York, and Susan Silbey, Sociology, Wellesley College, for providing office space. I owe a special thanks to the books series editors: Maureen Cain for suggesting the book project on penology to me, and Carol Smart for her invaluable editorial suggestions, her patience and her postmodern faith that this book would eventually emerge. I thank Adele Murdolo for her incisive comments on sections of the manuscript, for proof-reading and for everything else. And finally, I thank all my undergraduate and postgraduate students for supportively, or not, punishing me with critique.

As a contribution to the project of merging theory and practice in the field of penality, the royalties from the sale of this book will be donated to the Women Against Prison Collective in Victoria, Australia.

Introduction

This book started off as a different project. It was to have been a kind of sister book to Taylor, Walton and Young's *The New Criminology* (1973). Its task was to do for the study of punishment what that book had done for studies of criminality. In retrospect, *The New Criminology* was more of a cumulative critique of the old than a programmatic statement of the new, but it did put enough new critical perspectives together on what was then called 'deviance' to make a substantial contribution to the rupturing of the positivistic framework of crime's master discipline, criminology. Fifteen years later, when this book project was conceived, it seemed appropriate to take a similar critical approach to penological analyses of punishment, but to do so from a feminist perspective, thereby correcting Taylor, Walton and Young's masculinist bias – a bias which precluded any chance of their realising that 'fully social theory of deviance' which they thought they were marching towards. The time seemed to be ripe to move beyond a theoretical framework in which it could be concluded that:

> men are now consciously involved (in the prisons that are contemporary society and in the real prisons) in asserting their human diversity. The task is not merely to 'penetrate' these problems . . . . The task is to create a society in which the facts of human diversity . . . are not subject to the power to criminalise.
>
> (Taylor, Walton and Young 1973: 282)

Men? Asserting their human diversity? Freedom from the power to criminalise? By the late 1980s this would simply not do. The analytical framework of *The New Criminology* cried out for feminist revision.

My book project, which was provisionally and predictably titled *The New Penology*, was not to be deterred by the fact that the devastating critiques and paradigm-shifts launched by the new criminologies and post-criminologies in the 1970s and 1980s had not succeeded in displacing positivistic criminology from its place of hegemonic preeminence in both common sense and 'expert' discourses about crime in Western societies. Regardless of that 'failure', the goal was to build on the critical groundswell which had begun to problematise crime in the late 1960s, by widening the ambit of that challenge to include punishment and its master discipline, penology, and to do so from a feminist standpoint. This, then, was the initial plan, but the book resisted strenuously, refusing ultimately to deliver on such a little-sister, add-in-feminism correctionalist project, and after several time-consuming convolutions, it eventually emerged in a different form.

Over the past twenty-five years, a range of critical – that is, Marxist, poststructuralist and, less frequently, feminist – perspectives have been brought to bear on the subject of punishment and, in particular, on the question of imprisonment in Western capitalist societies. Considered together, these critical views constitute a formidable challenge to traditional ways of conceptualising punishment. To keep one's critical credentials intact, one does not step out today to discuss the penal question without being able to cite *Discipline and Punish* at will. A familiarity with the political economies of punishment which have proliferated over the last two decades is also a requirement for the informed critical analyst. And yet, for all the advances made, the new critical perspectives on punishment remain deeply flawed in a significant, but as yet barely acknowledged way – they are, with very few exceptions, profoundly masculinist. The problem is not simply that the new theorisations of punishment ignore women or treat them as footnotes to the main event – the punishment of men; they also overlook the question of gender, or better still, the deeply sexed nature of punishment regimes and, by extension, their own analytical frameworks.

Here feminist analysts have stepped into the breach, conducting their own independent studies of penal regimes imposed on women. Alternatively, feminist scholars informed by postmodern theories have seized hold of the insights of critical androcentric writers, especially Michel Foucault, in order to chart the impact of disciplinary power on female bodies. In this, they have followed a lead from the master himself to move away from penality in the strict sense. For what Foucault had in mind in *Discipline and Punish* was an analysis of penality in which the carceral circle widened to the point where the form of the prison disappeared altogether. His agenda was to map all the disciplinary mechanisms which operate throughout Western society. However, while feminist analysts have cultivated the disciplinary axis of Foucault's new schema, extending it to the question of the sexed female body, they have for the most part ignored his ideas about 'the punishment–body relation'. Thus, while Foucauldian feminist studies of disciplinary regimes imposed on women have a potentiality to break out of conventional conceptualisations of punishment

– to transgress the boundaries of customary punishment discourse by reconceptualising the object of analysis – punishment per se has remained imprisoned within a masculinist theoretical stronghold. This has resulted in a radical disjunction between two critical theoretical projects: the masculinist one of analysing the emergence of punishment regimes in the context of the state's power to punish, and the feminist one of mapping the differential impact of disciplinary power on lived female bodies.

Bearing all this in mind, this book project began, slowly but surely, to change its focal concerns. In the meantime, David Garland published *Punishment and Modern Society: A Study in Social Theory*, a text which might seem to have hijacked the space where my book should have been. In fact, Garland's theoretical and political agenda is very different from mine. Indeed, our approaches to the critical project – the interrogation and calling to account of punishment conceived as an object of knowledge – are diametrically opposed. Garland seems to believe that the critical project is exhausted. At least, he argues that it is time to move beyond an approach which emphasises the coercive aspects of punishment. Such 'power' perspectives are too one-sided. What is required in the 1990s is a synthesising approach, a balanced appraisal of diverse perspectives, an 'analytical pluralism' no less, which takes account of 'moral values and sensibilities' in Western societies. 'Social', even 'cultural' and evidently universalising, ungendered, non-racist and non-ethnocentric 'modern sensibilities' are here returned to the analytical fold. What we need now, according to Garland, is an integrative approach setting out the 'social' foundations and 'social' significance of punishment (1990a: 1–2). In my view, this kind of synthesising, post-critical perspective – one which overlooks a wide range of transgressive feminist approaches to the question of the social control of women in Western societies – has the effect of foreclosing the development of a properly-grounded and *fully* critical paradigm. Much more still needs to be done to assist punishment, conceptualised as an object of knowledge, to break out of the confining claustrophobia of penology's narrow, positivistic obsession with competing treatment programmes and penal ideologies, and also from idealist philosophy's relentless repetitions of the unholy trinity of retribution, deterrence and reform. Rather than succumbing to that post-critical synthesising urge, which is now venturing forth under the sign of 'the social', we need to question what it is which is 'social' about the supposedly 'social' historical and sociological analyses of punishment which have emerged over the last two decades – analyses which continue to ignore feminist interventions in the broad field of social control. The goal of this book then, is to pursue the critical project by pressing it into the service of those moving towards a theoretically-grounded feminist analysis of penality.

Over the last twenty years critical approaches to the penal question have done much to move punishment from the restricting confines of both penological and philosophical discourses to the more fertile fields of political economies of punishment and critical sociologies and histories of what came to be called, after Foucault, 'penality'. This movement was kick-started by the republication in 1968 of Rusche and Kirchheimer's ground-breaking effort to pin penal regimes firmly to the mast of a political economy framework. The year 1968, then, serves as a starting-date, inasmuch as most attempts to write political economies of punishment in Western societies acknowledge a debt to these two 'founding fathers'. These contributions to a critical understanding of punishment are considered in chapter 1. Chapter 2 reassesses the impact of the 'new' social histories of punishment regimes which emerged in the late 1970s and early 1980s. Chapter 3 pays tribute to the 'master' theorist of penality, Foucault, and reviews some of the Foucauldian approaches to punishment which followed in his wake. Chapter 4 turns to the question of the punishment of women, a question sadly neglected in masculinist accounts of penality. It focuses on studies of the imprisonment of women in Western societies. Chapter 5 assesses the potentiality of postmodern feminist interrogations of coercions placed on women's lives to transform our understanding of penality. Finally, chapter 6 tackles the vexed question of the relationship between theory and practice – that is, between the critical project which seeks to theorise penality in progressive ways, and those political movements committed to exposing and overturning harsh penal regimes wherever they exist.

1 Political economies of punishment

The year 1968 was a momentous one in the recent history of the politicisation and delegitimation of knowledge claims in the social sciences in the West. In particular, the fallout from the heady events of that year was to transform radically two of the disciplines most directly concerned with crime, punishment and social control – criminology and the so-called sociology of 'deviance'. Indeed, it ignited the movement which was to give birth to 'the new criminology'. The connectedness of the political struggles of the late 1960s with the transformation of these disciplines is well known. However, 1968 was critical for this knowledge field in another crucial but as yet largely unregistered way. The unsung, watershed event was the republication of a little-known 1939 text, Rusche and Kirchheimer's *Punishment and Social Structure*. Over the next two decades, this book was to achieve 'classic' status and, tellingly, the dubious distinction of being widely acclaimed as the 'seminal' text for critical analysis – especially Marxist analysis – within the newly emerging field of the sociological study of punishment. More, it is seen to have had a 'seminal influence' on that crucially significant movement from traditional, positivistic penology to the 'social analysis of penality' which would construct the penal realm as an object of knowledge in its own right (Garland and Young 1983: 5–7). Inasmuch as *Punishment and Social Structure* provides an important materialist interpretation of some of 'the master patterns' of social control in Western industrial societies (Cohen 1985: 13), this text has proved to be 'seminal' indeed. It has become the foundational text in the genre of prison writing which is the subject of this chapter, namely, political economies of punishment.

'FOUNDING FATHERS'

It is the rediscovery of *Punishment and Social Structure* in 1968, and not the text itself, which should be seen as the rupturing event enabling critical analyses of penality to emerge from the intellectual deadwood of traditional penology. When it was first published in 1939 in the United States it had little impact, remaining under-utilised and largely uncited by Western criminologists and penologists until it was re-published thirty years later. Moreover, the text itself may seem a curious choice as the key or foundation text for critical sociologies of punishment. As we shall see, the authors did not work on the book together or even consult each other. Consequently, the text is internally inconsistent and even contradictory. Indeed, Kirchheimer's chapters tend to undermine Rusche's carefully elaborated thesis, much to the latter's dismay. And as for the book's reputation as the foundation Marxist political economic account of punishment – Marx is cited once in the text and only fleetingly in the references. Yet in the 1970s, the Rusche–Kirchheimer thesis, as it came to be called, was to become the point of departure for a reconsideration of 'the penal question' within a determinedly materialist and political economic framework. Without question, the re-publication of *Punishment and Social Structure* in 1968 signified the emergence of a 'new concern with the formulation of a general, and genuinely political economic, theory of punishment' (Garton 1988: 311). More broadly, it opened the way for a new mode of critical sociological analysis which would liberate punishment from the restricting confines of penological and philosophical discourses.

To privilege *Punishment and Social Structure* as the starting-point for critical sociological studies of the penal realm is to invite controversy. No doubt it will be objected that there are other more deserving contenders for the honour of father – if father there must be – of a sociological analysis which takes punishment or 'penality' as a discrete object of knowledge. One possibility is Willem Bonger, the Dutch Marxist criminologist whose work, especially *Criminality and Economic Conditions* (1916), has received the ambivalent accolade of assuming 'the mantle of the Marxist orthodoxy' in the crime field 'if only because (with the exception of untranslated writers inside the Soviet bloc) no other self-proclaimed Marxist has devoted time to a full-scale study of the area' (Taylor, Walton and Young, 1973: 222). But it is precisely Bonger's concern with crime, specifically with how economic conditions in capitalist societies produce crime, which eliminates him as a candidate for founder of critical sociologies of punishment. Not only did he fail to transform punishment into an analytical field; his ideas on social control and penal law were undeveloped and failed to advance a Marxist theory of punishment (1973: 230–2).

The Bolshevik legal scholar, Pashukanis, deserves more serious consideration. As we shall see, his thesis in *Law and Marxism: A General Theory* (1978) about the emergence of the specific form of capitalist punishment, has received much critical acclaim from Marxist legal analysts over the past decade. Moreover, they have drawn on Pashukanis's work to elaborate a more precise Marxist theory of capitalist penal forms than the Rusche–Kurchheimer thesis allows. Yet if Rusche and Kirchheimer 'did not use and probably did not know of Pashukanis's work' (Melossi 1978: 75), it is also the case that critical analysis of his work in Western Europe and North America postdated that of Rusche and Kirchheimer. The 1968 re-publication of *Punishment and Social Structure* catapulted this German work to front-runner status in the field, while the Pashukanis revival was to await the 1978 English translation of *Law and Marxism: A General Theory*.

The third and final contender for line honours as founding father of critical sociological studies of the penal realm is that sine qua non of sociological exegesis – Emile Durkheim. While his work has traditionally been the key reference point for the sociology of punishment, it may seem paradoxical that Durkheim, a non-Marxist, has been seriously considered as a founder of a critical sociological approach to the subject. However, Marxist and other critical analysts have closely scrutinised Durkheim's work on crime and punishment for sociological insights and, somewhat surprisingly, several claim to have found some. For example, Taylor, Walton and Young reclaimed Durkheim as a 'radical', a worthy forerunner of the 'New Criminology', one who broke with the 'analytical individualism' of social contract theory and with positivism (1973: 67–73). But it is not only Durkheim's work on crime, in particular his concept of 'anomie' and his notion of the 'normality' of crime which has attracted the attention of critical scholars: there has also been a resurgence of interest in those aspects of his work dealing with the links between punishment and social structure.

Here David Garland is a prominent admirer. Notwithstanding his damaging critique of Durkheim's theoretical account of law, punishment and the state, Garland still finds a purchase in his work, and has set about the task of 'rehabilitating Durkheim'. It is a strange rehabilitation. On the one hand, he argues that Durkheim's 'positions' on the subject of the form, history and social significance of punishment are incoherent, even contradictory, and that, moreover, 'Durkheimian concepts arbitrarily close off certain crucial questions concerning punishment' (Garland 1983a: 37). He warns that Durkheim's conception of punishment as 'unitary, essentialist and of a singular and pre-given significance' forecloses empirical investigation and radically limits the questions which need to be asked about the complex nature of diverse penal practices and discourses. Indeed, anyone wishing to understand this complexity 'would be advised to look elsewhere' as punishment was 'not a serious object of analysis at all' for Durkheim.

To those looking for the theoretical tools to guide political intervention, one can only say that Durkheim's theory of punishment renders any such intervention all but unthinkable.

(Garland 1983a: 58)

On the other hand, while Garland concedes that there is 'little prospect of a reformed Durkheimian sociology of punishment', he nevertheless maintains that there are 'progressive and important elements in Durkheim's work' which make it 'an indispensable resource'. Most importantly, Durkheim's approach is seen to have been 'doggedly social and historical': he insisted on the social construction of penal technologies and his historical method was 'materialist' and 'non-functionalist' in that it sought to explain institutions in terms of their 'necessary conditions'. To quote Durkheim's famous 1899 essay, 'The two laws of penal evolution':

> To explain an institution, it is not enough to establish that when it appeared it served some useful end; for just because it was desirable it does not follow that it was possible. In addition, one must discover how the necessary conditions for the realisation of that goal came into existence.

(Durkheim 1973: 297)

Equally significant, Durkheim, according to Garland, understood punishment to be 'both positive and productive'. That is, Durkheim saw that punishment was not merely a negative response to crime; punishment actually constituted crime – defined what is criminal – and had positive social effects such as reinforcing solidarity by symbolically displaying the collective sentiments. Finally, Garland credits Durkheim's recognition of the crucial ideological and symbolic significance of penal law with opening up an important area of analysis in which punishment becomes 'a system of signs' (Garland 1983a: 58–9).

For Garland, the recognition of 'the positivity of punishment' – 'the necessary first principle of any social analysis of penality' – is Durkheim's most important contribution to the field. Moreover, he maintains that it is one which is 'rarely accredited, even when subsequently rediscovered' by Rusche and Kirchheimer and then later by Foucault (1983a: 59). Accordingly, by the time he came to write *Punishment and Modern Society*, Garland devoted two chapters to reworking 'the Durkheimian legacy'. Here Durkheim is accorded legendary status, but in a manner which appears to contradict Garland's earlier assessment of this founding father's failure to take punishment as a serious object of analysis.

> More than any other social theorist, Durkheim took punishment to be a central object of sociological analysis and he accorded it a privileged place in his theoretical framework . . .

(1990a: 23)

And

> Durkheim's questions about the moral basis of penal law, about the involvement of onlookers in the penal process, about the symbolic meanings of penal rituals, and about the relationship of penal institutions to public sentiment, are all questions which are worthy of our close attention, even when the answers which Durkheim suggests are not themselves convincing.
>
> (1990a: 27)

Finally, Durkheim's reading of punishment as a moral process 'opens up important aspects of the penal complex and reveals dynamics and dimensions which are not otherwise visible' (1990a: 47).

Garland, then, makes a strong case for Durkheim as founding father in the field of penality. Interestingly, Garland is supported in this view by Steven Spitzer, a leading Marxist sociologist of law. Spitzer also believes that Durkheim should be reclaimed. In his view, critical analysts, such as Steven Lukes and Andrew Scull, have failed to provide a 'positive appreciation' of Durkheim's contribution to the sociology of law and punishment. In particular, they have failed to recognise a number of important 'tendencies' in Durkheim's thought – tendencies which 'could contribute to a truly critical understanding of the dialectical relationship between "laws" and "societies"'. These 'tendencies' include Durkheim's attention to the positive and productive nature of legal controls (Spitzer 1984: 864–5). According to Lukes and Scull, Durkheim's focus on the 'negative and constraining aspects' of law 'precluded any systematic inquiry into its positive or enabling aspects' (Lukes and Scull 1983: 7). In contrast, Spitzer, following Garland, claims that Durkheim's recognition of the positive effects of punishment established a mode of analysis which others (again, Rusche, Kirchheimer and Foucault) would follow (Spitzer 1984: 866).

Spitzer's spirited defence of Durkheim's founding role in the sociology of punishment is all the more remarkable when juxtaposed with his earlier empirical critique of Durkheim's theory of penal evolution. Briefly, Durkheim proposed that changing modes of punishment are linked to transformations in the nature of social structure. As societies become more complex and differentiated – to Durkheim, as they evolve from 'mechanical' to 'organic' solidarity – penal sanctions become less severe. More specifically, repressive (penal) law which reinforces mechanical solidarity is replaced by restitutive (civil) law which facilitates organic solidarity. Durkheim also claimed that as society became more complex, individual crimes – crimes against the person – come to replace collective crimes such as sacrilege and blasphemy. And finally, he proposed that deprivation of liberty, which he equated with incarceration, tends to become the dominant sanction in complex societies (Durkheim 1964; 1973). However, subsequent research on penal evolution, Spitzer's included, has yielded findings which tend to contradict Durkheim's claims. In particular, Spitzer's study of penal evolution in forty-eight societies indicated that punishment did not become less severe as society became more complex. On the contrary, greater punitiveness is associated with higher levels of structural differentiation. Moreover, the evidence challenges the contention that offences against the collectivity disappeared as societies became more complex. Indeed, Spitzer found all of Durkheim's assertions about the evolution of penal sanctions wanting in empirical corroboration (Spitzer 1975a: 623–30).

Spitzer's critique was an important contribution to the debate about the validity and usefulness of Durkheim's work on punishment. Another debate has centred on Durkheim's suggestion that society's reliance on penal sanctions tends towards a state of equilibrium – that is, a corollary to his notion that crime is both normal and functional for social solidarity is that the extent of crime in any society will be maintained at a stable level. This has led to the development of 'homeostatic' models which attempt to account for the 'constancy of punishment' by, for example, suggesting that oscillations in imprisonment rates are a manifestation of a homeostatic or self-regulating punishment process (Blumstein and Cohen 1973: 199). The details of these debates and the lines of division between Durkheim's supporters and his critics need not detain us.[1] Suffice it to note that Spitzer concluded his critique of Durkheim's propositions thus:

> Whatever its shortcomings, Durkheim's approach to the study of punishment provides a valuable model for the study of social control. In linking the nature of control to the organisation of society Durkheim makes explicit what too many investigators ignore – the fact that punishment is deeply-rooted in the structure of society.
>
> (Spitzer 1975a: 634)

Others, as we have seen, are less sanguine about the usefulness of Durkheim, even a rehabilitated Durkheim, for the sociology of punishment. Most damning, Durkheim is seen by his critics to have foreclosed important sociological questions about law by interpreting social solidarity as a 'completely moral phenomenon' – in his view law was always 'derivative from and expressive of a society's morality'. Moreover, in the process of elaborating his functionalist and organicist conception of society, Durkheim ignored power. Consequently, the limitations of Durkheim's view of law do not derive solely from his major errors of historical interpretation; his whole theory is no longer convincing (Lukes and Scull 1983). As such it scarcely warranted continuing attention. As one critic argued, Durkheim's attempt to render 'moral evolutionary beliefs into sociological propositions' was unsuccessful, flying in the face of the empirical evidence for the relationship between punishment and social order; and furthermore, his 'moral evolutionary' approach failed to question 'sociologically' his own assumptions about 'repression' and 'humanitarianism'.

> A *truly sociological* account of punitive practices must explain not only why certain forms are predominant under given social conditions but must also explain the nature and form of the penal and moral ideologies which justify and promote them.
>
> (O'Malley 1983: 149–50; my emphasis)

My main concern in all this is not to enter a debate of the 'tis/'tisn't kind about the most impressively credentialled 'founding father' of the sociology of punishment, let alone about the most 'truly' sociological, nor is it to arbitrate between conflicting assessments of the worth of Durkheim's potential as a critical theorist in the field. Rather, it is to comment that we can concede that Durkheim's proposals, even or perhaps especially those which are the most empirically or theoretically suspect, have proven fertile ground for further research, without overstating his contribution. For however many insights he provided into the connectedness of punishment and society, he remained locked within a moral evolutionary schema which failed, ultimately, to disconnect punishment from crime. While punishment was not, in his schema, a merely negative response to crime, it was still dependent on and inextricably linked to it.

> Since punishment results from crime and expresses the manner in which it affects the public conscience, it is in the evolution of crime that one must seek the cause determining the evolution of punishment.
>
> (Durkheim 1973: 300)

Furthermore, if Durkheim's work on the evolution of penal forms can be dismissed as not 'truly' sociological, the 'materialist' historical method which Garland attributes to him can just as readily be dismissed as not properly materialist. For example, the 'necessary conditions' – for Garland, the 'material conditions of possibility' (Garland 1983a: 59) – which must be considered to explain an institution turn out to be nothing more than the existence of 'sufficiently spacious public establishments, run on military lines, managed in such a manner as to prevent communications with the outside' (Durkheim 1973: 300). Thus are material conditions reduced to spatial possibilities in the Durkheimian 'materialist' framework of analysis. Consequently, whatever advances Durkheim made in understanding the 'positivity' of punishment, the emergence of a properly materialist history – one which would take account of political economy, of power, of class, and of labour relations and one which would also effect the great disconnection of crime and punishment, thereby enabling punishment to become a discrete object of knowledge – had to await the publication of Rusche and Kirchheimer's *Punishment and Social Structure*.

RUSCHE AND KIRCHHEIMER

Rusche versus Kirchheimer

In 1931 Georg Rusche submitted a research proposal to the Frankfurt Institute of Social Research. This proposal, which was to form the basis for *Punishment and Social Structure* which Rusche would 'co-author' with Otto Kirchhemier, took the form of a programmatic essay promising a new form of sociological research in the field of crime and punishment. Rusche began by stating that the study of crime and of crime control was a 'fruitful field for sociological research' inasmuch as they both 'compel an explanation derived from social relationships'. Moreover, crime and punishment illuminate those relationships. But if a properly sociological analysis was to emerge, we needed to move beyond ahistorical criminological studies which were not grounded in either the 'basic principles of sociological knowledge' or economic theory. In Rusche's view, analysis of the 'social function' of crime and punishment could be pushed 'far beyond previous research' if a few 'simple axioms of economic theory' and an historical approach were adopted. In brief, what was required was an 'economic-historical analysis' (Rusche 1978: 2–3).

Rusche's 'simple economic axioms' were 'the principle of less eligibility' and the category of the labour market. The less eligibility principle is that if penal sanctions are to deter 'the lower social classes which are the most criminally inclined' – those whose class, poverty and demoralisation drives them to crime – they must be worse than the living conditions of this 'lower strata'. Penal reforms are 'limited by the situation of the lowest socially significant proletarian class which society want to deter from criminal acts' (Rusche 1978: 4). As he had argued in his 1930 commentary on prison revolts in America, prison reform efforts which attempted to go beyond the less eligibility principle are 'inevitably condemned to Utopia' because of the need to deter: 'this law, which applies with a mathematical precision', was thus the key to understanding punishment (Rusche 1980: 42). This principle therefore became Rusche's 'principle of investigation' – his 'simple heuristic maxim' – one which, as he explained in his research proposal, functioned in relation to the state of the labour market:

the labour market is the determining category. The situation of the working class is different in an economy in which a large reserve army of starving proletariat follows the employers and drives the wage . . . down to a minimum, than in an economy in which workers are scarce . . .

(Rusche 1978: 4)

That is, in societies where workers are scarce, punishment is required to make the unwilling work, but when there is a 'reserve army' penal policy will take the form of harsh corporal and capital punishments. There is then a correspondence between labour market conditions and penal modes such that when the offender's labour is valuable, 'exploitation is preferred to capital punishment, and forced labour is the corresponding mode of punishment' (1978: 4–7).

This economic theory of punishment was, however, inadequate to understand penal forms: they had to be placed in an historical framework. Rusche was insistent on this point. To understand penal systems, 'economy theory has to be supplemented by a historical analysis'. Furthermore, it had to be a particular type of historical analysis. The legal historian's 'evolutionary conception' of the development of penal forms from a supposed 'barbaric cruelty' to humanitarianism had to be discarded because it was inaccurate. Penal history has been much less linear than this evolutionary schema implies. The task at hand was

to study the historical relationship between criminal law and economic, the history of class struggle, and to utilise these interrelationships to analyse the present prison system.

(Rusche 1978: 5)

This, then, was Rusche's original proposal. The tortuous process by which this proposal was transformed into a manuscript, translated into English, edited and re-written by a co-author not of Rusche's choosing has been reconstructed elsewhere (Melossi 1980). Suffice it to say here that Rusche was most unhappy with the finished product. Commenting on Kirchheimer's contribution to the text, he complained that it contained 'a number of weaknesses, which did not belong to the book and that I deplore very much' (quoted in Melossi 1980: 58). Rusche did not elaborate on his objections, leaving it to his biographer, Dario Melossi, to draw inferences from the fragmentary records. Melossi believes that Rusche had good cause to complain, as Kirchheimer's alterations 'produced a work split into two parts'. He surmises that while Kirchheimer may not have altered Rusche's original Chapters II to VII of *Punishment and Social Structure*, he most probably did rework a last section which Rusche almost definitely wrote on the contemporary situation in American prisons and in Nazi Germany. The Kirchheimer chapters not only ignored the kind of socioeconomic considerations which were central to Rusche's original proposal; they also shifted the emphasis from a socioeconomic to a political explanation of changing penal practices. Moreover, he removed any reference to contemporary American developments. But if, as Melossi suggests, Kirchheimer significantly changed Rusche's manuscript, eliminating his economistic, apparently 'Marxist' reading of American penal practices in order to avoid offending American intellectuals (1980: 56–7), the ploy was ineffective. With the exception of Thorsten Sellin, American criminologists and penologists ignored the book when it appeared in 1939, leaving it to languish until rediscovered thirty years later.

And yet, notwithstanding the problematic nature of *Punishment and Social Structure* – a text split in two halves with the second failing to expound the thesis developed in the first – and despite Rusche's anguish at the alterations and the subsequent neglect of the text, it was destined to be widely acclaimed as a 'classic'. By the 1970s, following its re-publication in 1968, it had become 'a classic macrosociological study of imprisonment' (Jacobs 1977: 90), a 'classic statement' of economic determinism (O'Brien 1978: 512), and even 'the most notable' example of a text attaining 'classic status' in the field (Downes 1988: 2). Certainly, it had become *the* definitive political economy of punishment, 'seminal' being the most common – and perhaps the most revealing – accolade.[2] But of all the critical acclaim showered on *Punishment and Social Structure* since 1968, the most noteworthy was surely that of Foucault, who wrote the text which has become the most influential late twentieth-century text on the question of punishment. In *Discipline and Punish: The Birth of the Prison* (1977a), a book which has transformed our understanding of the field which he redefined as 'penality', Foucault called *Punishment and Social Structure* a 'great work' – one which had provided 'a number of essential reference points'. Most important, in Foucault's assessment, it had taught us to 'rid ourselves of the illusion that penality is above all (if not exclusively) a means of reducing crime' (Foucault 1977a: 24).

Punishment and Social Structure

Turning to the text itself, we find Max Horkheimer's 'Preface' in which he assures us that while Rusche 'was not available for the reworking of his manuscript', Kirchheimer had retained 'in essence' the underlying concepts of Rusche's 1931 proposal in Chapters II to VIII (1968: ix–x). Then follows Kirchheimer's 'Introduction' setting out the ground-breaking theoretical propositions which so excited Foucault and others. These propositions develop, at times in an attenuated form, Rusche's original proposal. First, methodological considerations are raised. Forms of punishment must be studied in an historical context, not in a theoretical vacuum. Indeed, the neglect of 'the sociology of penal systems' can be attributed to the methodological hegemony of penal theories which are incapable of explaining the emergence of specific methods of punishment. Moral or 'absolute' juridical theories and 'teleological theories' which focused on 'real or hypostasised social needs' were to be avoided because they have had 'a negative influence on the historical-sociological analysis of penal methods'. What was required instead was 'a critical historical analysis', an 'historical conception of penology' which focused not on the idea but on specific methods of punishment (1968: 3–4).

Another practice to be avoided – one which Kirchheimer associated with Durkheim – was 'to limit oneself to a mere schema of the succession of historical manifestations, a mass of data supposedly bound together by the notion that they reveal progress' (1968: 4). In his starkest methodological directive for the development of a 'more fruitful approach to the sociology of penal systems', Kirchheimer emphasised the need to 'strip from the social institution of punishment its ideological veils and juristic appearance' in order to describe it in 'its real relationships'. Most crucially:

> The bond, transparent or not, that is supposed to exist between crime and punishment prevents any insight into the independent significance of the history of penal systems. It must be broken. Punishment is neither a simple consequence of crime, nor the reverse side of crime, nor a mere means which is determined by the end to be achieved. Punishment must be understood as a social phenomenon freed from both its juristic and its social ends.
>
> (1968: 5)

Having laid down the methodological imperatives of a properly constituted sociological analysis of punishment, Kirchheimer proceeded to set out the book's now classic propositions:

> Punishment as such does not exist; only concrete systems of punishment . . . . The object of our investigation, therefore, is punishment in its specific manifestations, the causes of its changes and developments, the grounds for the choice or rejection of specific penal methods in specific historical periods.

Then followed the fundamental premise in this materialist conception of penality: 'Every system of production tends to discover punishments which correspond to its productive relationships'. The origin and fate of penal systems are thus 'determined by social forces, above all by economic and then fiscal forces' (1968: 5). The force of these claims is however, somewhat diminished by Kirchheimer's declaration that 'the mere statement that specific forms of punishment correspond to a given stage of economic development is a truism' (1968: 6). For example, it is 'self-evident' that prison labour is impossible without manufacture or industry. Kirchheimer also foreshadows his view – one which differs substantially from Rusche's labour market paradigm – of the transition from competitive to monopoly capitalism. For Kirchheimer:

> the transition to modern industrial society, which demands the freedom of labour as a necessary condition for the productive employment of labour, reduced the economic role of convict labour to a minimum.
>
> (1968: 6–7)

Now 'fiscal motives' come to the fore and, as a result, 'the fine becomes the typical punishment of modern society'. Thus does Kirchheimer conclude the introduction, anticipating his chapters on the 'modern' period where the category of the labour market, central to Rusche's thesis, disappears. We can only presume that had Rusche been able to complete the book, he would have gone on testing his thesis concerning the fundamental relationship between the state of the labour market and penal forms (Melossi: 1978: 78; 1980: 56).

The substance of the book, the narrative history of punishment and social structure, is thus marred by a radical theoretical disjunction. But at least in Rusche's section – chapters II to VIII – the state of the labour market does operate as the central determinant in the history of punishment. Furthermore, these chapters follow the narrative outline of Rusche's original proposal in which penal history is divided into 'three epochs' characterised by entirely different systems of punishment – penance and fines in the early Middle Ages; a harsh regime of corporal and capital punishments in the late Middle Ages and, his main focus, imprisonment from the seventeenth century. Rusche had posed the argument for economic determination forcefully in his proposal: the early medieval system of fines and penance 'corresponded to the needs of a thinly populated peasant economy' (Rusche 1978: 6). This claim is modified (courtesy of Kirchheimer?) in the book to: 'different penal systems and their variations are closely related to the phases of economic development' (1968: 8). Still, enough of the class analysis of Rusche's materialist framework is retained for us to recognise it as 'authentically' Ruschean.

Labour markets and penal history

As Rusche tells the story, an abundance of land and a labour shortage gave rise to a relatively lenient penal system in thirteenth-century Europe. By the fifteenth century, however, the beginnings of the development of a capitalist form of production led to a drop in wages, intense class conflict and an increase in crime amongst a newly emerging impoverished urban proletariat. Because there was now a labour surplus, labour, and therefore human life, was no longer valued. Consequently, punishments become harsher, with mutilations and death sentences increasing markedly over the sixteenth century (1968: 8–22). With the rise of mercantilism in the late sixteenth century, the conditions of the labour market again change fundamentally. New labour shortages and increased wages led capitalists to turn to the state to find new means to control and exploit labour. New forms of punishment – galley slavery, transportation and penal servitude at hard labour in houses of correction – therefore focused on enforcing labour. The emergence of new capitalist labour market conditions in the eighteenth century, however, forced further changes in penal forms. The prison now emerged as the dominant mode of punishment (1968: 24–5).

While houses of correction were established in the seventeenth century when labour market conditions were favourable to the 'lower classes', the emergence of an industrial reserve army led to the establishment of national prison systems in Europe in the nineteenth century based on the famous 'less eligibility' principle – 'the leitmotiv of all prison administrations down to the present time' (1968: 94). Conditions in the prison had to be worse than those of the 'lowest class' of labourers to force them to work. The advance of the industrial revolution in the early nineteenth century, especially in England, impoverished the proletariat and drove them to crime. This 'opened the way for new deterrence regimes' (1968: 112). As labour was no longer scarce, the unemployed were crowded into prisons which became places of torture instead of sites of labour exploitation. In the United States, on the other hand, labour market conditions were such that it was more profitable to turn prisons into factories and prisoners into productive labourers. American prison conditions were therefore generally less harsh in the nineteenth century (1968: 111–32).

Rusche's chapters, then, are couched within a firmly materialist political economic framework. Thus for example, the late sixteenth-century changes to methods of punishment based on exploitation of prison labour were 'not the result of humanitarian considerations', but of economic developments which revealed the potential value of human labour at the disposal of the state (1968: 24). Again, the adoption of a 'more humane method for the repression of vagrancy' – the house of correction – at the end of the seventeenth century was 'the outcome of a change in general economic conditions'. More precisely, it was 'part of the development of capitalism' (1968: 41 and 50). And consistent with the thesis in his research proposal, changes in penal forms are related to changes in labour market conditions. For example, the history of English transportation provided 'a clear and straightforward picture of the effects of changing social and economic conditions on criminal policy': it arose to relieve seriously overcrowded prisons 'at a time when the labour market was oversupplied' (1968: 122). Most important, he argues that the modern prison system emerged in the mercantilist period as a method of exploiting labour and training new labour reserves: 'The early form of the modern prison was thus bound up with the manufacturing house of correction'. More broadly, the 'exploitation of labour was the decisive consideration' in the control of local 'problem populations' (1968: 64–5). Thus from the early Middle Ages to the mid-nineteenth century – the period covered by Rusche – the state of the labour market is seen to have determined the form and severity of punishment.

This Ruschean narrative framework has been profoundly influential in the development of the political economic approach to the sociology of punishment.[3] First, Rusche established the periodisation which has shaped the direction of materialist prison histories. While his periodisation was not explicitly Marxist – there are no references to the famous primitive accumulation chapters in *Capital* – Rusche's penal history clearly connected the emergence of various forms of punishment to the different phases of the development of a capitalist mode of production. Moreover, the key historical periods are those in which imprisonment emerges as the mode of punishment preferred by the bourgeoisie – the seventeenth century for the establishment of houses of corrections, the early nineteenth century for the coming of the penitentiary. These periods become the focal points of future analysis in the political economy tradition. Second, Rusche provided this tradition with a mode of analysis – a historical materialist analysis, focusing on links between changes in labour market conditions and changing penal forms.

But much more than this, Rusche established the vocabulary of the political economies of punishment which emerged in the 1970s and 1980s. While sympathetic critics would complain that Rusche's analysis was flawed by an 'incomplete inscription of punishment into the scientific categories of Marxism' (Melossi 1978: 77), his conceptualisation of the punishment problematic in terms of the less eligibility principle functioning in relation to the labour market came to determine in advance the kinds of claims which would be made in this field. Systems of production and corresponding modes of punishment, labour markets, surplus labour, forced labour, problem populations and the reserve army of labour became the language of the new materialist analyses of punishment. Thus it could well be said that Rusche provided an 'implicit grammar' – the 'grammar of punishment theory' – within which work which was to be taken seriously and recognised by others in this field had to operate (Simon 1985: 931–5).

Indeed, it could be said that Rusche provided the 'rules of formation' (Foucault 1973: xi) which defined the proper objects of a political economy of punishment.

POST-RUSCHEAN DEVELOPMENTS

Within a decade of the 'rediscovery' of *Punishment and Social Structure,* the book was to become one of the most cited texts in critical sociologies and revisionist histories of penality. If in British-based work this reference is more likely to be in passing, or even dismissive (e.g. Philips 1983: 53–4), elsewhere the Ruschean revival has led to several dominant lines of inquiry. While the biggest impact has been in the United States where it has spawned an industry of doctorates and empirical studies testing the Rusche–Kirchheimer model, as it has come to be called, the labour market thesis has also been critically assessed in Europe, Australia (e.g. Braithwaite 1980; Garton 1982 and 1988) and Latin America (Muñoz Gómez 1987). The central analytical focus of these post-Ruschean political economies of punishment has been imprisonment, the historically specific mode of punishment associated in their accounts with the emergence of capitalism. Imprisonment, moreover, is seen to require 'special attention', not only because it is 'the penal sanction par excellence', but also because it is crucial that we question the idea that this punishment 'is a natural and eternal kind of sanction' (Muñoz Gómez 1987: 63).

These analyses have taken three dominant forms – histories of the origin of the prison and its relationship with the emergence of a capitalist mode of production in North America and Europe; theoretical elaborations of Rusche's labour market thesis to account for twentieth century penal developments such as fluctuations in imprisonment rates, and empirical studies of the relationship between unemployment and imprisonment in advanced capitalist societies. In all of these applications and elaborations of the Rusche–Kirchheimer model, subsequent analysts have identified several problems with its 'labour control hypothesis' (Spitzer 1979: 210). Indeed, the most considered criticisms have come from sympathisers with the Ruschean-inspired political economy project. Their most common charge has been that of economism, with its related sins of reductionism and functionalism. More specific criticisms have been directed at the problems created for the labour market thesis by the continued use of imprisonment and also by the complex nature of penality in advanced capitalist societies. In their attempts to deal with these problems, critical analysts have refined and reformulated Rusche's original format for a political economy of punishment.

Economism

First, let us consider the general charge of economism. This problem was identified as early as 1939, when *Punishment and Social Structure* was first published. While he could not imagine a 'more potentially fruitful project for research', Jerome Hall felt that the book fell short of being a major contribution to the field because its propositions about social structure and historical analysis

> simmer down to 'economic' influence – and 'economic' becomes sometimes the conditions of the labour market, occasionally methods of production, often the bias of dominant economic classes – usually the bourgeoisie.

Consequently, Hall found it impossible to determine just what their thesis was, although the 'most persistent current' seemed to be 'Marxist determinism' – 'a particularist ideology which leaves them open to criticism' (Hall 1939: 972). The more recent version of this criticism is that Rusche and Kirchheimer 'fall into economic reductionism' in maintaining that penal sanctions vary according to the needs of the economy to control the labour force, and that, in particular, the penal system is functional in relation to the needs of capital. Implicitly they assume that the state

> can always be counted on to perceive what the economy needs, and will invariably succeed in translating the perceptions of these needs into penal policy. Needless to say, there is no sociological principle that guarantees such a sequence of events.
>
> (Greenberg 1980: 203)

As Spitzer points out, there is a certain irony in the fact that Rusche and Kirchheimer fall into economic reductionism given their insistence on historical contingency and specificity. They assert that each system of production 'calls forth' particular punitive forms which reflect its economic 'needs', and while these needs are presented as historically specific:

> the hypothesis is still based on the assumption that an isomorphism exists between the productive demands of an economic system and the varieties of punitive control that emerge within that system.
>
> (Spitzer 1979: 224)

Even more ironically, Rusche and Kirchheimer themselves warn against a reliance on 'teleological theories' which focus on 'real or hypostatised social needs' (1968: 3). Yet although the needs which they outline are not universalised as in structural-functional theory, they nevertheless assume that punishment is 'an interlocking part of a functionally integrated system'

(Spitzer 1979: 224). Furthermore, the Rusche–Kirchheimer model's economistic and mechanistic positing of a direct correspondence between economic change and penal developments is seen as highly problematic in that the relationship between the economy and punishment 'is always indirect at best'. More accurately, it is

> mediated by a number of different structures, processes and contra-dictions that make it impossible to precisely deduce the anatomy of the economic order from a study of punishment or vice versa.
>
> (1979: 225)

Developing this critique, Marxist analysts claim that the labour market model may 'fit', if not explain, penal relations during the mercantile period, but they argue that its theoretical limits are clearly exposed when applied to advanced capitalist societies. With the advent of capitalism 'penal relations can, in no sense, be seen to be central to, or directly linked with, the process of production'. Rather, as Russell Hogg argues, the penal system must be understood as 'a fundamentally ideological-political appa-ratus under capitalism' and any relationship it has with labour market conditions 'cannot be posed as a direct one, unmediated by the super-structure within which it is located' (Hogg 1980: 69). More broadly, Hogg argues that the reductionism which lies at the heart of the Rusche–Kirchheimer theory can be seen in its

> adherence to a conception of penal relations as forming some discrete (if determined) level of the social formation throughout history, and the attempt to specify in advance its relationship to the economy.
>
> (1980: 57)

This reductionism has the unfortunate consequence of leading to 'untheorised shifts in explanation' in which the primacy of the economic is displaced by bourgeois ideology. For example, when prisons cease to be productive – the point at which a direct correlation between the use of imprisonment and the labour market is no longer plausible – Rusche and Kirchheimer drop the labour market thesis in favour of an explanation in terms of the bourgeois ideology of deterrence (Rusche and Kirchheimer 1968: 109–13). As Hogg explains, this is 'wholly inadequate' because 'the articulation of penal relations within a social formation cannot be specified in advance by theory'. What is required is a 'concrete analysis of penal relations within determinate social formations', and not simplistic general-isations about correspondences between penal forms and the economy (Hogg 1980: 57–8).

Melossi

The most comprehensive critique of the Rusche–Kirchheimer model from within the political economy perspective is found in Dario Melossi's introduction to the Italian translation of *Punishment and Social Structure*. In this bid to rescue the model from charges of economism and reductionism, Melossi raises a number of historical questions which it failed to explain adequately. One of the key problems is the persistence of imprisonment when the economic necessity for the institution no longer exists. We need to explain:

> the stubborn persistence of the prison institution after the creation of the surplus population by the industrial revolution had rendered it useless, at least by strictly productive criteria.
>
> (Melossi 1978: 77)

Rusche and Kirchheimer had argued that the early forms of the prison were introduced to provide forced labour during the mercantilist period, but the question of the use or non-use of coerced labour was hardly applicable to modern capitalist systems of production which are characterised by a permanent oversupply of labour. Like other critics, Melossi blames Kirchheimer for the weaknesses in the analysis here. For example, his claim that solitary confinement, a typical feature of the nineteenth-century prison when prison labour became unproductive, was an 'irrational' residue from an earlier period (1968: 137), has been criticised as effectively arguing that Rusche's thesis was not applicable to advanced capitalism (Platt and Takagi 1980: 91). Extending this critique, Melossi takes Kirchheimer to task for failing to confront the implications of fundamental economic changes which occurred in capitalist societies in the second half of the nineteenth century. Instead of extending the labour market thesis to the period 1880–1930 covered by his chapters, Kirchheimer shifted away from a socioeconomic analysis to a consideration of political institutions (Melossi 1978: 78), thereby abandoning Rusche's labour market thesis.

But more fundamentally, Melossi questions the capacity of the category of the labour market to account for the adoption of imprisonment as the dominant mode of punishment under capitalism. In his view, this category reduces 'that very complex phenomenon which constitutes the making of a bourgeois mankind by means of those social institutions that are ancillary to the factory'. That is, the category of the labour market obscures the importance of ideology: it cannot explain 'the deep connection' between 'the ideology of an epoch' and 'corresponding penal ideologies'. Because the concept of labour market cannot account for the introduction of the prison at a specific historical moment, let alone explain its continued existence, Melossi turns to 'the category of discipline which speaks to the specificity of bourgeois punishment'. Inasmuch as the bourgeois concept of discipline 'came to be the essence of capitalist work management', it is crucial that we focus on ideological forms of discipline and, in particular, the ideological function of the prison (Melossi 1978: 75–7).

In this connection, Melossi also argued for the need to take account, as Pashukanis did, of the rise of the bourgeois concept of time as the abstract measure of the value of commodities. In his view, Pashukanis's analysis of the way this concept made possible the notion that punishment in the form of deprivation of liberty could be made proportional to the crime, deepened our understanding of the origins of the prison. By positing a deep structural connection between the principle of proportionality in punishment advocated by late nineteenth-century reformers and the development of industrial capitalism, Pashukanis addressed the specificity of the form of the prison:

> Deprivation of freedom for a period stipulated in the court sentence, is the specific form in which modern, that is to say, bourgeois-capitalist, criminal law embodies the principle of equivalent recompense. This form is unconsciously yet deeply linked with the conception of man in the abstract and abstract human labour measurable in time.
>
> (Pashukanis 1978: 180–1)

In short, the inclusion of these bourgeois concepts of time and discipline was essential in any properly grounded materialist analysis of the prison. They provided an understanding of the 'inner structure of the prison' as integral to a broader bourgeois programme in a way which the labour market thesis could not: changes in the labour market simply did not 'penetrate to the core of the matter' (Melossi 1978: 75–7).

Significantly, Melossi argues that the economism of *Punishment and Social Structure* is not the result of a failure to consider ideological issues, as non-Marxists would have it. On the contrary, it stems from 'the incomplete inscription of punishment into the scientific categories of Marxism' (1978: 77). That is, it is inadequately Marxist. Indeed, Melossi argues that while American criminologists may have found Rusche's theory too 'Marxist', the evidence suggests that Rusche's economic theory was more traditionally liberal than Marxist – the central role which he gave to the category of labour market being a case in point (Melossi 1980). Had Rusche paid more attention to Marx's *Capital*, he would have come to a fuller understanding of the penal question, for Marx clearly explained how 'the mystery of modern prisons is discovered in the factory' – specifically in the factory discipline which was 'necessary to the wage-labour system' (Melossi 1976: 27–30). For Melossi, a properly-grounded materialist theory is one which places the parallel development of the factory and the prison in the context of Marx's theory of primitive accumulation.

Two comments are salient here. First, Melossi is not attempting a refutation of the Rusche–Kirchheimer thesis; his aim is rather to extend their argument and overcome the limitations of their model by broadening the concept of labour market to incorporate an analysis of capitalist discipline as it spread out of the factory and became the means of governing all capitalist social relations. In his view, the concepts of discipline and labour market are not contradictory: after all, the capacity of the working class to resist capitalist discipline is determined by its strength on the labour market. Furthermore, on the question of the continued existence of the prison, Rusche and Kirchheimer may appear to have assumed a steady decline in the use of imprisonment and a corresponding increase in the use of the fine in advanced capitalist societies. But Melossi argues that they did not take a definitive position on twentieth-century trends, and that, in particular, their observations on declining prison populations in some European countries in the late nineteenth century are not intended as theorisations of new developments. Thus, empirical studies which find different penal patterns, particularly in the United States, do not refute their model: they merely indicate that conditions differ.[4] Nevertheless, for all this, it is critical that they failed to analyse 'the function of reproduction of labour power' which is fulfilled by the prison, a function 'strictly tying' it to 'the form of the factory, and to discipline as the capitalist management of labour'. For Melossi, such an analysis is vital if we are to adequately explain the persistence of the prison – an institution which is obsolete 'in its deep structural core' – in post-industrial societies (Melossi 1978: 80–1).

Second, Melossi turns to historical analysis to address this key problem of the 'stubborn persistence' of the prison in modern capitalist societies. The crucial issue is to explain 'why prison?' – why it is that

> in every industrial society, this institution has become the dominant punitive instrument to such an extent that prisons and punishment are commonly regarded as almost synonymous?
>
> (Melossi and Pavarini 1981: 1)

Melossi came to the conclusion that the answer must be sought in history. In collaboration with Massimo Pavarini, he therefore set out – in *The Prison and the Factory* – to find the connections between the rise of the capitalist mode of production and the historical origins of the modern prison (Melossi and Pavarini 1981). Inasmuch as their analysis takes this historical form and also as it is indebted to Foucault, it is more appropriately discussed in chapter 2 along with other historical accounts of the parallel emergence of the prison and capitalist societies. Here we are concerned with exploring attempts to elaborate post-Ruschean theoretical models in order to account for twentieth-century penal developments – developments which, interestingly, Rusche himself realised might require modifications to his labour market theory (Rusche 1978: 7; Melossi 1978: 79).

Surplus populations, imprisonment and advanced capitalist societies

Within the political economy approach, it is the persistence of the prison under the vastly changed economic conditions of advanced capitalist societies which has been identified as the central problematic. Indeed, most of the effort to construct a more rigorous materialist analysis has concentrated on addressing this problem. The key question here is: what is the function of the modern prison? Post-Ruschean attempts to answer this question may be roughly divided into two broad streams. First, there has been a return to Marx's analytical categories, in particular his notion of the function of the 'relative surplus population'. Second, attempts have been made to reformulate the labour market thesis into hypotheses which are then subjected to empirical analysis.

First let us consider the return to Marx. The reclamation of Marx's concept of 'surplus value' has been made simplistically, as in Richard Quinney's unsubstantiated assertions that criminal justice is 'the modern means of controlling the surplus population' and that 'the prison population increases as the rate of unemployment increases' (1980: 145–9). However, theoretical elaboration of the concept of surplus population has also been undertaken at a more sophisticated level – for example, in Muñoz Gomez's analysis of the way the prison functions in dependent capitalist economies as a 'silo for part of the surplus population' (Muñoz Gómez 1988: 76), and most notably, in Spitzer's now classic conceptualisation of this group as 'problem populations'. In Spitzer's theory of 'deviance production', 'deviants are culled from groups who create specific problems for those who rule'. Consequently, one of the most important functions of systems of class control is 'the regulation and management of problem populations' which 'threaten the social relations of production in capitalist societies'. These problem populations become 'eligible for management as deviant when they disturb, hinder or call into question' capitalist appropriations of 'the product of human labour' (Spitzer 1975b: 640–2). Surplus production and surplus populations become the major problems under monopoly capitalism and with the emergence of state capitalism, control functions are increasingly transferred from civil society to the state. That is, 'the state is forced to take a more direct and extensive role in the management of problem populations' to ensure stability in advanced capitalist societies (1975b: 647). Spitzer thus shifts attention away from an exclusive focus on economic conditions and the condition of the labour market to questions of state regulation and control.

This conceptualisation of the surplus population as a threat to social order which forces the state to take on a controlling role has been further elaborated by Mark Colvin. Building on Spitzer's theory, he has focused attention on the 'contradictory latent functions' which the prison serves in the modern capitalist era – functions which he claims interconnect with the control of a surplus population. Colvin argues that internal conflicts within the prison as well as changes in penal policies reflect a larger conflict between the opposing interests of the monopoly and competitive sectors of capital over policies for controlling the surplus population (Colvin 1981). To test this claim, he deduces several hypotheses focusing on the effect of monopolisation on imprisonment rates and welfare rates. For example, he hypothesises that the greater the degree of industrial monopolisation, the lower the annual rate of new prison commitments and the higher the rate of welfare recipients. As is usually the case in such studies, the results of his empirical tests confirm his hypotheses – industrial monopolisation is a greater predictor of rates of imprisonment than crime rates (Colvin 1986).

The hypothesis-testing methodology adopted by Colvin is the dominant mode of inquiry used by the second stream of post-Ruschean analyses of modern penality. These accounts can be construed as attempts to construct more precise, empirically-grounded labour market theories (Garton 1988: 314) in order to explain the continued use of imprisonment in advanced capitalist societies. They most commonly take the form of testing hypotheses about correlations between levels of unemployment and rates of imprisonment on empirical data. Here Ivan Jankovic's study, 'Labour market and imprisonment' (1977) – the first application and extension of Rusche's labour market theory – is classic. Inasmuch as this study set the agenda for empirical research in the field, it warrants a close analysis.

Jankovic

Jankovic was one of the first Marxist analysts to recognise the significance of Rusche and Kirchheimer's work in the sociology of punishment. Most important, they had departed from the dominant, common-sense conception of punishment as 'an epiphenomenon of crime, a reaction by the state to the criminal's breach of the legal order', and the related assumption that the primary function of punishment was 'to revenge, prevent and decrease crime'. By showing how penal policies were shaped by economic and political considerations, they had, in his view, successfully broken 'the supposed bond between crime and punishment'. Jankovic's aim was to 'further transcend' this supposed bond by examining punishment 'as an independent phenomenon in its relationships with the social and economic structure'. More specifically, he was concerned to provide a 'better explanation' of the continued use of imprisonment in advanced capitalist societies than the Rusche–Kirchheimer thesis allowed – with its conceptual reliance on the exploitation of convict labour. For if, as they claimed, 'every system of production tends to discover punishments which correspond to its productive relationships', it followed that imprisonment must be meeting some needs of advanced capitalist economies. Significantly, however, the explanation was still to be sought within the terms of the labour market theory: Jankovic's aim was none other than to explore 'the applicability of the Rusche–Kirchheimer theory to contemporary Western societies' and to examine alternative connections between the use of imprisonment and the labour market (Jankovic 1977: 17).

Jankovic had two main criticisms of this theory. First, Rusche, or rather Kirchheimer, overemphasised the fine as the typical twentieth-century capitalist punishment. Second and more critically, they failed to provide an explanation for the continued use of imprisonment – a punishment which did not seem to correspond to the productive relationships of advanced capitalism. Their model worked well when applied to pre-capitalist societies in which the exploitability of forced, productive labour was clearly a crucial determinant of modes of punishment, but not in post-industrial societies which are characterised by an oversupply of labour. Jankovic therefore turned to Marx's analysis of the 'reserve army of labour' which enabled him to suggest that rather than seeing imprisonment solely as a means of extracting forced labour from convicts, imprisonment in capitalist societies could be explained as a mechanism by which the state regulated the size of the surplus labour force (1977: 18–20).

Importantly, Jankovic does not abandon the Rusche–Kirchheimer model which he sees as containing implicit hypotheses which could be 'operationalised'. The 'severity' hypothesis predicts that punishment will be more severe during economic crises and is restated by Jankovic to suggest that prison populations will increase as unemployment increases, regardless of the volume of recorded crime. Thus, this hypothesis is operationalised in terms of the relationship between imprisonment and unemployment rates. The second hypothesis – the 'utility' hypothesis – predicts that imprisonment will be used to remove part of the surplus population from the labour market. This is operationalised in terms of the impact of imprisonment on unemployment (1977: 21–7).

To test these hypotheses, Jankovic deployed a multiple linear regression technique on data pertaining to unemployment and imprisonment rates in the United States for the period 1926–74. He found that while the utility hypothesis was not supported by the data, the relationship between unemployment and imprisonment was 'positive and statistically significant', regardless of the volume of crime', except during the Great Depression. While Jankovic conceded that his failure to confirm the utility hypothesis detracted from the significance of his confirmation of the severity hypothesis, he insisted that his findings lent support to the Rusche–Kirchheimer thesis. Most importantly, they demonstrated that the relationship between unemployment and imprisonment is 'a direct one, independent of the changes in criminal activity' (1977: 28).

Quantitative political economies

Independently of Jankovic's study, David Greenberg – in yet another 'seminal' and certainly much-cited paper, this time on the influence of 'exogenous variables' such as the business cycle on 'oscillatory punishment processes' – also found inspiration in the Rusche–Kirchheimer model. Interpreting that model as suggesting that the unemployment rate is the most useful indicator of the state of the economy, Greenberg hypothesised that prison rates would increase during periods of unemployment. This hypothesis was strongly confirmed with his Canadian data for the period 1945–59 (Greenberg 1977: 648). Moreover, he found, as Jankovic did, that changes in the crime rate seemed to be unimportant. Comparing similiar findings in the United States for the period 1960–72, Greenberg therefore concluded that in both countries 'changes in commitments to prison can be explained almost entirely by changes in the unemployment rate'. At the same time, he did not think his research supported Rusche and Kirchheimer's thesis that penal policies are governed by labour market considerations 'irrespective of the problems crime posed for society'. While such a proposal was not contradicted by his data, he thought it was 'implausible' for the period under consideration. After all, it was 'farfetched' to assume that Canadian and North American judges 'orient their sentencing policies to the requirments of the labour market'. Nevertheless, in finding the capitalist business cycle as well as class and class conflict to be 'directly relevant to an understanding of the functioning of the prison system' (1977: 650–1), Greenberg supported Rusche's thesis in principle. More importantly, he helped open a way for the analysis of punishment to burst out from the limitations imposed by so-called 'homeostatic models' of the punishment process – models which aimed to verify the Durkheimian functionalist and consensual 'stability' hypotheses that society is a normatively integrated self-regulating mechanism (e.g. Blumstein *et al.* 1976). Greenberg thus placed variables 'exogenous' to 'the crime-punishment system' on the interpretative map (Greenberg 1977 and 1980).[5]

These post-Ruschean studies by Jankovic and Greenberg have set the pattern for what seem to be interminable empirical excursions into the correlation between unemployment and imprisonment rates. Hypothesis testing, some variant of least squares regression, and time-series data have become part of the post-Ruschean political economy package deal for adventurers in search of the holy grail of the economic determinants of the modern prison. This format has been followed in several Western countries. For example, acknowledging the influence of the North American mode of analysis, Steven Box and Chris Hale developed a 'complementary radical position' which does not deny the possibility that crime rates increase with unemployment, but which nevertheless asserts that 'unemployment levels have an effect on the rate and severity of imprisonment *over and above* changes in the volume of crime' (Box and Hale 1982: 22–4; their emphasis). Translating this claim into the inevitable hypothesis, they predicted that:

> both the frequency and severity of imprisonment will vary positively with the rate of unemployment when the level of crime and the numbers of persons formally available for imprisonment are controlled.
>
> (1982: 26)

Finding that their model appeared 'to fit' the data for England and Wales for the period 1949–79, Box and Hale claimed to have extended the arguments of the North American radical criminologists who had constructed the early models connecting unemployment and imprisonment rates (1982: 30).

For the most part, these studies have succeeded in documenting a relationship between unemployment and imprisonment. Occasionally they fail to discover one – most notably in Greenberg's study of Poland (Greenberg 1980). More frequently, there are internal disputes – for example, when Don Wallace rejected unemployment rates in favour of labour force participation rates in his analysis of the political economy of incarceration rates in the United States between 1971–77. Concerned to address the problems that attended Rusche's hypothesis when applied to late capitalism, Wallace insisted that there were various ways to 'operationalise' Rusche's labour market concept. In particular, he argued that labour force participation was a 'more theoretically and empirically reasonable indicator of prevailing labour supply' than unemployment rates. Moreover, it was 'faithful to the type of Marxian analysis pioneered by Rusche'. Again, the first step was to generate testable hypotheses. One was that prison rates 'vary inversely with labour supply, falling when labour is scarce and rising where there is a labour surplus'. The second step was to subject them to the now familiar multiple regression analysis. He found that overall, Rusche's thesis was supported (Wallace 1980: 61–4).

However, his critics claim that there is not 'a strong theoretical case for using labour force participation rates for examining the recession–imprisonment relationship' (Box 1987: 187). The problem, as Box points out (and this is a point to which we will return), is that many people, notably women, will be 'voluntarily' unemployed, and therefore not perceived as a threat to capitalist stability in times of economic crisis. Michael Lynch, on the other hand, has built on Wallace's theory to suggest that the rate of surplus value, which is a measure of labour's exploitation, is a more useful measure of labour market conditions than unemployment statistics (Lynch 1988: 329–34).

Lynch's study of arrest and prison admission data in the United States for the period 1950–80 is in many ways the apotheosis of the Ruschean-inspired quantitative, Marxist political economy approach to the penal question. Marx's theory of surplus value, surplus populations, multiple regression analysis, testable hypotheses relating prison admissions to the rate of surplus value and previous studies of unemployment rates are all brought together to provide support for Rusche and Kirchheimer who were the first to suggest that 'punishment was a reaction to the requirements of the system of economic production'. And once again, a conclusion is reached which is consistent with Rusche's original thesis: Lynch finds that in advanced American capitalism the rate of prison admissions was 'directly influenced by the rate of surplus value'. Moreover, this relationship was 'independent of any effect the level of crime might have on punishment' (Lynch 1988: 340).

The drive to transform Rusche's original propositions into hypotheses and to test them relentlessly on endless samples of empirical data, shows no sign of abating. The fiftieth anniversary of the publication of *Punishment and Social Structure* was celebrated by a special issue of *Contemporary Crises* in which the quantitative mode of analysis is still current. While Hale (1989) raises some important problems with this approach, James Inverarity and Ryken Grattet continue the tradition of deploying an elaborate multivariate analysis, this time to measure what they call the 'covariation between the volume of social control and the labour market'. Expanding the scope of empirical analysis, they seek to determine whether postwar United States time-series data indicate that the level of unemployment has corresponding influences on prison admissions, mental hospitalisations and welfare case-loads. Not surprisingly, they interpret their failure to find evidence of trade-offs occurring between imprisonment and other modes of social control, such as welfare or psychiatric hospitalisation, as supporting previous findings that 'unemployment rates directly affect imprisonment holding crime rates constant' (Inverarity and Grattet 1989: 351–2). Also, we now have a time series study indicating a significant correlation between variations in unemployment and the evolution of prison populations in twentieth-century France (Laffargue and Godefroy 1989).

Almost finally, we should note yet another North American attempt to extend the Rusche–Kirchheimer tradition, one deploying 'individual-level data' on 1,970 criminal defendants (rather than the usual aggregate-level data at the national or state level) in order to assess the impact of unemployment on incarceration decisions in 1982. In this adaptation of the Ruschean model, the aim is to focus '*directly* on the unemployment/prison relationship', in order to test the 'unemployment/prison hypothesis'. This hypothesis was supported, in particular, by evidence indicating how the unfortunately-named 'in/out' sentencing decisions of judges related to the defendants' employment status (Chiricos and Bales 1991: 702–3; their emphasis). More broadly, the study found that unemployment had a 'significant, substantial, and independent impact on the (in/out) decision to incarcerate' and that the impact of unemployment was strongest for young black men and violent crimes. Yet notwithstanding the adoption of a novel gender-aware approach – one which tests the unemployment/prison relationship with measures of unemployment which are age, race *and* gender specific – the researchers see their work as extending Rusche and Kirchheimer's labour market thesis, a thesis which, in a moment of gender-sensitive oblivion, they describe, in the usual way, as 'seminal' (1991: 719–20).

Finally, in the long list of researchers working in what seems to be an infinitely expandable genre, Gloria Lessan has attempted to move beyond the dominant mode of research in this field. Instead of focusing on the unemployment–imprisonment relationship, she considers other structural conditions, notably inflation, which 'generate marginalisation' as well as the state's 'placative control' or welfare system. Predictably, this desire to change the research direction generates yet another hypothesis. It is that:

in the face of unemployment and inflation the state will respond with more coercive control. To the extent that the state is entangled in a fiscal crisis, its use of coercive control is inversely related to the maintenance of placative control.

(Lessan 1991: 179)

Predictably too, the hypothesis is confirmed. Using annual time-series data from the United States for the period 1948–85, Lessan found that after she controlled for variations in violent crime rates, prison capacity and age structure, inflation rates and annual fluctuations in black and white male unemployment rates exerted an independent positive effect on imprisonment rates. Moreover, welfare had a 'nonsignificant' or negative effect on imprisonment. Once again then, the line of argument put by the 'conflict theorists', commencing with Rusche and Kirchheimer, is supported:

'coercive control increases with deteriorations in the economy' or, more simply still, 'the state responds to unemployment with more coercive control' (1991: 188–9). Thus, fifty years after it was published and over twenty years after it was re-published, *Punishment and Social Structure* continues to leave its mark on empirical analyses of punishment systems.

CRITIQUES

So much then, for the quantification of the labour market thesis which has become the trademark of post-Ruschean analyses of imprisonment in advanced capitalist societies. What are we to make of it? It should be said from the start – if it is not already obvious – that these studies are numb-ingly dull, and perhaps intrinsically so. From within the paradigm, Chris Hale has warned of the danger of 'taking our own statistical modelling too seriously'. As he sees it, the problem lies with using the technique of least squares regression – a method of analysis which 'seduces its users into utilising a language of causality' and which misses the complexity of penality (Hale 1989: 331–2). But the problem is deeper than this. It is as if the 'dull compulsion of economic relations', which Marx described so lucidly (Marx 1970: 689), has taken over its own analysis, coercing its Marxist executors into a tedious regurgitation of a tired old labour market formula. Certainly, the excitement and power of the original story which inspired the political economy of punishment – Marx's story of the process of capitalist accumulation, the criminalisation of the expropriated, the bloody laws against vagabondage – is dissipated in the relentless orthodoxy of a mechanical application of the Rusche–Kirchheimer model to different sets of empirical data. In short, studies in the political economy of penality are afflicted by the same deadening paralysis which characterises the repetitive discourses of positivistic penology.

Furthermore, the empiricist mode of analysis adopted by these studies is vulnerable to the criticism that it reduces theory to hypotheses which it then assumes can be tested by reference to an external 'real world' of empirical facts. By wrongly supposing the possibility of a direct access to a real world of 'facts' – in this case, unemployment statistics and prison admis-sions rates – this approach ignores the fundamental sociological insight that such facts are not 'simply given by reality . . . they are always the product of definite theoretical and ideological practices' (Garland 1983a: 38). It is at this level – at the level of theoretical exchanges about what constitutes the 'facts' of penality – that we can usefully begin our critique of the political economy approach. The continuing internecine disputes over the best way of measuring the surplus population or of controlling other variables need not detain us.[6]

Beyond economic functionalism

Political economy approaches to the 'the penal question' may be seen as regional applications of a more general theory, that of Marxist historical materialism. Melossi makes this explicit when he declares the history of prisons to be 'a particular chapter of a more general history' – for him, 'that of the making of the reproduction of the working class' (Melossi 1978: 81). Alternatively, these approaches to punishment may be seen as applications – in the field of penality – of some of the theoretical perspectives which have emerged within Marxist sociologies of law, the state and criminal justice. As such, they are vulnerable to all the criticisms which have been levelled at those theories from outside the Marxist paradigm, but also from within Marxist theorisations of the state – notably, the charges of economism, functionalism and instrumentalism. The details of these critiques have been thoroughly canvassed elsewhere.[7] But it is crucial to note that the dominant political economy approach focusing on labour market conditions is mired in outdated conceptualisations which have been thoroughly deconstructed by Marxist analysts working within structuralist and post-structuralist paradigms. It is to their specific criticisms of the 'classic' Ruschean-inspired models of punishment that we will now turn.

The related charges of economism, reductionism and functionalism re-emerge as the predominant criticisms of these models. As Spitzer has observed:

> the tendency to see punishment as explicable exclusively in terms of its direct economic functions is a problem for almost all of those explanations which can be classified as forms of the labour control hypothesis.
>
> (Spitzer 1979: 224)

That is, these studies have for the most part failed to loosen the functional relationship between punishment and economic organisation or to recognise that capitalist forms of punishment are 'rarely if ever direct expressions of bourgeois interests'. It is ironic – and also a gauge of the hazardous nature of a preoccupation with political economy – that Spitzer maintains that it is possible to 'retain a materialist focus without succumbing to the errors of reductionism and oversimplification' (1979: 225), for he too has been accused of making precisely those errors in his 'Marxian theory of deviance'. His analysis of 'deviance processing' has been pilloried as a 'classic example of teleological reasoning' in so far as it presents control systems as functional for capitalism – stemming from the 'needs' of the capitalist ruling class to control problem populations. Thus prisons are 'caused' by these needs (Horwitz 1977: 362–3). Spitzer can protest that Horwitz does 'serious violence to the Marxian model' by overlooking the decisive element in his explanation – 'the historically-based development of contradictions in class society' (Spitzer 1977: 364–5) – but the political economy of punishment continues to be plagued by the problem of causation created by determinist teleologies in which penal law is represented as functionally adapting to the needs of capitalism.

Again, this problem has been addressed within the Marxist paradigm. For example, in their critique of economistic explanations of crime control, Humphries and Greenberg insisted that explanations of change cannot be 'restricted to the analysis of the economy narrowly defined'. We also need to take account of the nature of the state, ideologies, class mobilisations and class fractions. Indeed, a mode of production is 'too limited a concept to tell us much about crime control'. Carefully avoiding the language of causality, they argue that penal ideologies are certainly related to stages in capitalist development, but it is questionable whether they could be 'deduced' from them. Social control systems, including punishment regimes, must now be understood in terms of 'social formations', which, as in Althusser, are composed of economic, political and ideological 'instances'. However, it is important to eschew the distinction made between independent variables (such as surplus populations) and dependent variables (the increase in prison populations) because: 'crime control is itself a part of a social formation, and thus the social formation cannot be considered as entirely prior to it, either logically or empirically'. Indeed, in their revised Marxist view, the mode of production itself is 'not entirely distinct from social control conceptually', as penal forms – for example, penal slavery and prison labour – can be 'part of the forces and relations of production'. It follows that analysts of penality face 'a complex problem involving joint or reciprocal determination, rather than unidirectional causality' (1981: 240–2).

This kind of critique has been developed further by Claude Faugeron and Guy Houchon in their commentary on the interpretative movement from penology to what they call 'a sociology of penal policies' (1987). Acknowledging Rusche's influence in moving analysis on from a 'microsociology of penal institutions' to a macrosociology of modes of punishment, they nevertheless warn that

> any attempt to explain the penal function in society by social structure runs the risk of becoming an idealist deviation which would amount to looking for an immediate relationship – practically a teleological relationship – between the class divisions of society and the results of penal mechanisms. Such an approach amounts to treating the penal machine as an unequivocal whole guided by a more or less clearly expressed will to discipline the proletariat, explaining almost everything in terms of the 'bourgeois culture' of the judges.
>
> (1987: 396)

In place of outmoded functionalist variations of the base–superstructure metaphor and instrumentalist linkings of the prison to the management of the working class for disciplinary purposes, they advocate focusing on 'intermediate levels' between class divisions and penal forms. These 'inter- mediate levels' should be understood in terms of 'balances in which power relations are not always where one expects them to be, and where pro- cedures have at least as much weight as ideologies' (1987: 398). These balances are negotiated at the level of public debate, within 'para- and peri-penal institutions' and also within criminal justice administration. What is required is a sensitivity to social mechanisms such as 'the law of interprofessional dynamics' and 'the operating law of the system' – laws which pertain to the operationalisation of penal policy – to 'penal policy concretely as it is made' (1987: 398–401). In this conception, procedural rules within the penal system – or, as they note Rusche suggested, the role played by welfare payments in modulating sanctions – are significant 'intermediate mechanisms' or variables which can explain the specific form taken by penal orders (1987: 416).

More sophisticated theorisations of penality have, then, moved us beyond the labour market and even beyond the mode of production. We have arrived at what has been depicted as 'a more valid type of comparative research' on penal sanctions than the kind which measures imprisonment rates – one which takes account of 'the whole ensemble of punishments' available at any specific historical time. To understand penality fully we need to consider competing systems of control such as psychiatry and juvenile justice systems. Moreover, it has now been suggested that the 'interchangeability of soft control with tough control measures' which has emerged over the last two decades, makes for a complex penal field which 'cannot possibly be grasped' by Rusche's labour market thesis, let alone by 'one single index' like the imprisonment rate (Schumann 1983: 270–1). It is this attention to complexity which has come to characterise Marxist theorisations of penality, especially modern forms of penality. A dominant theme is the significance of the non-penal sphere. Following Heinz Steinert who warned against overestimating the effectiveness of the criminal law which, he said, was 'a means of repression, but a second-order and rather marginal one in a functioning capitalist system' (Steinert 1977: 438–40), the current trend is to downplay the importance of criminal sanctions. Thus Spitzer suggests that:

> Regulations which are considered to lie outside the punitive realm may actually be far more important in establishing a structure of domination than the most visible and documented forms of legal coercion.
>
> (1979: 225)

Consequently, the study of punishment and social change must include analysis of contract law, tariffs, wage and immigration laws. Moreover, this is seen to be particularly necessary if we are to understand penality today, because forms of punishment in modern society – for example, welfare-orientated and therapeutic ones – 'complicate the study of social control' (1979: 226).[8]

The main thrust of this analysis is clear: economistic models will no longer suffice to explain penality. In particular, the prison, the persistence of which has been identified as the key problematic, demands an analysis which extends beyond economism. For while it could be argued that the prison 'neatly corresponded' to the plans of the dominant classes to educate the working class to the needs of factory discipline during the phase of primitive accumulation – especially in England – such a neat correspondence model is hardly applicable to advanced capitalist societies. On the one hand, it has to be acknowledged that the working class is not 'the exclusive or even the main victim of repression in penal institutions' (Ferrajoli and Zolo 1985: 77). The hardest hit today are rather immigrants and other socially marginalised groups such as the unemployed. On the other hand, 'detentive punishment in the form of direct repression and physical restraint appears to be losing its original capitalist function'. Indeed, the decline in prison sentences relative to other punishments suggests that confinement as a form of punishment is becoming an exceptional form of social control in some Western jurisdictions. But simultaneously with this weakening of the 'punitive–repressive function' of the prison, there has been an extension of penal interventions in society, a much-commented-on widening of the net of social control. Such observations have led some Marxist observers to the view that the penal system is becoming 'an ideological apparatus', its function being to pronounce guilty verdicts which for the most part have no effect except to stigmatise the accused. It is not that the prison will lose its function within late capitalist societies, but rather that the importance of the 'archaic penalistic prison structure' now lies in the 'ideologically stigmatising use of criminal prosecution' rather than direct repression. With the increasing differentiation of the social control system, prison 'appears to be confined to a generic legitimating role' (Ferrajoli and Zolo 1985: 77–8).

These Marxist analysts of modern penality have abandoned traditional categories in relation to bourgeois economy in their efforts to grapple with the complexity of modern penality as well as with the problem of the continued existence of the prison. Influenced by structuralist Marxist theorisations of a new importance for ideology, they have turned their attention to the relationship between penal and 'non-economic' forces and, in particular, to the ideological or legitimating function of the prison.

Without doubt, this move from instrumentalist to structuralist paradigms is a significant advance over crude economic determinism. However, very few Marxist analysts have followed through the implications of the new significance given to ideology for the study of penality, or developed the 'new notion of causality' suggested in revisions of the economism of the base–superstructure metaphor (Garland and Young 1983: 27–8). Once again, the most significant contribution has been made by Dario Melossi. As his analytical model is the most advanced within the political economy genre, it warrants a close analysis.

Melossi's Ruschean revival

It is fitting to conclude this section on recent post-Ruschean Marxist political economies of punishment with Melossi's work, for, as we have seen, he has done the most to revive interest in Rusche's original formulations in the field. In the mid-1980s, Melossi returned to Rusche's explanatory model and found it wanting in this significant way: it continued to posit crime as the intervening variable between economic conditions and punishment. For example, he detected a tendency in *Punishment and Social Structure* to 'read' the connection between improved living conditions in the early twentieth century and a decreasing prison population 'as though it were mediated by a decrease in crime rates'. Consequently, because Rusche (or was it Kirchheimer?) did not, in Melossi's view, fully challenge the 'legalistic bond' between punishment and crime, the sociology of punishment and criminal law could not be 'freed of its centuries-old subordination to the sociology of criminal behaviour'. However, according to Melossi, later studies applying Rusche's model – notably Jankovic's and Greenberg's – not only represented the relationship between social structure and punishment as analytically independent of the relationship between social structure and crime; they also demonstrated a 'significant association', indeed, a 'direct relationship', between economic conditions and imprisonment rates which was not mediated by changing crime rates (Melossi 1985a: 170–4).

The significance, then, of these Ruschean-inspired studies is that they made a crucial break with the analytically restricting 'legal syllogism' – the common-sense idea that punishment is simply the consequence of crime and that, if there is a need for sociological explanation, 'social structure explains crime and crime explains punishment' (Melossi 1989: 311). Melossi, however, wanted to take this research further. He wanted to discover whether we can use the finding common to American, British and his own Italian-based work of a statistically significant association between business cycle indicators and imprisonment indicators to build 'a causal model' of these relationships – one which would correct Rusche's economistic account. In particular, he was interested in theorising the relationship between the 'verbalisations' of criminal justice agents and the economy. In his view, the standard empirical studies did not provide

> a satisfactory account of the contemporaneous shifts in society toward verbalisations which becomes motives for more severe punitive action among agents of social control, at a certain point in time.
>
> (1985a: 178)

To replace the economic functionalism of the old model, he therefore suggested a new investigative strategy which establishes

> a 'discursive chain' between, on the one hand, the ways in which the social conflicts around the business cycle are rationalised . . . and, on the other hand, the vocabularies of motive which are available to the agencies of penal control as they account for their actions.
>
> (1985a: 178)

Following this strategy, and what he refers to as Greenberg's 'seminal intuition' that labelling processes are not restricted to immediate interactions (Greenberg 1977: 651), Melossi proceeded to develop 'a grounded labelling theory' – one which is concerned with the way 'variable social-structural elements', such as the 'political business cycle', impact on definitions of criminality (1985b). To cut short a long story about the changing verbalisations used by criminal justice agents which accompany the upswings and downswings of the political business cycle, Melossi adapted C. Wright Mills's 'vocabularies of motive' to suggest that a 'vocabulary of punitive motives' constitutes the crucial intervening variable between changes in economic indicators and changes in 'correctional variables'; or, more obtusely, between 'the unfolding of the political business cycle and that expression of the "law in action" represented by changes in imprisonment rates' (1985a: 187). Put simply, he argued that changes in punitive vocabularies used by law enforcement officials depend on oscillations in the ideological or 'moral climate', oscillations which in turn depend on the alternation of economic periods of expansion and recession. In hard times, for example, their verbalisations against crime are partly a response to an anti-crime public mood, which in turn is connected to the downswing of the economy (Melossi 1989: 320). Thus:

> the sources for an increase in severity of punishment should not be sought either in specific 'economic' functions, such as the control of an increasing mass of unemployed, or in specific motives of individual agents of social control.

Rather, they must be sought in the 'moral climate' which develops in hard times (1985a: 183).

While all this may seem a long way removed from Rusche's 'simple economic maxims', Melossi at least finds a 'symbolic' or pedagogic importance in Rusche's version of the less eligibility principle. Also, he remains committed to the original project of devising a 'causal model of variations in economic conditions and punitive policies' and he is still wedded to the hypothesis-testing methodology which he uses to revise and refine Rusche's model of the association between economic and penal changes. His ultimate goal is not an abandonment of that original project but rather a 'successful test' of the new causal model. Such a test would represent a major advance in sociological explanations of variations in punishment – explanations which would not be 'fettered by either legalist or economist assumptions' (1985a: 183–8). Finally, while Rusche may not have completely freed the concept of punishment from its 'legalistic subjugation to that of crime' (as others have claimed he did), *Punishment and Social Structure* did at least represent a challenge to the 'legal syllogism' – a challenge which questioned the very legitimation of 'the "State's" power to punish'. It therefore opened the door to all those sociological investigations of punishment which 'dare step beyond the role of obliging technocrats of an unquestioned legal syllogism' (1989: 321–3).

Clearly, political economies of punishment have come a long way since Rusche's labour market theory was rediscovered in 1968. Responding self-critically to charges of economism, reductionism and functionalism, analysts in the field have made considerable theoretical advances. For example, quantitative analyses linking imprisonment rates to unemployment rates have begun to explore the role of the state in regulating surplus populations. But this Althusserian 'moment' has also been subjected to internal critique, the most recent trend being to suggest that capitalist states 'appear to lack coherent social control strategies' (Inverarity and Grattet 1989: 366). Post-Althusserian superstructural-level Marxists, such as Melossi, have moved beyond functionalist conceptions of the state to consider hegemonic ideologies, movements in public opinion and 'discursive chain' reactions, the effect of which is to suggest the 'relative autonomy' of penality from the state as well as from economic determinations. Admittedly, Melossi's new causal model with its multiple interrelationships still seems to operate within a Marxist positivist tradition, but its sensitivity to ideological shifts provides it with an explanatory power extending well beyond the reach of economistic models. Unemployment levels, the centrepiece of the Ruschean approach, are now perceived to be merely one manifestation of economic crises which involve complex economic, political and ideological processes and 'the totality of capitalist social relations' (Hale 1989: 330).

Yet for all the modifications which this mode of analysis has undergone, it remains fundamentally flawed in two significant ways. First, while the identification of a range of social-structural variables has proceeded apace, explanations in this vein remain prisoners of what ultimately proves to be a disabling discourse – one which is so preoccupied with structural determinants and causal models that it is oblivious to the fact that, whatever its 'structural sources', punishment is ultimately experienced on a human level (Spitzer 1985: 579). That is to say, in most political economies of punishment, prisoners – the people who bear the brunt of all the punishment structures – are lost from view. Second and related, these accounts have remained profoundly masculinist: they not only ignore the fact that prisons hold women, they also remain oblivious to feminist challenges to Marxist categories of analysis. From a feminist perspective, the 'totality of capitalist social relations' – the end point of post-Ruschean analysis – thus turns out to be a very attenuated totality indeed.

The feminist challenge

While feminist interventions in the field of penality will be explored in chapters 4 and 5, it is important to consider here the specific ways in which, from a feminist perspective, political economy approaches leave much to be desired. First and most obviously, women appear only fleetingly, if at all, in these accounts. We catch sight of them briefly in the seventeenth- and eighteenth-century houses of correction – spinning or preparing textiles in the Amsterdam *spinnhaus* and the French *hôpitaux généraux*; being sexually abused in the eighteenth-century English workhouses.[9] Generally, however, the analysis is ungendered. Spitzer, for example, does not notice that the so-called 'problem populations', even the ones he characterises as 'social dynamite' – containing the 'more youthful, alienated and politically volatile' – tend to be composed overwhelmingly of men (1975b: 646).[10] Second, political economies of penality continue to be pitched in a deeply masculinist tone. It is as if the prison – quintessentially masculine because its populations are predominantly male – demands a masculine, more penile-than-penal discourse in which women prisoners are peripheral and feminism beyond consideration. Certainly, the persistent characterisation of work in this field as 'seminal' seems apposite, and where else would a reviewer describe a book (*The Prison and the Factory*) as a 'ball-breaker' (Ditton 1983: 74)?

Occasionally however, there are signs of a realisation that all is not well in this seemingly impenetrable masculinist fortress. Box and Hale, for example, are among the few working within the political economy paradigm to notice unemployed women and to develop gender-sensitive hypotheses which are cognisant of the fact that variations between imprisonment and unemployment will be stronger when taking a male population, especially a younger male population, into account (1982: 24–30). Belatedly, Melossi too has begun to suspect that elaborations of Rusche's theoretical model must discuss the so-called 'dual labour market':

> not only in terms of the distinction, on the side of demand, between monopoly and competitive sectors of the economy, but also on the side of supply, in terms of a labour force structured by race, ethnicity and gender.
>
> (1989: 316–17)

One can only hope that researchers in this field will follow his call to take gender, race and ethnicity into account. But this may be overly optimistic. As we have seen, some recent North American studies have begun to incorporate a gender dimension into their hypothesis-testing models by noting, for example, that the unemployment–imprisonment relationship is strongest for unemployed black men (Chiricos and Bales 1991). But there are few signs that this form of analysis will be extended to cover the question of masculinity, or even the pervasive evidence that the relationship between unemployment and imprisonment is profoundly gendered. Certainly, the suggestion of a critical analyst, commenting on the subjugation of women in the patriarchal monogamous family, that 'To be punished is to be treated like a woman' (Shank 1980: 35) would appear, on the evidence, to be beyond the imagination of researchers working within the discursive boundaries of political economies of punishment. And none of them has taken up Rusche and Kirchheimer's suggestion, based on their observation that women in the *hôpitaux généraux* were guilty of crimes punished by galley slavery in the case of male offenders, that the gradual rise of imprisonment was bound up in part with the need to provide special treatment for women (1968: 65–6).

More fundamentally, Marxist analysts of the political economy of punishment have ignored feminist critiques of their outmoded interpretative frameworks. Two decades of feminist interventions in the broader field of political economy – for example, in the domestic labour debate, the debate about gender and class as two relatively autonomous systems, the development of gender-integrated approaches to class and gender and the consideration given to relations of distribution as well as relations of production – have simply passed them by.[11] This is not the place to consider feminist theoretical encounters with unrepentant, unreconstructed, vulgar, masculinist Marxism. Suffice it to note, first, that a dismissive relegation of women to a footnote (e.g. Faugeron and Houchon 1987: 416–17) will no longer do; second, that women are not easily, and certainly not appropriately, subsumed within a political economy framework centred on labour market conditions; and, third, that a feminist political economy of punishment has yet to be written. Rather than speculate on whether it will be written as a chapter in the history of the working class or, more likely, a chapter in the history of women, it is more useful to search for clues as to the direction such a study might follow.

As we shall see in chapter 4, the 'classic' macrosociological text, *Punishment and Social Structure*, is not the starting point for feminist analyses of punishments imposed on women. Paradoxically however, John Braithwaite's testing of the Rusche–Kirchheimer model in the context of Australian penal history in the late nineteenth century suggests intriguing possibilities for feminists. Impressed by Rusche and Kirchheimer's 'compelling' arguments about the economics of imprisonment, he concludes that the decline in imprisonment rates in the states of Victoria and New South Wales between 1850 and 1920 corresponded with 'the demise of serious labour shortages in Australia and the concomitant destruction of the profitability of prison industry' (1980: 203). While Braithwaite's study has been criticised for failing to consider the impact of declines in serious criminal offending on imprisonment rates in the two states (O'Malley 1983: 158), another crucial aspect of his work has been overlooked. Critical of Marxist accounts which ignore 'the female criminal', Braithwaite analysed women's imprisonment rates. He found that in Victoria women's imprisonment rates decline during periods of economic crisis, whereas male imprisonment rates show sharp increases. He comments:

> The obvious explanation for the fact that female imprisonment rates have not increased during the crises of Australian capitalism is that women, particularly in the 1890s and 1930s, were not fully integrated into the capitalist market in labour, but were participants in a separate (domestic) market.
>
> (1980: 204)

Surmising that the role of women in keeping the family together becomes more crucial during hard times when the men might be unemployed, he predicted that women would be 'even less likely to be incarcerated during economic crises' (1980: 203–4). A properly-grounded – that is, Marxist *and* feminist – political economy of punishment would do well to pursue these suggestions.

In this connection, it is of more than passing interest to note that in 1973 Taylor, Walton and Young, the triumvirate of self-proclaimed 'New Criminologists', lamented that 'a political economy of social reaction' – that is, of social reaction to criminal behaviour – had not yet been written. Twenty years later, we have moved some way towards formulating one, thanks largely to the rediscovery and subsequent refinements of Rusche and Kirchheimer's text. But just as the New Criminologists assumed that they could arrive at 'a fully social theory of deviance' (1973: 274) without considering women, let alone gender, so analysts working towards more sophisticated political economies of punishment have, for the most part, assumed that they could do so without considering that women are punished too. In this vital respect, their accounts are woefully inadequate.

Still, for all their faults, for all the numbing dullness of their prose, the monotony of their methodological imperatives and the tedium of theoretical posturings which tend to obscure rather than clarify the nature of penality, political economies of punishment deserve credit on several counts. First, they have opened up to critical sociological inquiry a field which was formerly colonised by correctional penology and its misleading teleologies of 'progressive' penal evolution. Second, they have reclaimed punishment as an object of knowledge from the restricting analytical frameworks constructed by idealist philosophies of deterrence, retribution and reform. Within these idealist frameworks, questions of power, politics, ideology and domination had been displaced by an obsession with penality as a 'moral object'. Now, thanks largely to the theoretical elaboration of political economies of punishment, questions about the power to punish have moved to centre stage, pushing to the background the philosophical preoccupation with 'the eternal moral dilemma of "the right to punish"' (Garland 1983b: 85). Third, they have reconnected punishment to social and economic structures and, in the process, provided a firm materialist foundation for progressive research and political interventions in the field. Finally, they have come to understand that ideologies are material practices having material effects on penal practices.

In chapter 2, we will explore the 'new' social histories of penality in which ideology comes into its own. But before we do, it is worthwhile reflecting that as they move into the dizzy heights of seemingly autonomous superstructural 'effectivities', Marxist analysts of penality seem to lose their way. At least, something gets lost in the analysis. As the focus shifts to ideologies, discursive chains, vocabularies of punitive motive and non-discursive economic structures, the more traditional social structures, modes and relations of production and labour markets – the very same economic factors which Rusche took as his investigative starting point in his 'economic-historical' analysis – fade from view. Whether the economy is determinant in the first or last instance, or whether it has a determinant role at all, are issues which political economies of punishment have yet to resolve. Georg Rusche must be rolling in his grave.

2 'New' histories of punishment regimes

The writing of this chapter has been overtaken by a number of significant yet disparate publishing events which have transformed its purpose. Once it may have been appropriate to speak glowingly and in much detail of the proliferation over the last twenty years of so-called 'new social histories' of punishment. History, after all, especially this 'new' or revisionist social history, has done much to transform our understanding of the emergence and form of modern punishment regimes in the West. There was a time, as recently as the late 1980s, when the task of this chapter would have been straight-forward. The project would have been to examine critically the new 'master' theories of transformations said to have occurred, especially since the late eighteenth century, in the 'master patterns and strategies for controlling deviance in Western industrial societies' (Cohen 1985: 13). These transformations and, indeed, the master patterns themselves are the ones unearthed and meticulously charted by the self-proclaimed 'social' or revisionist historians of penality since 1970. Perhaps it would even have been fitting to lionise these accounts – notwithstanding their fatal masculinist flaws. But now such a project seems redundant. The main problem is not that the revisionists themselves have revised their own accounts, refining and rewriting their 'social' analyses of penality to their hearts' desires; nor is it that these accounts have been reproduced, critiqued from masculinist as well as feminist standpoints, and even tabulated (e.g. Cohen 1985: 16–17) in countless texts. Over and above all this, these accounts now have to face up to the challenge posed by post-colonial critics who have demolished the pretensions of Eurocentric history (however revisionist and 'social' it purports to be) to make universalising theoretical and historical claims about institutional and social practices, let alone about 'master patterns'. For such claims, we now understand, are nothing more than 'white mythologies' (Young 1990).

So: how do the revisionist historical accounts of penality stand up to this the latest challenge to their transgressive credentials? While post-colonial writers have not yet scrutinised these accounts, their critique of Western Eurocentric history must, by extension, include its new as well as its 'old' punishment histories. What would post-colonialists make of the now not-so-new 'social' histories of punishment regimes which claimed the radical high ground in the 1970s? Presumably not much, although surely they would concede that these histories did at least specify their geographic focus in England, France or North America. What is worrying, however, is the universalising tendency apparent in the privileging of Western institutional forms and periodisation which extends to speaking of 'master' (read again: Western) social patterns of penal control. The language of 'master' imprints surely creates the impression that the new historians of Western punishment systems saw their work as revising not simply Western penal history but rather 'the histories of prisons in *most* countries', as one revisionist so indiscreetly put it (Ignatieff 1983a: 75; my emphasis). Surely too, the few passing references to non-Western penal systems would not save the new histories from being relegated to the Eurocentric waste basket.[1] Moreover, if all this is not enough, David Garland has recently provided such a detailed overview and rigorous critique from within a Western analytical framework of the key neo-Marxist and other social histories of punishment that any further elucidation would seem to be superfluous (Garland 1990a). What then is left of the 'new' social histories of the 1970s which is worthy of comment today, let alone in a chapter in a book purporting to be a feminist intervention in the field?

This may seem to be a strange way to have started this chapter – with an intimation that it has all been said before – and an even stronger intimation of the devastation wrought by post-colonial attacks on the writing of Eurocentric history. In the light of these trenchant critiques, it would appear to be excessive to regurgitate once more the revisionist social histories of changing modes of punishment written within just such a Eurocentric framework ten to twenty years ago. Surely the effect would only be to compound the problem of the saturation of the market in revisionist historical literature. Certainly, it is difficult to recapture the excitement – the shock of 'the new' – of the new social history at *that* historical time, the time when it was indeed 'new'. But that is precisely the task of this chapter: its mission is to reclaim the sense of paradigm-shifting import which the new social history injected into the study of punishment regimes, and at the same time to rescue that history from both the condemnation of the critics and the condescension of its own post-revisionist modifications.

HISTORY? WHICH HISTORY?

Over the last two decades, history has become the privileged site of contestation in the field of penality. Where once a 'technicist penology'

(Garland and Young 1983: 10–11) – one preoccupied with a positivistic assessment of the efficacy of different penal measures – ruled the field, now history has become the discipline par excellence in this field. Today one does not step out to debate questions of punishment, much less penality, without supporting historical evidence at one's fingertips. But the discipline of history is itself a hotbed of dissent, splintered by debates over content, periodisation, interpretation and, more fundamentally, over the issue of the kind of history which is required for an understanding of past and present punishment regimes. This brings us to the first key question – that of categorisation. If history is essential, which history do we mean?

The categorical question

Since the 1970s, it has become standard practice to divide histories in this field into three categories: traditional or administrative history, traditional Marxist history and social or revisionist history, which is also referred to as social-control history. While an outline of the first two kinds of history will be sketched below, our main concern will be with the last group of revisionist or social histories. Notwithstanding internal divisions, a continuing process of reworking earlier positions and a refusal to speak of 'a unitary "revisionist" school' (Cohen and Scull 1983: 2), it has now become acceptable to refer to revisionist histories of punishment. Sometimes different or more complex categorisation systems are utilised in order to highlight divisions within the standard categories. For example, a theoretical and political distinction has been made between social-control history and what has been called 'traditional "revisionist" history' (Muraskin 1976: 559). In this construction, one of the classic 'revisionist' accounts, David Rothman's *Discovery of the Asylum* (1971) is pitted against the social-control school, as exemplified by Tony Platt's *The Child Savers* (1969). But this is unusual. Most commentators cluster all the social histories together. Admittedly, some accounts are difficult to place. For example, some analysts categorise Melossi and Pavarini's *The Prison and the Factory* (1981) as an economistic elaboration of the Rusche and Kirchheimer thesis, while others place it in the social history or 'neo-Marxist' camp, inasmuch as it draws on the work of non-economistic and even post-Marxist analysts, notably Foucault.

But where should we place Foucault? Not only was he against classification, he was against his work being classified as social history (Foucault 1981). Furthermore, in the introduction to the second volume of his *History of Sexuality* (1987), he states that, while his works are studies of history, he was not an historian. Certainly many historians would concur: Foucault's reception by historians has hardly been one of unmitigated acclaim (e.g.

Megill 1987). Still, *Discipline and Punish*, his intervention into penal history or rather into the field he redefined as penality, is usually counted as one of the key revisionist historical texts, along with Michael Ignatieff's *Just Measure of Pain* (1978) and Rothman's *Discovery of the Asylum* and *Conscience and Convenience* (1980).[2] For this reason, reference will be made in this chapter to his impact on social histories of punishment. However, in certain significant ways, Foucault is not properly categorised as a revisionist or social historian. Moreover, for reasons to be examined later, his contribution to the field of penality is so momentous that it warrants a separate chapter.

Traditional versus 'new' histories

Who then are the social or revisionist historians and would the new social history please stand up? Before we address the specific question of what counts as social history in the field of penality and also the more general question of just what, exactly, is 'social' about the new social history, it might be useful to contrast it with the traditional histories which it sought to replace, or at least, revise. The revisionists sought to break with two forms of traditional history – on the one hand, orthodox, mainstream or administrative history, and on the other hand, traditional Marxist history as exemplified by Rusche and Kirchheimer. This latter tradition, as we saw in chapter 1, was self-conscious about its method and politics: the aim was to explore the historical relationships between penal laws, labour markets and class struggle within the framework provided by a Marxist political economy. In contrast, what the revisionists referred to as orthodox or mainstream history tends to present itself as 'The' history, or indeed 'History', as if it were beyond being called to account. Accordingly, it is not explicit about its agenda, assumptions or methodology. We therefore have to resort to revisionist characterisations of mainstream history in order to comprehend just what it was that the new social historians wanted to challenge.

Self-styled revisionists working in the broad field of social control have characterised mainstream histories as 'reformist', meaning that they present past and present reformers and their reforms as progressive: for example, changes in penal practices and the management of madness are depicted in mainstream histories as 'inherently progressive' (Cohen and Scull 1983: 1–2). They also label these histories as 'teleological', meaning that they treat history 'as a progress from cruelty to enlightenment' and assume that events, including penal events, 'moved towards their "proper" modern end' (Ignatieff 1983a: 76; Philips 1983: 51). From a revisionist perspective, mainstream penal history usually takes the form of a dull narrative of administrative and institutional changes in penal practices in

Western jurisdictions since the Middle Ages, concentrating especially on nineteenth-century developments. It is a history without passion, power or conflict. Such a history is typified by the momentous tomes of Sir Leon Radzinowicz, the doyen of traditional, positivistic criminology in the United Kingdom. Revisionist critics have noted the usefulness of the wealth of empirical material presented in Radzinowicz's first four volumes of the history of English criminal law. They have even conceded that this, the high water mark of administrative history, is essential reading in the field. All this is acknowledged, notwithstanding the fact that it was written from 'the administrative point of view' and from the perspective of a linear reform-as-progress 'Whig view of history', one which ignores the social control aspects of reforms and which fails to analyse 'how these moves by the state were seen and felt from below, by the people most affected by them' (Philips 1983: 52–3). And as for the last volume in the series – the momentous volume five, a history of English criminal law and its administration from 1750, co-authored with Roger Hood – which traces the emergence of penal policy in the United Kingdom from the 1830s to 1914, a critical reviewer has acclaimed it as 'the most important work ever written on the history of British penal policy'. In the same breath however, this critic can inform us that it has 'major limitations as history' (Wiener 1987: 83 and 94).

Foremost amongst administrative history's catalogue of errors – as listed by the revisionists – is its treatment of penal policy as 'a self-contained and self-explicable sphere' best understood retrospectively from a late twentieth-century professional perspective. By presenting penal policy as responsive to changing penal needs, Radzinowicz and Hood neglected the wider social and political context of the making of penal policy, especially 'the subtle network of power relations in which criminal policy was embedded'. In this connection, they were also far too dismissive of 'social control' interpretations of Britain's penal past. As a result, they adopted an 'overly "pragmatic" and teleological' perspective, one which omits to see British criminal policy 'as an integral part of social, political and cultural history' (Wiener 1987: 85–96). Clearly then, a different kind of history is required. Radzinowicz and Hood do provide a thorough account of Victorian and Edwardian penal policy. They assess the legacy of the transportation system, provide an account of the construction of the system of penal servitude, and chart the steadily declining crime rates at the close of the nineteenth century, the declining use of punishments such as transportation, flogging and executions, the diminishing reliance on a deterrent prison system, the shortening of prison sentences as well as the turn-of-the-century experiments with radical new transformative policies for young potential recidivists, habitual offenders, vagrants, chronic inebriates and the 'feeble-minded'. They also cover the emergence of probation, juvenile courts, and the development of the fine, restitution and compensation. But for all that, the most that can be said about such administrative, teleological history is that it is 'a work of chronicle rather than interpretation', one which has produced 'a quarry of data that will be mined for years to come' (Martin 1988: 407).

What then is it that data-intensive administrative chronicles have left out? What is the interpretation which is required, and by whom? What is the point of reference for these dismissive critiques of the massive tomes of empirical historical penal detail produced by one of the leading figures of positivistic criminology? The answer to the last question, which must be addressed first, is the social or revisionist history of punishment produced in the 1970s. This history was part of the wider movement which came to be known as the new social history and which encompassed a number of fields – the prison, mental health, public welfare, juvenile justice, the urban school and hospitals. What these 'new' histories had in common was a concern to highlight the politics of the history of reform in these various fields of the study of social control. More particularly, they set about exposing the political bias of administrative or 'reformist' history's presentation of past reforms as a story of progress. As Ignatieff amongst others explained, the effect of reformist history was justificatory: it suggested that contemporary social control institutions were the outcome of just such a history of progress, and that they could be 'improved by the same incremental process of philanthropic activism in the future'. He continued:

A reformist historiography thus served a liberalism of good intentions, which in turn seemed to legitimise dubious new initiatives – psychosurgery, chemotherapy and behaviour modification – as legitimate descendants of the reforming tradition.

(Ignatieff 1983a: 76)

The aim of the new social or revisionist historians, then, was to question the legitimacy of past and present 'reforms'. As such they were present-orientated. Furthermore, the new histories were themselves politically loaded: they were the product of what Ignatieff refers to as 'the libertarian, populist politics of the 1960s' (which, he omits to specify, took place in particular locations, notably the United States and Western Europe). The mission of this new Anglo-American and Eurocentric historiography of social control was to politicise history: it was, as Ignatieff put it, 'avowedly political' (Ignatieff 1983a: 76). Its practitioners were driven by a desire to intervene against repressive state-run institutional regimes such as prisons and psychiatric hospitals and on behalf of their inmates.

Later, we will focus specifically on the new social penal history, but for now we need to provide a sense of what, exactly, was 'new' and 'social' about the new social history which emerged in the late 1960s in the West. To understand what was new about social history in the late 1960s, it is important to realise that what might now be called traditional social history had become a recognised field of inquiry only in the 1960s. Yet by the early 1970s, social history had already generated a dissenting or 'new' position within the ranks of self-defined social historians. The signficance of this internal conflict between old and new social history is frequently lost in retrospective accounts of social history. For example, looking back from the 1980s, Mark Poster recalled that social history revolutionised the discipline of history with its new methodologies borrowed from the social sciences and its new objects of study such as 'population, the city, the family, women, classes, sports and psychobiography'. But he criticised social historians, without distinction, for failing to theorise their 'empiricist positions'. In his view, Marxist and non-Marxist social historians alike ignored 'the theoretical presuppositions of their work' (Poster 1984: 70–1). In another retrospective glance, Peter Stearns declared that it was 'impossible to define social history adequately by discussing it in terms of period or area', but he suggested that it could at least be identified (albeit vacuously), as a field which was 'continually exploring new facets of the social past' (Stearns 1980: 208 and 211). Becoming slightly more specific, Stearns recalls that social history had been written in the United States before 1960 on topics related to 'the behaviour and material culture of large numbers of people under the impact of industrialisation and urbanisation' – 'social' here apparently referring to a large group of people. In the 1960s, however, a 'new enthusiasm' was fuelled by a drive 'to deal historically with topics, such as the family, ordinarily left to sociology'. In his view,

> the primary impulse was twofold. . . . First, in a memorable phrase, history was to be seen 'from the bottom up', through the experiences and perceptions of ordinary rather than extraordinary actors in the past. The clearest general definition of social history in the United States focuses on its concern with the general membership of a society, and not just individuals among the elite. Second, not only the mass of people but also the framework of their daily lives – their families, artifacts, community life, their births and deaths – was to be studied in order to fill out the historical characterisation of a period.
>
> (Stearns 1980: 212)

Bland though this characterisation is, Stearns at least managed to emphasise the growing importance in the 1970s of a new 'history-from-the-bottom-up' or history-from-below approach, one which was concerned with 'lower-class groups' such as slaves, servants and the working classes, and also with the question of social control.

> Social-control approaches have been used with particular success in histories of education and of custodial institutions, considerably revising conventional assumptions that the beneficence of reform-minded administrators could be taken for granted . . .
>
> (1980: 216)

According to Stearns (whose distancing tone here marks him as a traditionalist social historian), these bottom-up histories took a variety of forms, some stressing class divisions and conflict, a few adopting a Marxist model, based on Antonio Gramsci's theory of hegemony, while others rejected 'a rigorous class conceptualisation' in order to focus on the capacity of 'client populations' and other marginalised groups to develop 'semi-independent' yet adaptive subcultures which allowed for 'some independent basis for reaction to larger systems and processes' (1980: 216–17).

Lost in this flat account is any sense of the 'quantum leap in the quality and quantity of work' done in the field of social history in the 1970s when critical historians began to re-examine the 'interrelationships between the modern state and its apparatus of social control' (Cohen and Scull 1983: 1). Nor, more broadly, does Stearns provide any sense of the violent dissensions over the purpose of social history which rocked the discipline at that time. There is no sign here that, by the late 1970s, critical social historians like Tony Judt had come to the conclusion that social history was in a state of crisis, that it had become little more than

> a gathering place for the unscholarly, for historians bereft of ideas and subtlety. The writings thus produced are without theoretical content, a failing disguised by an obsession with method and technique. They represent collectively a loss of faith in history.
>
> (Judt 1979: 66)

From this critical perspective, social history, obsessed as it had become with quantifying long-term patterns and amorphously-defined trends such as modernisation, had lost sight of historical, that is, political events. Most crucially, it had forgotten that 'history is not just about politics, it *is* politics', politics understood in the broad sense of the ordering and preserving of power. For this disgruntled critic, one significant consequence of this divorce of political from social history was

> the insulting denial to people in the past of their political and ideological identity. Consciousness of any kind, particularly that relating to class, is

glossed over or paraphrased, so that human society in the past takes on an oddly impersonal, neo-hegelian quality. Strangely, then, modern society fails at its first hurdle – the proper and sympathetic account of *people*.

(Judt 1979: 68: his emphasis)

Interestingly, Judt singled out the editor of the *Journal of Social History* – unnamed in the text of his scathing indictment of social history, but identified in a footnote as Peter Stearns – as one of the worst offenders. Stearns's brand of social history was, in Judt's view, precisely the sort of 'history with the politics left out' which was 'inimical to the very enterprise of social history' – the sort which had transformed social history into 'a sort of retrospective cultural anthropology'. The only hope for rescuing social history from this crisis lay with those historians who remained 'committed to the proper pursuit of history' and who understood that a return to 'the centrality of politics, properly understood', would bring 'a recognition of the full identity of people in the past' (Judt 1979: 71 and 87–8). What, though, was meant by 'politics, properly understood' and how did the 'new' or critical social historians want to set about politicising social history? It was all very well for left critics to condemn what they saw as the 'political crisis of social history' and to declare that 'history is primarily the story of who rides whom and how' (Genovese and Genovese 1976: 219): the difficult task was to move beyond polemic and get on with reworking the job specifications of social historians in various fields of inquiry.

The shock of the new

In the field of penality or social control, the goal of rewriting history from a new or critical perspective was to be accomplished on several fronts as revisionist historians set about reconnecting the study of crime and punishment to the state. The contours of some of these new social histories of punishment will be mapped later. At this point it is essential to try to reclaim some of the transformative impact of the 'new' social history which pushed its way noisily and self-consciously on to the historical and political agenda in the United States and Western Europe in the late 1970s. Certainly, it is difficult to recapture an excitement which has been lost over time in this now much-traversed field. Perhaps all that can be done is to make an emphatic declaration: social history, or rather 'true social history' – 'the history of the historically inarticulate lower classes of society' written, of course, with the politics left in (Philips 1983: 55) – transformed the discipline of history and, crucially, our understanding of processes of social control instigated by the state in the West. In short, the new 'master' stories of punishment have been instrumental in transforming the study of punishment into a more sophisticated analysis of penality.

However, their impact should not be exaggerated. On the one hand, administrative history, as exemplified by the last volume of *The History of the English Criminal Law*, proceeds as if social history never occurred. In a brusque aside, Radzinowicz and Hood dismiss in a footnote what they refer to as 'the Asylum Theory', identified as 'a "term of art" used by modern criminologists to refer to a trend in penal policy based on a large scale use of incarceration to promote objectives of reform and cure' (1986: 220). In this way, they not only misrepresent and caricature social history's focus on social control, they also imply that there is no need to engage with the central arguments of the new histories of punishment which were written, as it happens, in the period between the publication of the fourth volume of Radzinowicz's history in 1968 and the fifth in 1986. Evidently, the significance of the insights and paradigm shifts produced by the new social history in the 1970s has passed administrative historians by. From where they sit, comfortably in ivory towers, the din of revisionist haggling over critical interpretations of the penal past is mere background noise, unworthy of comment. On the other hand, it seems to be business as usual for traditionalist Marxist historians. With a few exceptions, notably Melossi and Pavarini (1981) who single out Foucault's work as highly compatible with the Marxist project, they continue to produce political economies of past punishment regimes couched in the terms of a historical materialism which is largely untouched by revisionist hands. To this extent, Marxist historians of punishment share with mainstream administrative historians a disdain for the insights produced by the new social histories in the 1970s.

So much then for distinguishing traditional history from the new. A simpler way of demarcating the old from the new is by means of a date. Once again, the momentous year 1968 springs to mind. Admittedly, this may not be the historical moment which analysts informed by post-colonial critiques of the writing of Western history would choose.[3] But it needs to be recalled that the new Western history of the 1970s was focused, albeit unself-consciously, on Western institutions. Furthermore, in relation to the specific question of punishment, the new history was provoked by what was widely perceived to be a deep crisis in Western prison systems in the late 1960s. It was a time when critics of Western institutions saw a pressing need to ask 'some basic questions'. For example, the Italian criminologists Melossi and Pavarini felt obliged to question 'the very phenomenon of prison'. They explained what happened when they did:

we were surprised to discover – and this discovery affected the way of thinking to which we had subscribed until then – that despite the existence of a great number of studies within various political approaches, no one had clearly posed a question which began to appear increasingly central to us: *why prison?* Why is it that in every industrial society, this institution has become the dominant punitive instrument to such an extent that prison and punishment are commonly regarded as almost synonymous?

(Melossi and Pavarini 1981: 1; their emphasis)

In various and sometimes conflicting ways, the new histories of Western punishment regimes written at this time of penal crisis sought to address this central problematic: why prison? In this connection, it was no accident that Rusche and Kirchhmeimer's *Punishment and Social Structure*, the theoretical starting point for many of these new punishment histories, was republished in 1968. It too was born of the crisis within Western penality which was to transform ways of thinking of punishment in those jurisdictions affected by it. The year 1968 then, can be taken as the watershed year demarcating old from new histories of Western prison systems.

THE NEW (SOCIAL) HISTORY OF PUNISHMENT

Models and boxes

By now, this chapter should have conveyed two somewhat contradictory themes – a sense of the excitement generated by the new social history, but also a sense that the new post-1968 stories of correctional change, most of which concentrated on the emergence of the prison in the nineteenth century, have been told, revised, critiqued, classified and even categorised into boxes. Stanley Cohen, for example, has divided up the various histories of the emergence of the prison into three models or boxes – the 'uneven progress' model, the 'we blew it' version of history and the 'discipline and mystification' model, alternatively known as the 'it's all a con' view of correctional change. Each of these models contains four 'sub-plots' which Cohen characterises as:

(i) a master theory of how correctional changes or reforms occur in general; (ii) an account of why this specific historical transformation occurred . . .; (iii) an account of how the reforms embodied in this transition actually 'failed'; and (iv) the contemporary political moral of the whole story.

(Cohen 1985: 15)

As Cohen tells *his* story, the 'progress' model is the conventional view of correctional change, one 'based on a simple-minded idealist view of history' in which ideas form the motor-force for change. In this model, changes are seen to have occurred when a 'reform vision' is put into practice. It is this belief-in-progress type of history, characterised above as administrative history, which was challenged by the revisionism of the 1970s. Cohen divides up the revisionists into two camps, or rather, his second and third models. The second ('we blew it') model is based on a less idealist view of history than the progress model, but ideas and intentions are still taken seriously, this time, however, not as 'the simple products of humanitarian impulses or advances' but as 'functional solutions to immediate social changes'. Cohen chooses Rothman's histories of penal developments in nineteenth- and early twentieth-century North America as the most influential version of this model. Rothman's much-told stories about the 'reform' of penal regimes in response to a perceived 'social' need for order emphasise the ways in which reform goals were undermined in their implementation. They are stories with 'a heavy moral lesson for contemporary liberalism' – a lesson about naive optimism in reform in the face of pragmatic obstacles to change. But reform is still possible, so long as we monitor closely the ways in which 'convenience' undermines the original vision or 'conscience' (Cohen 1985: 17–21).

Finally, Cohen dumps the rest of the revisionist histories into his third ('discipline and mystification') box. These stories, identified by their cynical 'it's all a con' view of correctional change, reconstruct nineteenth-century prison history in materialist rather than idealist terms. Notwithstanding some significant differences in emphasis, they all tell tales about the imposition of a new control system which 'served the requirements of the emerging capitalist order' by disciplining the working class and mystifying 'everyone (including the reformers themselves) into thinking that these changes were fair, humane and progressive'. Again, for all their differences, these stories assume that the 'motor force of history lies in the political economy'. At one end of the range of stories are the more 'orthodox' Marxist tales, typified by Rusche and Kirchheimer's account of punishment systems conforming to specific modes of production, or Melossi and Pavarini's emphasis on the functional connections between the prison and capital's need to discipline the proletariat. Here the changing exigencies of capitalism – changes in the mode of production, fiscal crises, phases of unemployment, the requirements of capital – determine punishment regimes. At the other end is the 'somewhat "softer" version of this model' represented by Ignatieff's *Just Measure of Pain*. This version is 'softer' in Cohen's view because it rejects economic reductionism and so-called 'left functionalism' (1985: 21–3). Instead, Ignatieff insists on 'the complex and autonomous cluster of religious and philosophical beliefs' which led reformers to conceive of the penitentiary in the 1780s. As Ignatieff himself explains:

I put an unfashionable emphasis (for Marxists at least) on the role of reformers and on their system of beliefs because I think it is their role and not any functional necessity of the economic system which explains why the penitentiary was adopted as the particular solution to the crisis in punishment after 1776.

(Ignatieff 1982: 66)

Yet although beliefs are important in this explanatory schema, Cohen still places Ignatieff's account in the disciplinary box because of its interpretation of reform activity as 'expressing a new strategy of class relations'. This account remains materialist and disciplinary because of its emphasis on property crime, the role of the prison in containing the labour force, class antagonisms and the success of the nineteenth-century reformed prison in controlling the working class (Cohen 1985: 23–4).

If Cohen has no problem placing Ignatieff in the disciplinary box, Foucault is another matter altogether. *Discipline and Punish*, in Cohen's view, almost defies categorisation in that it

veers between a materialist connection between prison and emerging capitalism and an idealist's obsession with the power of ideas. But he must belong to this category (or a category of his own) because of his theory of relentless discipline, his ridicule of the whole enterprise of liberal reform and his total rejection of conventional notions of success and failure.

(Cohen 1985: 24)

Thus, with a bit of effort, Foucault can be squeezed into the discipline box. Cohen's succinct summary of Foucault's famous history of discipline and punishment make it clear how:

The 'Great Incarcerations' of the nineteenth century – thieves into prisons, lunatics into asylums, conscripts into barracks, workers into factories, children into schools – are to be seen as part of a grand design. Property had to be protected, production had to be standardised by regulations, the young segregated and inculcated with the ideology of thrift and success, the deviant subjected to discipline and surveillance. The new disciplinary mode which the prison was to represent, belonged to an economy of power quite different from that of the direct, arbitrary and violent rule of the sovereign. Power in capitalist society had to be exercised at the lowest possible cost (economically and politically) and its effects had to be intensive and extended – 'relayed' throughout the social apparatus.

(1985: 25)

Such a history, focused as it was on the dispersion of power throughout society and, indeed, on the emergence of a 'disciplinary' or 'carceral' society, obviously belonged in the 'disciplinary' box, if it belonged anywhere.

So much then for Cohen's summary of the dominant modes of historical interpretation available today: we can pick between progress, 'benevolence gone wrong' or 'relentless discipline'. There are of course other summaries of revisionist explanations for the transformation in Western punishment systems at the close of the eighteenth century. However, Cohen's truncated account of the revisionist historiography of changes in 'the master patterns and strategies for controlling deviance in Western industrial societies' – which he tabulates conveniently under the heading 'Master changes in deviancy control' (1985: 13–17) – provides one of the most concise summaries. While Cohen alludes briefly to critical evaluations of the models, he did not see his task as that of arbitrating between them. His goal was rather to present an overview of 'the revisionist package', one which he presents as having implications for understanding contemporary control systems. Indeed, as he makes clear, it is only by understanding those great transformations in penal systems in the early nineteenth century that we can begin to comprehend the changes taking place today (1985: 28–30).

We are now in the thick of what might be called a deep play of interpretative exegesis. Immersed as we are in a secondary account of revisionist punishment histories, it may seem as if we have become captive to precisely that kind of redundant retelling of stories which this chapter had hoped to avoid. Is there any escaping this trap of regurgitating what has been told, revised and even recanted, many times before? Or must any attempt at assessing the significance of the new history necessarily be enmeshed in what are by now well-established modes of categorising the new revisionist punishment histories of the 1970s? Are they all boxed up, Cohen-style, with nowhere to go? Fortunately, we do not need to remain imprisoned within the classificatory cages built by previous commentators. In order to break out, what is required is a recollection that our purpose here is to recapture the theoretical and political significance of the new history for transforming our understanding of penality. One way of doing so is to provide a sense of its reception by other analysts. Stanley Cohen's response, detailed above, is a case in point; David Garland's more recent one is another (1990a). But perhaps a better way of reclaiming that sense of paradigm-shifting import conveyed by the new histories at the time that they were written is to turn to their creators' assessment of what they were about and, more crucially, what difference they think they made.

A revisionist's own overview

Ignatieff's now classic revision of his own revisionist history, *A Just Measure of Pain*, provides one such assessment (1983a). In so far as this critique offers a comparative overview of the new social histories of punishment as well as a 'public recantation' of 'the faults' in his own contribution (Ignatieff 1982: 66), it warrants a close analysis. Ignatieff begins his critique by conflating revisionist history with social history and reminding us that this history, which proliferated after the radicalisation of politics in Western nations in the 1960s, covered a broad range of institutions such as the asylum, the urban school, the welfare system, the juvenile court as well as the prison. In relation to the prison, he singled out a trilogy of 'major' revisionist works: Rothman's *The Discovery of the Asylum*, Foucault's *Discipline and Punish* and, of course, his own work. As mentioned earlier, Foucault's work will be considered in the next chapter, but it is convenient to set out here Ignatieff's account of the points of convergence between his three exemplars of revisionist prison history. His self-styled 'schematic summary of the revolution in discipline as the revisionist account would have it' (1983a: 82) can serve as mine, as there is little point in providing yet another overview of these by now well-established histories of the 'master patterns' of penality.

According to Ignatieff, he, Rothman and Foucault all subscribed to the view that nineteenth-century reform programmes were inextricably connected to strategies of power which could only be understood if the history of the prison was 'incorporated into a history of the philosophy of authority and the exercise of class power in general'. They also all agreed that there was 'a revolution in punishment between 1780 and 1850'. Such a statement typifies the approach of Eurocentric historians who allow Western institutions to stand for all, and to perceive changes in those institutions as occurring on a global scale. Amending this error, it becomes apparent that what Ignatieff means is that the revisionists, however much their explanations may have differed, concurred in the view that a transformation occurred between 1780 and 1850 in European and North American punishment regimes. For 'each society'—by which he means England, France and North America – the revisionists noted the following key developments in this period: 'the decline of punishments involving the public infliction of physical pain'; the emergence of imprisonment as the dominant penalty for serious offences, and the coming of the penitentiary as 'the bearer of reformers' hopes for a punishment capable of reconciling deterrence and reform, terror and humanity'. More specifically, the new prisons 'substituted the pains of intention for the pains of neglect' and 'the rule of rules for the rule of custom'. As well, they 'put an end to the old division of power between the inmate community and the keepers' and 'enforced a markedly greater social distance between the confined and the outside world' (1983a: 77–81).

Where the revisionists differed was in their various explanations of this transformation in punishment in the West. Again, Ignatieff provides a useful summary. It is well to bear in mind that his critique is basically a response to criticism of the revisionist histories that they over-schematised a very complex penal story and reduced the reformers' intentions to 'conspiratorial class strategies of divide and rule'. Against this, Ignatieff concedes that the revisionists' accounts, his own included,

> contained three basic misconceptions: that the state enjoys a monopoly over punitive regulation of behaviour in society, that its moral authority and practical power are the binding sources of social order, and that all social relations can be described in the language of subordination.
>
> (1983a: 77)

In thus pulling back from the more alarmist class-control readings of the original revisionism, Ignatieff sets up his claim to offer a more balanced and reflective post-revisionist account of penal developments.

The most interesting section of the critique set outs Ignatieff's self-critique – his reassessment of his and Foucault's explanatory schemas. In both these schemas, the penitentiary was represented as part of 'a new strategy of power' aimed at the control of the illegalities of the working classes between 1780 and 1850. Beneath the reform rhetoric lay a reality of carceral networks of asylums, prisons, workhouses and reformatories. Here a new disciplinary ideology became a key 'strategy of class relations' as the disobedient poor were pressured into submitting to a new industrial order. Ignatieff however, is at pains to distinguish his own account, which emphasised 'the religious and philanthropic impulses behind institutional reform' and the humanitarianism of the reformers, from Foucault's more cynical account of the same institutional developments. Ignatieff's 'model of the reform of character' in the penitentiaries was 'one of symbolic persuasion'; Foucault, on the other hand, stressed 'disciplinary routinisation'. Still, they concurred in the view that there was a connection between 'this new strategy of power' which combined discipline with humanity and 'the social crisis' of early nineteenth-century Europe. For both, the 'recurrent surges of distress-related crime, pauperism and collective pauper unrest' form the background to the 'institutional revolution' in France and England. Now however, Ignatieff has become alert to the 'dangers of social reductionism' in the control models which he and Foucault had deployed to explain the new power strategies of mass imprisonment and the creation of a police force. In particular, interpreting the emergent carceral network as an institutional response to breakdown in labour market discipline will no longer do. Such an explanation does not get to the heart of the interpretative problem, namely, 'why authorities chose the particular remedies they did, why they put such faith in institutional confinement', rather than in corporal or capital punishment in response to the perceived breakdown of social control (1983a: 86–9). He might have added that these questions, probably more than any others, underlie much of the conflict between critical historians over the interpretation of the political significance of the emergence of the prison as the dominant mode of punishment in the West in the nineteenth century.

In his revised view, Ignatieff still sees a divide-and-rule strategy behind the efforts to quarantine criminals from the working class, but he is less certain that this strategy actually worked to create a criminal class separate from the working class, as Foucault had assumed. Anticipating his main argument that the new historians exaggerated the power of the state, Ignatieff displays his new-found moderation in the following passage.

> Certainly repeated imprisonment did isolate the criminal from his own class. But it is a serious overestimation of the role of the state to assume that its sanctioning powers were the exclusive source of the social division between criminal and respectable. The strategy of mass imprisonment is better understood in class terms as an attempt by the authorities to lend symbolic reinforcement to values of personal honour which they themselves knew were indigenous to the poor.
>
> (1983a: 91)

That is, support for punitive sanctions against serious criminal offences crossed class lines: they were not imposed from above on an unwilling populace. Further to the question of class power, Ignatieff now concedes that the adoption of 'the institutional solution', and of the penitentiary in particular, 'cannot be explained in terms of their supposed utility in manufacturing social divisions within the working class'. Now he would emphasise the reformers' belief in reform through discipline. The 'religious vernacular' of their reform arguments was much more significant than Foucault and the other social historians had realised. It testified to their commitment to a 'drama of guilt' for each individual offender which was institutionalised in the prison system (1983a: 92).

Next, Ignatieff turns to a related question – 'the problem of agency': 'Whose interests did the new institutions serve? In whose name were the reformers speaking?' It is Ignatieff's revised view that the social histories of the 1970s were especially faulty on these questions of agency. Foucault in particular was hazy about just who, exactly, 'directed the carceral archipelago'. Caught as he is in a paradigm of disciplinary power extending throughout society, Foucault has trouble identifying 'the privileged sites or actors that controlled all the others'. In all those disciplinary discourses which emerge to run around in a seemingly free and ungrounded fashion, it is difficult to identify the historical agents of the strategies Foucault describes. Occasionally, the 'bourgeoisie' makes an appearance, but it is never pinned down to specific social groups. And where is there any conception of the ruling class as the key historical agent behind the emergence of the carceral archipelago, and the making of the penitentiary in particular? Here Ignatieff comes to grips with the limitations of his own work, noting that it had been criticised

> for using 'middle class' as a synonym for 'ruling class' in a period in which it would be more accurate to speak of a bewilderingly complex competition for political power and social influence by different class factions, professionals, industrialists, and merchants, aristocratic magnates, and small gentry farmers.
>
> (1983a: 94)

His own historical evidence, he now concedes, suggests that the ruling class was not 'a collective social actor' at the time of the construction of the British prison system. It is his more refined position that:

> One can speak of a ruling class in the sense that access to strategic levers of power was systematically restricted according to wealth and inheritance, but one cannot speak of its acting or thinking as a collective historical subject. One can only ascribe historical effectivity to identifiable social constituencies or individuals who managed to secure political approval for penal change through a process of debate and argument in society's sites of power.
>
> (1993a: 94)

Contradiction, argument and conflict over penal policy within the ruling social groups are now to be emphasised over class and control themes. Interestingly though, it is Foucault's work, with its emphasis on 'an all-embracing disciplinary *savoir*' or world view, which is presented as more at fault in these respects than Ignatieff's: it is Foucault rather than Ignatieff who fell into the rationalist and conspiratorial traps of presenting the development of penal policy as 'an unfolding strategy of carceral *savoir*' (1983a: 95).

As for the functionalist trap of assuming that the new nineteenth-century penal system functioned just as its designers intended – to control the populace – Ignatieff concedes, at least initially, that his work was as much at fault as Foucault's. Both relied on a 'social control' model of the prison's function which assumed that capitalist society required the intervention of a state-run system of repression. Further, both assumed that this system worked effectively. In this his most important concession, Ignatieff admits that he as much as Foucault overstated the role of the state and the penal sanction in particular in reproducing exploitative capitalist social relations. More simply still, they overemphasised 'penal force'. Indeed, they over-emphasised the whole question of force. At this point however, as he turns to question the role of force in the maintenance of social order, Ignatieff once again directs his attack exclusively against Foucault. *Discipline and Punish* is faulted for describing all social relations, including the family, in terms of power, domination, discipline and subordination. Apparently, Foucault fell prey to 'a fashionable current of thought' in the 1970s, notably feminism, or more especially 'the feminist critique of patriarchal domination' – a critique which, in Ignatieff's considered view, has

> 'over-politicised' family social relations, neglecting the collaborative and sacrificial elements of family attachment and over-emphasizing the power aspects of family interaction.
>
> (1983a: 98)

Leaving aside, for the moment, the singularity of the charge that Foucault was unduly influenced by feminism, the main drift of Ignatieff's critique is that in locating the family on a continuum of disciplinary institutions with the prison, and by describing family and other social relations as relations of domination, Foucault has neglected our 'human capacity' for sociability, voluntarism and 'order-seeking behaviour'. The implication is clear: it is time to go beyond social control explanations with their language of power and carceral archipelagos and their 'state-centered conception of social order'. What we need now is a more balanced understanding which gives roughly equal weight to the coercive and the consensual dimensions of human behaviour. To accomplish such a balance, Ignatieff insists that we will need to reassess critically the role of the state in reproducing social order. But he has already made up his mind: 'the new social history of law and punishment in the 1970s exaggerated the centrality of the state, the police, the prison, the workhouse and the asylum'. The way forward, according to the new post-revisionist Ignatieff, is to look more at informal rituals and practices, to locate the prison 'within a whole invisible frame-work' of sanctions and regulation throughout society, and to retreat from the alarmist state-centred interpretations offered by the new social histories of the 1970s (1983a: 96–101).

So much then for Ignatieff's overview of revisionist punishment histories and his disavowal of his own pre-1980 position. It is to be hoped that it has served the purpose of filling in some of the complexities and nuances left out of Cohen's abridged, boxed-up version. There are of course many other summaries and overviews of the new histories, but none, with the exception of David Garland's which is considered below, offers that self-reflexive gloss which is the distinguishing characteristic of Ignatiefff's famous retraction. Pausing at such length on his reply to his critics has enabled us to bypass the criticisms themselves – criticisms which focus predominantly on the control themes of revisionist history (e.g. DeLacy 1981). It has also served to illustrate just how far a 'radical' historian is prepared to retreat when the feminist implications of his control interpretation become apparent to him. The question of control, particularly social control, is an important one to which we will return, but let us now turn to a consideration the broader issue of the revisionists' contribution to a new understanding of Western punishment regimes.

ASSESSING THE NEW SOCIAL HISTORY

Social context, power and control

In all the criticism directed at the revisionist histories of punishment, some of which will be considered here, we should not lose sight of two of their most fundamentally significant and far-reaching effects. The first was to provide a greatly enhanced understanding of the contingency of penal forms. Whether they remained faithful to Marxist categories of analysis, or moved so far along the spectrum of revisionist explanation as to be no longer recognisable as Marxist, or even as wedded to a political economy of punishment, the new histories had this much in common: they all provided a sense of the pivotal importance of social context, that is, of contextualising prison regimes. Admittedly, there was no consistency in their deployment of 'the social'. Indeed, most of them failed to clarify just what was 'social' about their new histories of punishment. Even those purporting to provide a social history were remiss in this regard. Ignatieff, for example, simply advised his readers that the starting point for his social history of the penitentiary in Great Britain was the 1770s, 'when the vision of the "total institution" first began to take shape out of two centuries of accumulated experience with workhouses, houses of correction, and jails' (Ignatieff 1978: 11). Apparently Ignatieff did not feel the need to elaborate on the meaning of 'social history'. He was content with conveying an implicit meaning of social or historical context, one which included two hundred years of 'waves' of experiments with 'modes of total discipline'. Nowhere is the 'social' of *A Just Measure of Pain* explicitly defined. We are informed only that the penitentiary fulfilled a 'larger social need' than the control of crime; that it was a response to 'the whole social crisis of a period', and that it was 'conceived as a machine for the social production of guilt' (1978: 210–13).

But where in all this are the people whom social history was supposed to write in? It is all very well to begin with an account of the convict's daily routine in Pentonville and to even name an inmate, one George Withers (1978: 3–11), but the 'bottom-up' perspective, which was supposed to define the new social history, quickly fades behind the focus on the control strategies of the ruling groups. Perhaps by the time Ignatieff and the other revisionists came to write their histories of the great nineteenth-century transformations in penal forms, the social of social history was taken for granted. From a more critical perspective, 'the social' of the new social history functions in the same way as Beverley Brown has suggested in another context: as 'the magic bullet' to show up the errors of previous conceptualisations – in our case, of administrative history. With the invocation of 'the social' in penal history, the idealist notions of progress and reform may be banished in the name of social origins, social change and social control. Thus 'the social' or even 'society' comes to stand as the cure for Whig history's idealist errors.[4] Still, for all that can be criticised about this loosely-constructed 'social', the contextualising strategy of the new social history was a considerable advance on the dreary, linear change-as-progress assumptions of traditional history.

The second major contribution of revisionist punishment history was to emphasise the politicality of history. Notwithstanding their divergent agendas, these new histories can all be seen as regional applications of the critical new historical understanding of the late 1960s that history must be written from an explictly political perspective. Ignatieff's fighting concluding words to *A Just Measure of Pain* make this political commitment of the revisionist historian clear:

> As Foucault and others have proved, history . . . has a discrete but important role to play in combating carceral power and the coercive structures of thought that underpin it. It can explicate the genesis of structures of scientific argument about human nature and deviance and can establish the connections between this structure and the imperatives of class rule. Above all, it can help to pierce through the rhetoric that ceaselessly presents the further consolidation of carceral power as a 'reform'. As much as anything else, it is this suffocating vision of the past that legitimises the abuses of the present and seeks to adjust us to the cruelties of the future.
>
> (Ignatieff 1978: 220)

Ignatieff, as we have seen, was to draw back from some of the central political claims of his social history, but he did not recant his belief in the political significance of penal history and its role in breaking up the suffocating vision of the past, in questioning the rhetoric of 'reform' and in confronting carceral power. For Ignatieff as for the other revisionist historians of punishment systems, history had to be precisely that politicised story which the new social historians were demanding in the late 1970s.

At this point, our analysis of the new social history could take a number of different directions. First and most immediately, we should turn briefly to the question of politics and power – 'carceral' or 'disciplinary' power – noting how it returns us to the issue of control, or rather 'social control', the dominant theme of the new social histories of punishment. As should be clear by now, social control interpretations of nineteenth-century reform measures and institutional developments came into their own in the 1970s. Indeed, by the early 1980s the concept of social control had become 'the dominant paradigm for describing not simply reform movements, but interclass relationships from the 1830s through the progressive era' (Mayer 1983: 17). Since then, however, the concept has been subjected to quite a battering across the political and theoretical spectrum, as Ignatieff's retreat from his earlier commitment to a control framework makes clear. In Marxist as well as non-Marxist quarters, 'social control' has been lampooned as tautological, vacuous and functionalist (e.g. Stedman Jones 1983; Mayer 1983; DeLacy 1986). At one level, the question has been asked: 'What is social about social control?' (Fine 1986). At another, the kind of history which a reliance on this broad amorphous concept produces has been condemned as 'ahistorical history' – as history which cannot effectively account for specific changes at specific times (Mayer 1983: 22). Certainly, social control themes are still being raised in accounts of past and present penal regimes. For example, Melossi has recently attempted to develop a theory of social control in which the state is represented as 'nothing more than a powerful rhetorical device' or 'a dependent conceptual variable', one dependent on the social construction of meaning, or rather on 'the social control of meaning'. It follows that we can no longer 'picture the state' as 'the author of control'. Rather, 'the current state is the state of social control'. In developing these themes, Melossi came to reject his earlier Marxist-framed work on the prison as an 'ancillary' institution which performed the role of reproducing capitalist social and economic relations in the nineteenth century. In this his post-Marxist moment, Melossi carries social control to new theoretical pastures which lie beyond the reach of a 'state-concept' (Melossi 1990: 153, 168 and 172).

But we are getting ahead of our story. Suffice it to note here that historians, including revisionist historians, have been reluctant to resort to a 'social-control' explanation of changing legal and penal forms (Philips 1983: 59).[5] Others have explictly refused it (DeLacy 1986). However, the self-imposed task of this chapter is not to defend the concept of 'social control' but rather to reclaim from later critiques a sense of the theoretical breakthrough which was made in the 1970s when the new histories began to explore the interrelationships between emergent modern Western states and their control systems. Whether those systems were described in terms of 'social control' is not the crucial issue.

What we need to do at this stage is to pause to take stock and direct our attention to the key questions. First, what are we to make of the social history of punishment and second, how should we organise our response to it? In a recent overview, David Garland arranged these critical penal histories along a kind of continuum, ranging from orthodox Marxist to neo-Marxist studies of punishment. Not surprisingly, he takes Rusche and Kirchheimer's text as the benchmark of traditional Marxist analysis, its orthodoxy signposted clearly by its reliance on the classic categories of political economy, modes of production, the labour market and class struggle. In Garland's categorisation of the new histories, Melossi and Pavarini's *The Prison and the Factory* (1981) should be read as an extension of the orthodox Ruschean thesis that labour-market conditions directly affected prison regimes. Looking for relief from what he describes as reductive economistic themes, Garland moves on to the neo-Marxist accounts which are concerned to locate penality within the ideological and political field, instead of viewing it narrowly in economic terms, and which thus offer 'a more nuanced and subtle account of the part played by penality in the negotiation of ruling-class hegemony and the maintenance of social order' (1990a: 111). Here he places the work of Pashukanis, Douglas Hay, Ignatieff and his own book *Punishment and Welfare*, which he describes as yet another of those accounts which are concerned with the question of 'how penal policies are forged by particular social movements within the constraints of larger social structures' (1990a: 126).

At this point, it may seem as if we are once again flirting with the danger of regurgitation, this time with Garland's assessment of revisionist punishment history. Do we really need to engage with yet another overview of this much-revisited history? The answer is: no, if such an engagement takes the form of a simple rehash of another critical assessment; yes, if the goal is to problematise modes of categorisation in order to reclaim the interpretative power of the new histories from the condescension of its later critics.

Garland's post-revisionist synthesis

That Garland's book *Punishment and Welfare* (1985) focused on the development of new penal-welfare institutions in Britain in the late nineteenth and early twentieth centuries, serves to remind us that the new history was not exclusively concerned with the coming of the penitentiary.

Written several years after the classic social histories of Rothman, Ignatieff and Foucault, *Punishment and Welfare* is nevertheless properly classified as new social history inasmuch as it raised what might be called historically-informed social questions. First, 'how is penal change possible and how does it come about?'; second, what is the relationship between punishment and social structure, or, better still, between 'forms of social organisation' and 'forms of penality' – 'penality' being defined here as 'the whole of the penal complex, including its sanctions, institutions, discourses and representations' (Garland 1985: vii and x)? This terminology immediately gives it away that this text was written within a Foucauldian framework. But, as Garland later explained, the book addressed a question which was Marxist in orientation, namely, 'how a changing mode of production gave rise to political and ideological developments which had direct consequences for social and penal policy' (1990a: 126). *Punishment and Welfare* was new social history in another key sense: its aim was to examine the central features of the contemporary British system of penality by means of a critical historical analysis of the system which preceded the modern one (1985: 1). Finally, like the revisionist histories of the 1970s, Garland's self-defined 'history of penal strategies' had a political agenda: to provide a framework in order to confront policy questions in Britain's welfare state.

Reflecting back on his account of the transition from the Victorian mode of penality to the modern British penal-welfare system which he claims emerged after 1895, Garland is content to reiterate his argument that a distinctively new penal-welfare apparatus emerged between 1895 and 1914. As he summarises the argument, the 'new penality' was linked to 'a new set of institutional strategies which came to be called the Welfare State':

> Its distinctively positive approach to the reform of deviants, its extensive use of interventionist agencies, its deployment of social work and psychiatric expertise, its concern to regulate, manage, and normalise rather than immediately to punish, and of course its new 'welfarist' self-representation – all these characteristics combined to link the new penality into the new set of social strategies, ideological forms, and class relations which emerged at this time.

Such an interpretation, Garland concedes, could be read as a Marxist:

> The Marxist implications which one might draw from this study would point to the links between particular modes of production and modes of penality, the tendency of legal and penal categories to correspond to the dominant pattern of economic relations, and the supporting role which penal ideologies play in constructing a hegemonic form of social domination.
>
> (1990a: 128)

But Garland is emphatic that the main thrust of his historical analysis of the new penality in Britain was not that economic processes determine penal outcomes but rather that 'penal outcomes are negotiated' by a range of decision-making agents, frequently with conflicting agendas, within the limits imposed by broader structural imperatives. Thus the focus of analysis should be 'the medium of human action', in particular 'conjunctural political' and specific struggles, rather than any deterministic mode of production (1990a: 128).

Clearly, Garland is at pains to distance his analytical framework from the Marxist model. He is willing to concede that wider economic, legal and ideological forces 'will produce pressure towards specific kinds of penal practice' but he retreats from any causal analysis. Marxism, he insists, can only provide a partial account of penal changes. Indeed, he goes so far as to suggest that

the most obvious limitation of *Punishment and Welfare* as a *historical* account, is its tendency to view penal change only from the point of view of its implications for class domination and the control of the poor. In doing so, it replaces the analysis of *cultural* forces by an analysis of *ideological* forces . . .

(1990a: 129: his emphasis)

It is Garland's considered view that such a class-bound perspective overstates the political implications of penal measures. While a Marxist framework helps us to theorise penality's relationship to class-divided societies, it misses the other – as yet unnamed but evidently 'cultural' – determinants and significances of penal measures.

By 1990 then, Garland had modified his 1985 punishment-and-welfare position in a way which is reminiscent of Ignatieff's earlier and more famous 'recantation'. His great retreat from a social-control framework or 'power' perspective in favour of a 'more multi-dimensional framework' (1990b: 1) will be discussed further in the next chapter. After all, it is Foucault's 'power perspective' even more than the economistic accounts of the Marxists which he has most clearly in his sights, and to which he devotes the most critical attention. Here it is relevant to note that Garland concludes his overview of the various Marxist and neo-Marxist accounts of punishment with a summary of their arguments which might not be recognisable to the writers themselves. For this five-point summary manages to dilute their historical accounts of punishment regimes, robbing them of the power of their arguments and pushing their key analytical categories so far into the background that the accounts are no longer identifiably Marxist or even neo-Marxist. Gone are the familiar Marxist benchmarks – the theory of surplus value, modes of production, class divisions, ruling-class strategies of domination and even the primacy of the economy. Instead we have the 'benefit' of Garland's summary account of these critical perspectives in which penality is converted into 'a state-controlled apparatus of repression and ideology' which operates as 'an instrument of governance by one class' (which one?) against another. Broader ideological, political and economic struggles also affect penality, according to the summary account, and penal practices are even connected to the 'ideological commitments of the ruling bloc'. As well, punishment contributes to the legitimatory role of law and is linked to other social policies which regulate the poor and other 'problem' populations. Indeed, penal practices are shaped above all 'by the condition of the lower classes and other strategies adopted towards them by the governing elite' – that is, by 'wider strategies of rule' (1990b: 130).

In Garland's view, these are the five important points which have been developed by Maxist and neo-Marxist analyses, but what he finds most striking about them is that they do not need to be expressed in Marxist terms and are therefore not tied to that framework. It follows that, if these the most significant 'Marxist' findings about penality 'are not essentially "Marxist"', then they can be made to be more compatible with non-Marxist perspectives on punishment (1990a: 130). And if this is the case, Garland is well on the way to achieving his goal of forging a new synthesis of punishment studies in which punishment is reinstated as a fundamental object of social and also 'cultural' analysis. As he explains, his new project is to explore the penal realm 'in all its different aspects' by reopening 'basic questions about punishment's social foundations' and charting its functions and effects. But his ultimate goal is nothing less than that of uncovering

> the structures of social action and the webs of cultural meaning within which modern punishment actually operates, thereby providing a proper descriptive basis for normative judgments about penal policy.
>
> (1990a: 10)

This represents a significant shift in direction away from the social control focus of the revisionist histories of the 1970s and his own history of the emergence of Britain's penal-welfare complex in the late nineteenth century. In contrast to those sociologies and histories which have sought to explain punishment in terms of social-control functions or to analyse it in relation to other strategies, such as welfarism, as his own *Punishment and Welfare* did, or as an effect of ideologies or of economic and political relations, as the new social history did, Garland now wants us to understand punishment 'as a set of cultural practices'. To this end he insists that analysts should seek out 'the pattern of cultural expression as well as the logic of social control' (1990b: 10). As Mark Finnane explains, Garland now wants to stress 'the centrality of punishment as a cultural institution in its own right', one which should be perceived not simply as an 'effect' of other relations but rather 'as an agent in social structures, creating meanings, constructing cultural and political differences, expressing the psychological dispositions of social actors' (Finnane 1991: 107). Garland believes that what is required to achieve such a project is an analytical framework which is 'more flexible and multi-dimensional' than that suggested by analysts such as Foucault. Whereas Foucault's aim was the more limited one of highlighting the power dimensions of punishment, Garland's is to understand 'the social institutions of punishment . . . in *all* their complexity' (Garland 1990b: 12; my emphasis).

Clearly, Garland's agenda is very different from mine. His is to usher in a new sociological understanding of punishment as cultural agent which will move us beyond the interpretative battle between the revisionists of the 1970s, who stressed the coercive, disciplinary and class dimensions of penal regimes, and their critics who have sought to re-emphasise the humanitarianism of the reformers and the 'consensual' or widely-accepted nature of the penal changes they introduced. My agenda is the more modest one of rescuing the new social histories from the crustacean bed of two decades of criticism, and coercion–consensus balancing acts, which have culminated in a synthesising overview such as that attempted by David Garland. Or, in the event that they cannot be rescued, my project becomes the even more modest one of reclaiming some of the conflict and passion of the new history which gets lost in the warm, murky, synthesising schematisations of this post-revisionist age.

RECLAMATION ACTS?

The politics of (Western and masculinist) 'social' history revisited

If nothing else, revisionist histories of punishment regimes were faithful to the clarion call of the dissenters within the ranks of social history to politicise all fields of inquiry calling themselves 'social'. They not only put the politics back into history; they ensured that historians would squabble over the interpretation and meaning of past penal forms for years to come.[6] But for all the controversy and passion that they injected into the study of punishment, the controversy over the revisionist histories remained a local squabble in two significant senses. First, the scope of the new histories was restricted to Western penal systems. The revisionists however, rarely noticed that their studies were so limited: they claimed to be reconceptualising the historical analysis of punishment *tout court*. Occasionally, an effort was made to draw on material from non-Western societies.[7] But more commonly, the focus was exclusively

Western. As Harding and Ireland argue, this has significant implications for an assessment of the new history. Most crucially, the unacknowledged preoccupation with Western penal forms has had the effect of narrowing the analytical framework to state legal systems. As a result there has been, as Harding and Ireland point out, 'a strong tendency to present a paradigm of punishment in the form of a state institution' and 'it is significiant that state, in this context, is primarily understood in a Western sense'. In this view, it is the Eurocentric bias of the revisionist studies which led to the state-centred focus which Ignatieff, for one, later came to regret. Because they concentrated on the model of Western industrialised capitalist nations, the revisionists overemphasised the power of the state to punish, thereby ignoring the forms of punishment located elsewhere, in particular in so-called 'stateless' societies. Thus, a critique of the Eurocentric bias of punishment studies leads, in this instance, to a plea for a retreat from 'conventional' state-focused studies and the recognition of 'the wide diaspora of penal institutions' in 'society as a whole' – the 'penal totality' no less. The political agenda here is to insist that there is a 'widely spread punitive impulse throughout society as a whole' (Harding and Ireland 1989: 16–17, 23–36). But what is of interest to us is that in the process of making their case for a focus on 'popular penality' or 'non-state penality', Harding and Ireland dump all the major revisionist histories – those of Foucault, Ignatieff, Melossi and Pavarini, Garland – into the 'conventional' bag, along with Rusche and Kirchheimer's traditional Marxist account, inasmuch as they remained state-centred. As they see it, the problem with such a state-focus is that it overemphasises the coercive side of punishment, when what is required is 'a more balanced perspective of the totality of penal practice' (1989: 67–72).

Clearly, their preoccupation with forming a 'balanced' view indicates that Harding and Ireland's critique of the revisionist social control studies is a product of the 'consensual' Western interpretative paradigm, and not of the far more radical post-colonial challenge to Western epistemologies. Still, they make a crucial point, one which could provide the starting-point for a post-colonial theoretical analysis of punishment. It is Harding and Ireland's insight that the drive to transform punishment into an object of analysis is a peculiarly modern Western one. Indeed:

> the reflective and critical intellectual tendency to view punishment as a *problem*, requiring justification, analysis, and study is predominantly reflective of an *angst* that appears to have developed in Europe some two or three hundred years ago . . .

Moreover, what distinguishes modern Western discourse on punishment is the development of a radical critical position, which challenged not only the operation of specific modes of punishment . . . but more fundamentally, the normative framework within which punishment was carried out . . .

(1989: 74–5)

Paradoxically then, a radical critical position such as the one taken by the new history contributed to the process of transforming punishment into a specific sphere of knowledge, but at the same time it has delimited this sphere within the restricting parameters of modern Western culture.

As Harding and Ireland point out, this blinkered Eurocentric vision leads to some serious misjudgements about penal practices, notably incarceration. They provide a very relevant example – that of Melossi and Pavarini's Marxist thesis (1981) about the relationship between the origin of the modern prison and the rise of the capitalist mode of production. This thesis rests in part on the assumption that imprisonment did not exist as a form of punishment in pre-capitalist societies. The problem with this assumption is that, as in other Western punishment studies – revisionist and traditional alike – it is based on a study of imprisonment in Western Europe and North America. The use of imprisonment in non-capitalist or predominantly non-industrialised Third World countries falls outside the scope of the analysis. The findings drawn from these Eurocentric studies, whether they are written from a Marxist or non-Marxist perspective, are tantamount to tautologies: they start by locating imprisonment 'within the temporal and spatial confines of capitalist social structures' and, not surprisingly, they 'discover a system that reflects the conditions of such a society' (Harding and Ireland 1989: 195–6).

As if this were not enough to sink the pretensions of the revisionists to have radically challenged punishment historiography, another caveat must be placed on any remaining enthusiasm for their 'new' social histories. This second caveat is that they ignored women and, in this significant respect, were not so 'new' after all. Just as in traditional accounts of past penal regimes, there is a formidable silence about the historical realities of the punishment of women in the revisionist penal stories. Occasionally, women inmates of workhouses and prisons rate a mention, but always in passing or as a footnote to the main agenda: the imprisonment of men. The implicit assumption is that penal regimes impacted uniformly on male and female offenders. Gender considerations simply fell outside the scope of the revisionist re-writing of 'the master patterns' of penal history. Belatedly, the revisionists themselves picked up this fatal flaw. Class and power had figured strongly in their accounts, but gender, they finally acknowledged, had been sadly neglected. The solution seemed to be to extend the analysis to a consideration of 'differentiation by gender' (Cohen and Scull 1983: 11), as if 'adding' gender would keep feminist monitors at bay.

Feminist incursions into the masculinist analytical field of penality, including work which engages critically with revisionist punishment history, will be considered in chapter 4. But we should note here the methodological inadequacy of the suggestion that gender be added to the revisionist histories of the 'master' patterns of penality. It was the fate of these histories, and of the new social history in general, to have a very flawed vision of 'the social'. Even as they opened up new dimensions of the social, feminist historians were asking: what is 'social' about the new social history? From a feminist perspective, conventional masculinist social histories are simply scandalous. As late as 1985, the Australian feminist historian Kay Daniels expressed surprise that historians could continue to 'write histories of whole societies without ever thinking about the place of women at all'. Interestingly, she gives as an example an Australian convict history in which the convicts are all men: 'it is male convicts who rebel and the punishments discussed are generally *their* punishments – the punishments of male convicts' (1985: 27–9: her emphasis).[8] As for the new social history which had emerged over the past two decades, Daniels felt that it had the potential to make a useful alliance with feminism if historians could overcome the stumbling block that social history had not proved to be 'sympathetic to either women or to feminism'. Indeed, much of it was 'explictly anti-feminist' (1985: 34 and 38).[9] Her examples are not germane to the study of punishment, but one at least implicitly anti-feminist social historian of punishment springs to mind: Ignatieff, as we have seen, was appalled by what he considered to be the undue influence of feminism on his fellow social historian, Foucault.

Reflecting on the relationship between social history and 'her-story', Joan Scott has also been critical of masculinist social historians who assume that gender difference can be explained within its existing explanatory framework, thereby failing to see gender as 'an issue requiring study in itself' (1988a: 22). Certainly, this is true of the social historians of social control – that is, when they noticed gender at all. Without exception, they appear to have been oblivious to the very idea that gender is 'a useful category of historical analysis', let alone to the implications of that suggestion (1988b). Of course, it is easy to condemn the naivety of past epistemological paradigms from the advantage of conceptually-developed hindsight. When the new social history burst on to the intellectual scene, feminist scholars like Joan Scott were still developing their sophisticated gender-sensitive analytical frameworks. Writing in the 1970s, before the development of poststructural critiques of fixed binary oppositions such as male/female, the revisionist historians were trapped within masculinist paradigms in which 'the social' was equated with 'men' (as in the notion of the prison as a 'factory of men') and 'gender', if it was thought of at all, was a synomym for women (as in, add in a few examples of women inmates). It is therefore hardly surprising that the revisionists were as remiss as mainstream historians when it came to theorising gender. Without access to complex gender analyses, their framings of the 'social' could not benefit from an understanding that 'gender' is used 'to designate social relations between the sexes' – that 'man' and 'woman' are socially relational categories. If only they could have realised that gender is both a 'constitutive element of social relationships' and also a 'primary way of signifying relationships of power' (1988b: 32 and 42) when they came to write their 'social' histories of penal regimes. A comprehension that gender is not simply a social relation but a relation of domination could only have enhanced their conceptualisations of the operation of carceral power.

The 'social' analysis of penality will be greatly enriched when a feminist scholar writes a critique of the new social history of punishment in the mode of Joan Scott's superb deconstruction of gendered representations in E. P. Thompson's profoundly masculinist *The Making of the English Working Class* (1988c). But that feat will have to await another book. It suffices to note here that feminist critiques of masculinist studies which purport to represent 'the social' have exposed a flaw which is fatal to any attempt to brush up the transgressive credentials of the new social histories of punishment produced in the 1970s. Any history, especially self-defined 'social' history, which fails to theorise gender relations is surely beyond reclamation.

Revisiting the rediscovery of 'the birth' of the prison

Can anything now be saved of the new social history? In its defence, it might be helpful to recall that the ultimate goal was to ask some very basic questions about punishment with a view to disturbing the taken-for-granted inevitability of punishment regimes. Specifically, the revisionists wanted to know: why prison – why is it that today 'prison and punishment are commonly regarded as almost synonymous?' (Melossi and Pavarini 1981: 1). More broadly, the goal was to politicise punishment by historicising it – by demonstrating not only its historical contingency but also its role in the class politics of discipline and control. As we have seen, it was the emerging predominance of penal confinement in early modern societies and, in particular, the establishment of penitential regimes in early nineteenth-century Europe and North America which caught the imagination of the social historians. Three of the most cited punishment histories – Foucault's *Discipline and Punish: The Birth of the Prison* (1977a), Ignatieff's *A Just Measure of Pain: The Penitentiary in the Industrial Revolution, 1750–1850* (1978), and Melossi and Pavarini's *The Prison and the Factory: Origins of the Penitentiary System* (1981) – all dealt with the coming of the penitentiary. Produced during the penal crises in the West in the 1970s, all three histories bear the revisionist stamp, but only the last, at least according to one reviewer, was properly 'materialist'. Only *The Prison and the Factory* managed to locate the institution in 'the material conditions and not only the ideas' of the relevant periods – the early sixteenth-century to mid-nineteenth-century Europe and late seventeenth-century to mid-nineteenth-century North America. Moreover, it was the only one to be 'theoretically informed by Marxism' (Mandel 1982: 848).

It is precisely for this reason – the fact that *The Prison and the Factory* is seen as Marxist rather than 'social', and theoretical rather than historical – that some critics do not include it in their overviews of revisionist punishment history. Yet, in so far as it engages with Foucault's disciplinary themes and shares with his and other critical histories of the 1970s a political concern about contemporary prison systems, this text is an appropriate choice as exemplar of the revisionist rediscovery of the birth of the prison – a rediscovery informed by a political desire to research the historical determinants of the contemporary penal crises in the West. In *The Prison and the Factory*, Melossi and Pavarini sought to overcome what they identified as the central problem with Rusche and Kirchheimer's traditional Marxist account of punishment – the persistence of the prison into the twentieth century, notwithstanding changing economic conditions. Their solution was to refine Rusche and Kirchheimer's account of the parallel emergence of the prison and capitalism via the concept of discipline. In this construction, the prison is presented as ancillary to the factory, with discipline as 'the functional connection' between them (Melossi 1979: 91).

> The history of segregated institutions and of their prevailing ideology can be reconstructed from capital's fundamental need to extend its command: The history of their ancillary nature can be traced to the factory, which is no more than the extension of the capitalistic organisation of labour above and beyond the factory . . .
>
> (Melossi and Pavarini 1981: 45)

The capitalist disciplinary practices which spread out from the factory to the 'ancillary' institutions gradually came to be seen as a means of reproducing capitalist social relations. Thus, the persistence of the prison under the changing economic conditions in the second half of the nineteenth century can be explained in terms of a continuing need to socialise the labour force to industrialised capitalist production.

In brief, Melossi and Pavarini argue that the early European and North American prisons were 'an essentially bourgeois creation' aimed at instilling obedience. Moreover they worked: they functioned to discipline the work-force in the interests of the capitalist class. This supposed functional fit explains why imprisonment emerged as the dominant mode of punishment under capitalism. According to this Marxist interpretation,

> the revolution in punitive forms, which had slowly developed out of the origins of the capitalist mode of production up to the developed liberal capitalism of the nineteenth century meant that ... prison was defined as the dominant form of punishment, bourgeois punishment *par excellence*.
>
> (1981: 95)

This attempt to improve on the Rusche–Kirchheimer thesis by confronting the 'economic and ideological specificities of bourgeois punishment' may have won Melossi and Pavarini 'the theoretical high ground' (Garton 1988: 315), but this is not to suggest that their account is convincing. On the contrary, there has been much dissent about the origins of the modern penal system, which has been associated – at least in Marxist and social histories – with the birth of the prison. Uncertainty as to the precise birthdate of the modern prison has left critical accounts of the emergence of bourgeois punishment vulnerable to quite a savaging. Indeed, much of the historical critique of these accounts has been directed to the question of periodisation, or more especially to the question of what should be decreed as the decisive moment at which the prison emerged.[10] Was the prison born between 1770 and 1840 as Foucault would have it? Or was the decisive moment much earlier, around the time of the transition to capitalist social relations as Rusche and Kirchheimer claimed, or more exactly at the time of the establishment of bridewells or houses of correction in Elizabethan England (Melossi and Pavarini 1981: 11–16)? Or should we locate the origins of the modern penal system with its 'actual formation' much later at the turn of the twentieth century, as Garland does (1985: 4–5)?[11]

These questions do not need to be resolved here as they fall outside the scope of this book.[12] However, we might note in passing that this desire to locate the precise moment of the birth of the prison is symptomatic of a universalising tendency such that, however much they profess to be analysing specific punishment regimes, it is *the* prison whose birth is being recorded. Our goal in this chapter is to recapture some of the interpretative power of critical punishment histories without getting caught up in the internecine debates for and against the specific claims of analysts writing under the rubric of 'the new social history' of punishment. To fall into such a trap would be akin to labouring at a treadwheel, such is the thoroughness with which questions about the emergence of modern penal systems, and the prison in particular, have been canvassed. All we need note is that attempts like that of Melossi and Pavarini to construct a Foucauldian-influenced Marxist history stand as a testimonial to the power of what has been, indisputably, the most influential of the revisionist histories, one which defies any bid to confine it here.

On the other hand, it could also be said that *The Prison and the Factory* encapsulates the faults of the Marxist variety of new history.[13] It is Eurocentric in its focus on Western punishment systems; it is masculinist in its failure to consider gender, and it is functionalist in its 'needs-of-capitalism' assumption about the apparent 'fit' between the disciplinary logic of capitalist production and the disciplinary logic of the early penitentiaries. In addition, its methodological eclecticism – its attempt to merge Foucault's theoreticist genealogical methodology with the empirical imperatives of social history within a Marxist framework – leads to tensions in its argument.[14] As well, there is a tension between the somewhat different theoretical frameworks of its two authors. Whereas Melossi's approach is materialist in that he ties European penal developments to the changing needs of capitalism, Pavarini emphasises ideological issues such as the contradictions in the bourgeois world view between the legal equality of workers in the marketplace and their subordination in the factory (Mandel 1982: 849). Moreover, while their account is bold and schematic in its attempt to 'impose intelligible order on a complex history', and while it manages to draw attention to neglected control features of the precursors to the prison, it fails to deliver on the required historical evidence for its claims. For example, it is enlightening to propose a particular social function for the English bridewells – that of disciplining the labour force – but in her detailed history of the bridewells Joanna Innes has noted problems of 'chronological fit' between the emergence of these institutions and the Marxists' theory of social change. It is all very well to argue that the bridewells were well suited to the system of labour relations in the early modern period, but unfortunately the Marxist timing is out: the bridewells 'arrived too late in the day' to facilitate fundamental changes in the organisation of production (Innes 1987: 44–8).

What is most problematic about *The Prison and the Factory* however, is that it fails in its self-imposed task of explaining why imprisonment became the form of punishment germane to capitalism. It will not do to invoke Pashukanis's 'contractual–bilateral thesis of prison punishment' as Pavarini does. According to this thesis, imprisonment, because it represents a 'deprivation of a quantum of liberty' measured in time, becomes the punishment par excellence in a commodity-producing society. In this view, 'loss of liberty represents the most simple and absolute form of "exchange value"' (Melossi and Pavarini 1981: 184–5). But as Jankovic argues, the most 'simple and absolute' form of exchange value under capitalism is represented by money. It follows that fines, rather than imprisonment, should have developed into *the* capitalist punishment. Furthermore, their argument that prisons function to produce a disciplined workforce is not a sufficient explanation of the birth of the prison under capitalism because the discipline could have been imposed outside the prison. Besides, while the text constructs a theoretical model of the prison as a 'factory of men' – a 'factory producing proletarians', and thus as a paradigm of bourgeois society[15] – the historical evidence suggests that prisons are more likely to produce 'lumpenproletarians', not disciplined workers (Jankovic 1983). Melossi and Pavarini then, may have set out with the laudable intention of discovering 'why prison', but, in the view of Marxist and non-Marxist commentators alike, they failed to deliver. What then are we to make of this, and the revisionist attempts in general, to account for 'the birth' of the prison? On the plus side, they did draw critical attention to the parallel emergence of the prison and the capitalist mode of production. On the down side, they failed to account for this in a convincing fashion and, in particular, had trouble getting the historical evidence to fit the social, political and economic function required by their theoretical imperatives. Thanks to the revisonists, we now know that the emergence of the prison as the dominant penal sanction was a crucially important development in the West, but we are still awaiting the development of a satisfactory explanatory framework in which to place it.

In this connection, it is relevant to note that revisionist accounts of the birth of the prison met with a mixed reception from Marxist analysts. While some have been willing to engage with the changing conceptual landscape by accommodating ideological and political determinants of penal regimes, others have continued to produce political economies of past penal regimes with barely a fleeting glance at the new social history. For example, Humphries and Greenberg, influenced by the findings of Ignatieff and other revisionist historians, constructed a Marxist framework for theorising 'the dialectics of crime control' which incorporated an assessment of the nature of the state, popular ideologies and even divisons within classes. In their view, 'a mode of production is too limited a concept to tell us much about crime control' and therefore should not be treated as the independent variable in a Marxist theory of historical change in crime control.

> Indeed, the mode of production is not entirely distinct from social control conceptually, for crime control can be . . . part of the forces and relations of production (consider penal slavery, prison labour, factory discipline).
>
> (1981: 241–2)

Other Marxist analysts have also been prepared to engage with the claims of the new social historians, especially those of Foucault, sometimes with impressive results. Spitzer's Foucauldian–Marxist account of the rationalisation of crime in capitalist society is a case in point. This study blends a Marxist analysis of the political economy of capitalist society with Foucault's thesis about the emergence of a disciplinary technology in a way, moreover, which pays attention to pre-capitalist societies in China, Japan and Inca Peru (Spitzer 1983)[16].

Some Marxists however, are less sanguine about the intrusion of non-Marxist conceptualisations into prison history. For example, in a study of the emergence of the New York State prison system, Gil Gardner has called a halt to revisionist incursions into the Marxist analytical framework. In his view, the revisionist histories of the 1970s had a detrimental influence on Marxist prison history which has followed them too far down the 'political–ideological' path. According to Gardner, the solution to the problem of economic reductionism which besets Rusche and Kirchheimer's traditional Marxist approach is not to switch our attention to 'political–ideological' dimensions of imprisonment. Rather, what is required is a critical reassessment of their labour-market thesis and, more generally, of the 'political–economic' dimenions of punishment. More specifically, he argues that

> the essential element in understanding prison history is an emphasis upon an empirical analysis of the relationship between imprisonment and the development of the mode of production – *independent of labour market conditions and the related motives of profit and the need to train or re-socialise labour.*

> (Gardner 1987: 89; his emphasis)

From this unreconstructed Marxist perspective, any work straying from economic orthodoxy by suggesting that penal changes could be read off from changes in the labour market irrespective of changes in the mode of production has to be faulted. Misguided by revisionism, Marxist prison analysts – Melossi and Pavarini included – have taken the wrong penal turn (1987: 90–1).[17]

So much then for the impact of revisionist punishment history on existing historiographical frameworks. On the one hand, administrative historians proceed as if the new history was not written, while Marxists like Gardner wish fervently that it never had been. On the other hand, it is undeniable that revisionism helped to transform punishment into an object deserving of critical appraisal by those willing to listen. However, the tedious internecine debates which it has generated between Eurocentric, masculinist historians of various persuasions over questions of theoretical interpretation have been overtaken by post-colonial and feminist critiques. For all the passion which it generated in the 1970s, the divisive issues of that time – the relationship between humanitarianism and coercion, the relative importance of ideological and economic determinants – pale into historiographical insignificance in the face of larger epistemological and political questions about the framing of the penal, or now 'penality', question.

CONCLUDING REMARKS

The various strands of analysis which collectively have been called 'the new social history' have played a key role in cultivating a critical interest in past and present penal regimes, at least in the West. Without these historically-based critical accounts, punishment would have remained an atheoretical and apolitical object of analysis, captive to empiricist sociologies and linear administrative histories. It is largely because of them that punishment has been politicised. Of course, some might disagree about the importance of politicising history. For example, we have been warned of the dangers of overpoliticising history: the 'veritable anarchy' of 'usable pasts' which is produced by a surfeit of perspectives, allegedly commits us to an infinite relativism (Tomlins 1985: 145–6). From this perspective, a politics on penality cannot be read off from any particular critical historical account of past punishment systems. But prison history is irredeemably interventionist. Just as the desire to transform the study of punishment into the social analysis of penality has been, and should be, accompanied by 'a healthy appreciation of the need to discuss policy' and to 'intervene in the practical', so the desire to write critical, theoretically-informed histories of punishment must be 'irrevocably tied to practice' (Garland and Young 1983: 5). That is, in the end we have to take sides.

In the final analysis, it may not be possible to salvage the new social histories of punishment from the wreckage of two decades of critical appraisal. From a critical perspective today, the texts of the revisionist heroes of the 1970s, tarnished as they are with the mark of a universalising Eurocentric and masculinist bias, are simply beyond reclamation. And yet for all their limitations, they did have the tremendously significant political effect of making punishment an object of knowledge and of thus providing a way to challenge the operation of specific modes of punishment. Previously, accounts of punishment systems proceeded as if penal power was a natural phenomenon, beyond critical inquiry. Punishment per se was taken for granted and changing penal forms were treated as inevitable, progressive developments. Now, thanks largely to the irreverent proddings of the revisionists, history has revealed punishment to be a social and political process, one irrevocably stained by the disciplinary manoeuvres and control strategies of the rulers, if not by the blood, pain, suffering and resistance of the ruled who, strangely, do not figure as prominently as one might expect in histories professing to be 'social'. The new social history of the 1970s may have focused far more deftly on the control strategies of the rulers than on the notoriously difficult-to-record resistances of the 'inarticulate' ruled, but it achieved this much: it ensured that punishment history can never be less than the story of who rides whom, and how.

3 The Foucault effect: from penology to penality

> First of all, many thanks to François Ewald for organising this conference on Michel Foucault, whose work is of such immense scope and so much alive. This is not, however, a commemoration. We are not guardians of the temple and there was no religion, just the will to knowledge.
>
> (Barret-Kriegel 1992: 192)[1]

> they don't understand what I am saying. . . . And in the moment when they cannot say: what he is doing is unacceptable, they say: what he is saying is false. But in order to say this they are obligated to lie and to make me say what I am not saying.
>
> For this reason, I don't think there's much to discuss concerning these words poured on top of my own.
>
> (Foucault 1989a: 192)

Blandine Barret-Kriegel's disclaimer notwithstanding, there was, and still is, a religion. The Foucauldian industry, with its production line of seemingly endless textual glosses on the grand master theorist of penality (and of discipline and power, sexuality and subjectivity, to name a few of his interests), has reached such epidemic proportions that it could well be called a religion. Certainly, the speakers at the international conference where Barret-Kriegel gave a paper on Foucault's contribution to a theorisation of the police state may not have consciously acted as guardians of the temple, but the effect was similar. Moreover, the proceedings of that conference have been published in French, and now English, along with countless other collections of articles on and interviews with Foucault, such that it was recklessly premature to title one of these *The Final Foucault* (Bernauer and Rasmussen 1988), when he is very much alive and anything but finalised. All these texts could be said to stand as so many testimonials to the power of his work or, if they were published after his death in 1984, as commemorations to an intellectual messiah. To provide the most relevant example, *Discipline and Punish*, his masterpiece on the transformations of Western punishment regimes, is widely accorded the status of a Bible, prompting Stanley Cohen to comment that 'to write today about punishment and classification without Foucault, is like talking about the unconscious without Freud' (Cohen 1985: 10). Indeed, such is the acclaim that Cohen's judgement is cited ad nauseam, as if it were a mantra. Foucault's place is thus secure in the sacred hall of philosophical deities. And yet while the adulation or, conversely, critique and condemnation (idolatry?), show no sign of abating, we can imagine Foucault refusing all 'these words poured on top of my own', just as he refused those of the communists in the late 1970s. We can imagine too that he would refuse them on the same dismissive grounds: simply, 'they don't understand what I'm saying.'

My concern in chapter 2 was to provide a sense of the exegetical effect of the revisionist histories of the 1970s on the study of punishment – that is, to suggest the pivotal importance of their contribution to that multi-dimensional and hence multi-layered interpretative deep play in which 'penality' now finds itself. As I indicated there, *Discipline and Punish* has been indisputably the most influential of the revisionist histories of punishment. Whether they have been for or against Foucault, analysts interested in taking a critical or informed approach to punishment today have had to come to grips with this crucial text which, as David Garland says

> has quite fundamentally changed the way in which intellectuals think about punishment and penal institutions. . . . Virtually by itself, it has transformed a field of inquiry that was narrow, technically focused, and of little intellectual consequence into a flourishing, interdisciplinary area that has become a central concern for sociologists, historians and criminologists.
>
> (Garland 1986: 866)

Furthermore, it was this text which put 'penality' on the interpretative map in such a compelling manner that by the early 1980s 'the social analysis of penality' was beginning to replace penology as the most pertinent field of inquiry into punishment. Foucult may not have bothered to provide a precise definition of 'penality', but those calling for the social and political analysis of penality were clear that what was now required was a shift away from empiricist penological enquiries to studies of the 'social foundations' of the practices and institutions of punishment (Garland and Young 1983).

The purpose of this chapter is to provide a sense of Foucault's place in this critical movement away from traditional ways of studying punishment. This is hardly an original plan. Foucault's impact on sociological, historical and even penological approaches to the penal question has been acknowledged, and less convincingly refused, over and over again. Indeed, one way to study the 'Foucault effect'[2] on the analysis of punishment would be to list the major works of his followers and detractors and to delineate the main lines of interpretative divergence, laboriously charting the whole host of confluent or conflicting readings in the process. The goal would be to continue in the vein of Allan Megill's work on 'the reception of Foucault' – renouncing any claim to convey 'the inner dynamic' of his work and resting content with using its reception 'as a surrogate for the work itself' (Megill 1987: 117). Instead, this chapter takes an entirely different approach, one which begins by returning to the author himself in a bid to recover what he had to say about punishment from what he would dismiss as merely 'words poured on top of my own'. Ironically, some of the excessive verbiage is his own, for Foucault had so much to say, clarify and revise, that something akin to an archaeological excavation is necessary to recover what we might refer to, perversely, as the original Foucault. Nowhere is this more apparent than in the field which he redesignated 'penality'. Still, the aim here is to recapture what might be called, again perversely, the essential Foucault, by revisiting his texts and, more pertinently, his clarifications of his intentions, methodology and goals in relation to the question of punishment, and to do so as far as possible without the mediation of the commentary of either the temple guards or their enemies.

Of course, this is an impossible task. Foucault's detractors join self-defined Foucauldians to intrude rudely at every point, declaring that such a plan is unacceptable, or false, or simply wrong-headed, premised as it is on the unlikely assumption that Foucault's words could speak for themselves. Worse still, my project could be denounced as un-Foucauldian. After all, Foucault was one of the first to pronounce the death of the author, a demise marked in his view by poststructuralism's – or was it structuralism's?[3] – concern to determine 'the functional conditions of specific discursive practices'. Certainly, it was *his* concern in 'What is an author?' to refuse the authorial function: the establishment of 'a genealogical table of exceptional individuals' was something he himself had never attempted (Foucault 1977b: 114). And speaking of mantras, he takes his from Samuel Beckett – 'What matter who's speaking, someone said, what matter who's speaking?' – in order to underline his hostility to the privileging of the author and his (always already *his*) meanings (1977b: 115–17). After all, 'books or texts with authors' are but 'objects of appropriation', subject to a 'penal code' no less, which assigns to books

> *real authors*, other than mythical or important religious figures, only when the author became subject to punishment and to the extent that his discourse was considered transgressive.
>
> (1977b: 124; my emphasis)

Was Foucault being prescient here, forecasting his own elevation to that much-disclaimed status of real author, over and above that of an important religious figure which, as I have suggested, he also became? Surely the most avowedly hostile anti-Foucauldian would not dispute his transgressive or even 'transdiscursive position', as author of a theoretical tradition 'within which new books and authors can proliferate'. Surely his enemies would concede that he, along with Freud and Marx, was one of the great 'initiators of discursive practices' who produced 'the possibility and the rules of formation of other texts', thereby establishing 'the endless possibility of discourse' (1977b: 131). Surely no-one would disagree that Foucault himself came to occupy the higher ground of 'real author', one who has been very much subject to punishment (in the form of punitive critiques) precisely because his discourses have been so transgressive of conventional paradigms.[4]

Actually, none of this matters. It is immaterial to my concerns here that Foucault put so much energy into evacuating the site of the author, even inciting the death of the author, and yet emerged as one himself. Nor does it concern me that he would protest at the idea of seeking the 'truth' of his position by turning to his clarifications of his ideas about punishment. I am not interested either in retaliating by basking in the irony that someone committed to an anti-author position could spend so much time modulating his own authorial voice. Nor does it matter that Foucault would presumably approve of my ultimate aim, which is to pay homage to *Discipline and Punish* by utilising it for my own transgressive purposes, thereby acting on his dictum that the only valid tribute to thought 'is precisely to use it, to deform it, to make it groan and protest'. And finally, if the guardians of the temple wish to protest that I have been 'unfaithful' to the master's text, may I say with Foucault that 'that is of absolutely no interest' (Foucault 1980a: 53–54). What matter who's protesting; really, what matter who's protesting?

PART ONE – FOUCAULT ON FOUCAULT ON PUNISHMENT

Discipline and Punish

A prelude: those who are familiar with *Discipline and Punish*, or with the countless reiterations of its central theses which abound in the secondary literature,[5] may be dismayed to hear that I intend to plunder this much-utilised text again, choosing anew from its feast of analytical offerings, as if I were the first to discover it. They may be further dismayed to learn that I intend to do so at some length. But it seems to me that this can be easily justified, for *Discipline and Punish* is by far the most significant of all the social histories of punishment and indeed, of all the transgressive texts on this subject – if the significance of a text is measured, as it should be, by its power to reconceptualise a field of analysis. This much said, let us begin with what Foucault had to say about the project of *Discipline and Punish* in the text itself. At first, this project seems clear enough. The aim of the book – which is surely self-evident in its subtitle: *The Birth of the Prison* – is to chart the redistribution of what he calls 'the economy of punishment' in the West in the early nineteenth century. To be more precise, it is to chart the transformation of forms of punishment in Europe and the United States between 1757 – when, as he tells the story, torture as a public spectacle was all the rage – to 1837, by which time 'modern' penal codes had introduced the discipline of prison's timetabled brand of punishment. More specifically, he singles out 'the disappearance of torture as a public spectacle' as his main focus. The political agenda of *Discipline and Punish* also seems to be crystal clear. It appears to fit into the standard revisionist agenda of the 1970s, that of challenging the conventional picture of the progressive evolution of penal forms over time. In Foucault's revisionist view, too much had been made of what he calls 'a process of "humanisation", thus dispensing with the need for further analysis' (1977a: 7).[6] The task was to replace the progressivist perspective with a critical account of the 'great institutional transformations' of the years 1760–1840, the period in which penalties became 'essentially corrective' and individualised, in order to understand their implications for the emergence of 'modern penality' (17).

Again, Foucault is clear: he was not interested primarily in the past. His goal was to write 'the history of the present'. Indeed, he insists that he had learnt the crucial lesson that punishment in general and the prison in particular belong to a 'political technology of the body' not from history but from 'the present' – that is, from the prison revolts in France in the early 1970s. On reflection, it seemed to Foucault that the prison movements which occurred in the West in the post-1968 period had aims which were not 'merely material': they were 'about the body and material things'; they were 'revolts, at the level of the body, against the very body of the prison'.

> What was at issue was not whether the prison environment was too harsh or too aseptic, too primitive or too efficient, but its very materiality as an instrument and vector of power; it is this whole technology of power over the body that the technology of the 'soul' – that of the educationalists, psychologists and psychiatrists – fails either to conceal or to compensate, for the simple reason that it is one of its tools.
>
> (1977a: 30–1)

Already then, by the end of the first chapter, Foucault has introduced the terms of a more complex form of analysis, one in which, for example, materiality is given a new meaning centring on the body. Also a new object of knowledge – 'penality' – is introduced, but not defined. Signs of this complexity appear within the first few pages. Very quickly, the object of analysis shifts from punishment to 'the punishment–body relation'. Under the old penal regime, physical pain or 'the pain of the body itself' was 'the constituent element of the penalty'. Now, within the new penality, the prisoner's body 'serves as an instrument or intermediary' for a penalty which takes the form of a deprivation of a right. 'The body, according to this penality, is caught up in a system of constraints and privations, obligations and prohibitions' and punishment, once 'an art of unbearable sensations' has become 'an economy of suspended rights', in which 'a whole army of technicians' – warders, doctors, chaplains, psychiatrists, psychologists, educationalists – take over from the executioner. Modern punishment, which had emerged by the mid-nineteenth century, is best read as a '"non-corporal" penality' (11). Not that the body disappeared from the penal frame. Punishment as torture, as 'a technique of pain', may have ceased:

> But a punishment like forced labour or even imprisonment – mere loss of liberty – has never functioned without a certain additional element of punishment that certainly concerns the body itself: rationing of food, sexual deprivation, corporal punishment, solitary confinement.
>
> (1977a: 15–16)

However, 'penality in its most severe forms no longer addresses itself to the body', but rather to what Foucault calls 'the soul'. That is, punishment now acts 'in depth on the heart, the thoughts, the will, the inclinations' of the prisoner (15–17).

This notion of the soul of the criminal is critical in that it is claimed that the soul is not only the object of 'modern penality'; it is an object susceptible to the 'scientific knowledge' provided by psychiatry and criminology. Such knowledge is invoked in order to judge not just the crime but rather the soul of the criminal. A determination of guilt is now transformed into 'a strange scientifico-juridical complex' involving a 'whole set of assessing, diagnostic, prognostic, normative judgements concerning the criminal' (18). That is, the court's sentence is no longer a legal decision that lays down punishment; the judgement now involves 'an assessment of normality' (20–1). Judges now judge 'something other than crimes' and the 'whole penal operation' has taken on 'extra-juridical elements and personnel'. It follows that the focus of historical analysis should not be on the supposedly increasing leniency of punishment since the eighteenth century. The goal should be rather to study the ways in which 'a whole new system of truth' becomes embedded in the exercise of criminal justice, or alternatively, the ways in which a body of knowledge, techniques and 'scientific' discourses becomes entangled with the 'power to punish'. Thus *Discipline and Punish* is to be a study of 'new tactics of power' or rather,

> a correlative history of the modern soul and of a new power to judge; a genealogy of the present scientifico-legal complex from which the power to punish derives its bases, justifications and rules, from which it extends its effects and by which it masks its exorbitant singularity.
>
> (1977a: 22–3)

Alternatively, its aim is to analyse 'the metamorphosis of punitive methods on the basis of a political technology of the body in which might be read a common history of power relations and object relations' (24).

Here we encounter a more difficult mode of analysis which, despite our best intentions to let Foucault speak, has us reaching for the secondary literature for an explication. In one of the most lucid accounts, David Garland singles out three interrelated concepts which Foucault uses to study punishment and other structures of domination – power, knowledge and the body. As he explains, Foucault perceives the human body as

> the ultimate material that is seized and shaped by all political, economic, and penal institutions. Systems of production, domination, and of socialisation fundamentally depend on the successful subjugation of bodies.
>
> (Garland 1990a: 137)

The docile, obedient body is produced by concentrating on the 'soul' which, Garland explains, is a concept used by Foucault to refer to what psychologists usually call 'the psyche, the self, subjectivity, consciousness, or the personality'.[7] The power to punish, an important manifestation of what Foucault calls 'a micro-physics of power' is brought to bear on this soul. Furthermore, the relationship between forms of power and the bodies or souls which are caught up in them 'involves a third element' – knowledge – or rather 'power–knowledge', which Garland describes as a 'kind of conceptual shorthand' for the interconnections between power and knowledge which take place in the control field. The successful control of bodies or souls requires knowledge such as that provided by the 'sciences of man' – the social sciences which developed in the eighteenth and nineteenth centuries. In Garland's succinct summary, Foucault's three-pronged conceptual framework reorders the history of punishment 'as a set of developing relationships between power, knowledge, and the body'. Furthermore,

> the implicit claim seems to be that power–knowledge–body relations constitute the irreducible basis of society and the historical process: bodies caught up in power–knowledge relations form a kind of physical

substratum which serves as a foundation for social relations and institutions. As for the intellectual developments which take place in legal theory or in the programmes of penal reformers, and even the wider changes which we see as the growth of individualism and the 'humanisation' of sensibility – all of these provide only a surface history, as far as Foucault is concerned. Rather than being the causes of penal and political change, these are merely the effects of more profound developments at the level of power– knowledge–body relations. In rendering the history of punishment as 'a chapter of political anatomy', Foucault is not offering one interpretation to be added to others; he is claiming to unearth the elementary structures on which all else is based.

(Garland 1990a: 139)

I have sacrificed a lot for the sake of clarity here. Not only have I resorted to a somewhat lengthy commentary from a temple guardian in a section which was supposed to be devoted to the words of the master; we have also got ahead of the story as it unravels in *Discipline and Punish*. But it is a momentary lapse. Returning to the text, we find Foucault throwing more light on his project by setting out several rules for studying the power to punish. These rules include conceptualising punishment as 'a complex social function', involving not only the 'repressive effects' or 'punishment aspects' of punitive mechanisms, but also a range of 'possible positive effects'; analysing punitive methods 'as techniques possessing their own specificity in the more general field of other ways of exercising power'; understanding the interconnection between punishment regimes and the 'human sciences' and, finally, determining whether the 'entry of the soul on to the scene of penal justice, and with it the insertion in legal practice of a whole corpus of "scientific" knowledge' reflects changes in the way the body itself is invested by power relations. In brief, the aim is to study penal changes in terms of 'a political technology of the body' (23–4).

In case all this seems novel or even strange, Foucault insists that he is merely developing the approach taken in Rusche and Kirchheimer's *Punishment and Social Structure* which, he claims 'provides a number of essential reference points' for his own analysis. Most important, it taught us to 'rid ourselves of the illusion that penality is above all (if not exclusively) a means of reducing crime'. Rather, we must analyse 'concrete' and specific punishment regimes, seeing them as 'social phenomena'. More particularly, Foucault admires the way Rusche and Kirchheimer related different punishment systems to different systems of production. However, he adds his own interpretative gloss to their economistic analytical framework:

systems of punishment are to be situated in a certain 'political economy' of the body: even if they do not make use of violent or bloody punishment, even when they use 'lenient' methods involving confinement or correction, it is always the body that is at issue – the body and its forces, their utility and their docility, their distribution and their submission.

(1977a: 25)

In brief, he wants to inscribe a history of punishment within a 'history of bodies' – a history, that is, of the 'political investment of the body' in power relations. Indeed, in next to no time, Foucault is speaking not of punishment but of 'the political technology of the body', the 'micro-physics of power', 'micro-powers', 'power–knowledge relations' and finally, simply, 'power–knowledge'. Pulling this all altogether, he wants to write 'a history of the "micro-physics" of the punitive power' which will be simultaneously, 'a genealogy of the modern "soul"'. Why? Because the soul is 'the effect and instrument of a political anatomy; the soul is the prison of the body' (26–30).

So much then for the seemingly straightforward, but increasingly complex, first chapter. What follows is an account of the birth of the prison, or what he prefers to call 'the micro-physics' of the punitive power. In brief, it is a story about the declining use of torture (the demise of 'the spectacle of the scaffold'); the shift in penal focus in the nineteenth century to the soul of the criminal; refinements in the mechanisms of power and surveillance to control individuals and populations (the birth of a 'new political anatomy'); the formation of 'the disciplinary society' and finally, the 'carceral archipelago'. As we will see, Foucault would say this is all fiction, and many historians and other hostile commentators would agree, but it is fiction heavy with interpretative messages. It is fiction, moreover, which lays claim to breaking new ground in the theorisation of punishment and, for this reason, demands a close inspection. Moreover, such is the power of this text that it demands our close attention precisely at those points where it breaks new theoretical ground. For example, Foucault agrees with Rusche and Kirchheimer that changes in penal forms are connected to changes in systems of economic production, but in his view they missed the significance of the 'truth–power relation' which lies 'at the heart of all mechanisms of punishment' (55). On the other hand, Foucault informs us that the thesis about evolving humanitarian concerns is wholly wrong as changes in penal forms must be accounted for in terms of changing technologies of power:

What was emerging no doubt was not so much a new respect for the humanity of the condemned . . . as a tendency towards a more finely tuned justice, towards a closer penal mapping of the social body.

(1977a: 78)

Take the example of the eighteenth-century penal reformers: as he sees it, they were concerned not so much with the cruelty of punishment as with a 'badly regulated distribution of power'. Their aim was to set up 'a new "economy" of the power to punish'. Accordingly, their criminal law reform programmes should be read as 'a strategy for the rearrangement of the power to punish' which will make it 'more regular, more effective, more constant and more detailed in its effects'. Moreover, the newly emerging 'juridical theory of penality corresponds in fact to a new "political economy" of the power to punish' (79–81). In this construction, 'reform' was a sign of a desire

> not to punish less, but to punish better; to punish with an attenuated severity perhaps, but in order to punish with more universality and necessity: to insert the power to punish more deeply into the social body.

> (1977a: 82)

New strategies of power then, and not new sensibilities, explain the birth of the prison. Furthermore, Foucault also rejects theories suggesting that the prison was the evolutionary end point of 'the great models of punitive imprisonment' set up in Europe and the United States in the late sixteenth, seventeenth and eighteenth centuries – for example the Amsterdam Rasphuis, the Flemish workhouses, the English houses of correction, Philadelphia's Walnut Street prison (120–6). The explanation for the emergence of 'the coercive, corporal, solitary, secret model of the power to punish' (131) in the early nineteenth century must be sought elsewhere – in the transformation of the disciplinary methods deployed in monasteries, armies and workshops into 'general formulas of domination' in the seventeenth and eighteenth centuries. It is in the fascination with 'projects of docility' – techniques for subjugating bodies or imposing on them 'a relation of docility–utility' – that Foucault locates the formation of a new power to punish (136–7). To understand penal change at the end of the eighteenth century, we must look to the formation of 'a policy of coercions' which produces 'subjected and practised bodies, "docile bodies"'. These penal changes were but an effect of the birth of a 'new political anatomy' in which the body becomes the target of new mechanisms of power which he calls 'disciplinary power' or simply 'discipline' (138).

Discipline, a specific technology of power which functions as a 'coercive link with the apparatus of production' (153–5) is not simply a key concept in Foucault's analytical framework: it occupies centre stage and all of Part Three in *Discipline and Punish*. Disciplinary systems establish 'a whole micro-penality' of time, behaviour and the body. Disciplinary punishment is 'essentially corrective': that is, preoccupied with training and 'normalising' those subjected to it. It is characterised by a 'normalising judgement' which exceeds the bounds of 'judicial penality' – the traditional penality of the law (177–3). Disciplinary techniques are not merely negative or repressive; importantly, they are also productive – they produce 'domains of objects and rituals of truth' and, in the process, they constitute individuals (194). Moreover, they do this inside and outside institutions, for disciplinary techniques are spread throughout society by means of 'the panoptic schema' – a mode of surveillance based on Bentham's famous cellular architectural design, the Panopticon. While Foucault recognised that the panoptic plan was never fully realised, its significance lay in the way in which it functioned as a 'generalisable' model of power which defined power relations 'in terms of the everyday life of men'. The Panopticon was 'polyvalent' in its applications, serving to reform prisoners, 'but also to treat patients, to instruct schoolchildren, to confine the insane, to supervise workers, to put beggars and idlers to work' (205). More, it epitomised the transformation of Western societies from the sovereign power of absolute monarchies to disciplinary power.

> The movement from one project to the other, from a schema of exceptional discipline to one of a generalised surveillance, rests on a historical transformation: the gradual extension of the mechanisms of discipline throughout the seventeenth and eighteenth centuries, their spread throughout the whole social body, the formation of what might be called in general the disciplinary society.
>
> (1977a: 209)

If panopticism is clearly recognisable as a model of power or as 'the general principle' of a political anatomy whose object is 'relations of discipline' (208), discipline itself is ambidextrous, even multi-talented, and certainly elusive.

> Discipline may be identified neither with an institution nor with an apparatus; it is a type of power, a modality for its exercise, comprising a whole set of instruments, techniques, procedures, levels of application, targets; it is a 'physics' or an 'anatomy' of power, a technology.
>
> (1977a: 215)

Moreover, discipline may be deployed in a range of institutions – the prison, houses of correction, schools, hospitals and the family – such that 'one can speak of the formation of a disciplinary society' and of 'an indefinitely generalisable mechanism of "panopticism"'. In Foucault's scenario, modern Western society was created through the deployment of a cluster of procedures for controlling individuals – surveillance, classifications, examinations – procedures which had been perfected in the armies, monastries and schools over the previous three centuries. Indeed the development of this disciplinary technology was the condition of emergence of our society 'of surveillance' (215–17).

Crucially, the formation of this disciplinary society must be connected to broad historical processes in the economic, 'juridico-political' and scientific fields. Taking economic processes into account is especially important as it enables Foucault to adjudicate the boundaries between his disciplinary interpretative framework and more familiar political economies of punishment. In his understanding, the emergence of discipline 'corresponds to a well-known historical conjuncture' – the one characterised by large population increases in the eighteenth century ('the large demographic thrust') and 'the growth in the apparatus of production' (more commonly known as changes in the mode of production). It is here that we might expect an encounter with Marx, but it is a fleeting one. Foucault simply wants to say that 'the accumulation of men' which the disciplinary project makes possible cannot be separated from the accumulation of capital. Technological changes in the division of labour 'sustained an ensemble of very close relations' with the emergence of disciplinary power. One is not prior to the other: they are mutually reinforcing processes. Thus:

> The growth of a capitalist economy gave rise to the specific modality of disciplinary power, whose general formulas, techniques of submitting forces and bodies, in short, 'political anatomy', could be operated in the most diverse political regimes, apparatuses and institutions.
>
> (1977a: 221)

Political anatomy, apparently, is not only compatible with political economy: it actually enhances the Marxist analytical framework which was oblivious to the significance of disciplinary power.

As for 'juridico-political' considerations, Marxists may be relieved to see 'the bourgeoisie', no less, appear at last, albeit briefly, on the Foucauldian stage. At last, the 'panoptic modality of power' seems to have some kind of connection with a dominant class. Admittedly, the connection is not direct, but there is nevertheless an intrinsic link between the rise of the bourgeoisie as the politically dominant class in the eighteenth century and the emergence of disciplinary power. For hidden beneath the 'legal fiction' of the 'formally egalitarian juridical framework' which masked the rise to power of this new class were 'systems of micro-power that are essentially non-egalitarian and asymmetrical' – the disciplines, no less. These disciplines, moreover, should be seen as 'a sort of counter-law' which 'distribute along a scale, around a norm, hierarchise individuals in relation to one another and, if necessary, disqualify and invalidate' (223).

This has powerful effects, because although the 'juridicism' of modern society seems to limit the exercise of power,

> its universally widespread panopticism enables it to operate, on the underside of the law, a machinery that is both immense and minute, which supports, reinforces, multiplies the asymmetry of power and undermines the limits that are traced around the law.
>
> (1977a: 223)

But what has all this to do with punishment? Well, as it happens, Foucault returns at this point to the question of punishment, saying that the prison ('with all its corrective technology') has to be 'resituated', theoretically speaking. Where?

> ... at the point where the codified power to punish turns into a disciplinary power to observe; at the point where the universal punishments of the law are applied selectively to certain individuals and always the same ones; at the point where the redefinition of the juridical subject by the penalty becomes a useful training of the criminal; at the point where the counter-law becomes the effective and institutionalised content of the juridical forms.
>
> (1977a: 224)

At this point one might feel tempted to abandon this increasingly convoluted plot and to skip over the section describing the ways in which scientific knowledges are implicated in all this – the way in which the 'sciences of man' (psychology, psychiatry, pedagogy, criminology) are entangled with the disciplines. But then we would miss Foucault's characterisation of modern penality as involving altogether new elements introduced by the 'penetration' of scientific knowledges, with their 'terrible power of investigation', into the judicial system. Such knowledges problematise the criminal 'behind his crime' and render punishment into 'a correction, a therapy, a normalisation' involving the measurement, assessment, diagnosis, cure and transformation of individuals (226–7). In other words, the power to punish is no longer a simple judicial exercise: now disciplinary techniques intrude at every point of the sentencing and penal process. Moreover, it is precisely this development – the generalisation of disciplinary power – which accounts for the birth of the prison:

> Is it surprising that the cellular prison, with its regular chronologies, forced labour, its authorities of surveillance and registration, its experts in normality, who continue and multiply the functions of the judge, should have become the modern instrument of penality? Is it surprising

that prisons resemble factories, schools, barracks, hospitals, which all resemble prisons?

(1977a: 227–8)

Leaving the question of discipline aside, we move on to Part Four, the section on 'Prison', where Foucault returns to more recognisable punishment themes. Here he also returns, again briefly and elliptically, to Marxist themes when he announces that the birth of the prison is not only an event within penal history; it is also an important moment in the history of 'those disciplinary mechanisms that the new class power was developing: that in which they colonised the legal institution' (231). However, the reference to class power is brief as Foucault is much more interested in problematising the 'self-evidence of the prison', in analysing how its

double foundation – juridico-economic on the one hand, technico-disciplinary on the other – made the prison seem the most immediate and civilised form of all penalties.

(1977a: 233)

Not that he is claiming that the prison was an entirely new institution. Certainly, the penality of detention was 'a new thing' at the turn of the nineteenth century, but the form of the prison antedated 'its systematic use in the penal system'. The coming of the penitentiary should be seen as 'the opening up of penality to mechanisms of coercion already elaborated elsewhere' (231) – notably, in disciplinary institutions such as workshops, armies and schools.

It is in this section too, that Foucault elaborates his now famous thesis about the relationship between reform and the prison. The prison did not antedate the reformers; rather, prison 'reform' is 'virtually contemporary with the prison itself: it constitutes, as it were, its programme'. From the beginning, the prison was caught up in reform programmes, 'whose purpose was apparently to correct it, but which seem to form part of its very functioning'. Thus, the prison should not be seen as 'an inert institution'. Rather,

The prison has always formed part of an active field in which projects, improvements, experiments, theoretical statements, personal evidence and investigations have proliferated.

(1977a: 234–5)

The prison then, is not an institution; it is rather part of 'an active field' or an 'unceasing discipline' (236). Moreover, it is not concerned primarily with offenders or even convicts but with another object altogether – 'the delinquent'.

This brings us to Foucault's famous thesis about prisons producing delinquency. The penitentiary substitutes the delinquent for the convicted offender, by re-educating him, treating him as 'a biographical unity, a kernel of danger, representing a type of anomaly' (251–4), requiring the intervention of scientific knowledges such as psychology and criminology. But lest it be thought that all that is being suggested here is the tired old cliché that 'prison fabricates delinquents', Foucault adds that

> it also fabricates them in the sense that it has introduced into the operation of the law and the offence, the judge and the offender, the condemned man and the executioner, the non-corporal reality of the delinquency that links them together and, for a century and a half, has caught them in the same trap.
>
> (1977a: 255)

That is, the penal focus has been transferred from the 'branded, dismembered, burnt, annihilated body of the tortured criminal' to 'the individuality' of the delinquent, 'the little soul of the criminal' which has remained the focus of penal attention ever since the early nineteenth century (254–5). More exactly, this occurred during the period between 1750 and 1820 when 'penal detention replaced public execution as a calculated technique for altering individual behaviour' (264).

Importantly too, Foucault's thesis about the production of delinquency connects to his equally famous problematisation of the generally received view that the prison system has been a failure. Noting that the prison was denounced from its inception as a failure, he comments on several already familiar ways in which the prison could not but fail to produce delinquents – for example, 'by throwing the inmate's family into destitution' (268). But Foucault takes the analysis of the supposed 'failure' further:

> Is not the supposed failure part of the functioning of the prison? Is it not to be included among those effects of power that discipline and the auxiliary technology of imprisonment have induced in the apparatus of justice, and in society in general, and which may be grouped together under the name of 'carceral system'?
>
> (1977a: 271)

That is, if the prison has survived for so long and if 'the principle of penal detention has never seriously been questioned', it must be that the carceral system had 'very precise functions'. Then follows his famous reversal of the problem of the prison's failure. Instead of trying to account for this failure, we should reverse the problem and ask

> what is served by the failure of the prison; what is the use of these different phenomena that are continually being criticised; the maintenance

of delinquency, the encouragement of recidivism, the transformation of the occasional offender into a habitual delinquent, the organisation of a closed milieu of delinquency.

(1977a: 272)

What lies behind the apparent failure of the prison system? Simply this – the penality of the prison provides a way of handling and distinguishing illegalities. It is a strategy of unspecified 'dominant groups' to distinguish 'illegalities' – the exploitation of legal loopholes by dominant groups – from 'popular illegalities', such as popular protests against taxes, 'fair price' revolts and resistance to conscription. It is these popular illegalities which must be transformed into delinquency in the carceral system (272–7).

Thus, rather than seeing the prison as a failure, Foucault hypothesises that it has 'succeeded extremely well in producing delinquency' – in producing the delinquent as 'a pathologised subject'. The carceral system has 'substituted the "delinquent" for the offender, and also superimposed upon juridical practice a whole horizon of possible knowledge' of the offender (277). By fabricating this 'enclosed, separated and useful illegality', one which enables 'the dominant class' to control the population, the prison has guaranteed its own longevity. Delinquency had so many uses – the identification of a troublesome population, colonisation, the patrolling of prostitution, the provision of a pool of *agents provocateurs* to control political groups and workers – all for the 'profit and power of the dominant class' (277–80). Thus at bottom, the 'discipline–penality–delinquency system' was functional for the dimly-defined but always already strategic dominant groups (290).

And finally, skipping to the end of *Discipline and Punish*, we find Foucault fixing 1840, the year of the opening of an institution for juveniles, as the 'date of completion of the carceral system' (293) or, alternatively, as the 'point of emergence' of a new power to punish which is still with us today (296). What distinguished this juvenile institution, a 'model in which are concentrated all the coercive technologies of behaviour', was its regime of training – its practices which 'normalised by compulsion the conduct of the undisciplined or dangerous' with the aid of the new scientific knowledges, in particular psychology. For Foucault, the 'appearance of these professionals of discipline, normality and subjection surely marks the beginning of a new stage' for it was they who were entrusted with 'the supervision of normality' (295–6). Furthermore, inasmuch as this juvenile institution contained non-offending juveniles as well as young offenders, it exemplified a whole series of institutions which 'well beyond the frontiers of criminal law, constituted what one might call the carceral archipelago' (296–7).

With the assistance of this much-cited notion of a carceral archipelago, introduced to signify 'extra-penal incarceration', Foucault vaults the walls of the prison in order to chart the spread of disciplinary power throughout society. It is by means of the 'carceral archipelago', an ever-widening carceral circle which moves out from 'penality in the strict sense', that the 'penitentiary technique' is transported from the prison 'to the entire social body' (298). It is by this means, too, that 'the two long, multiple series of the punitive and the abnormal' are now linked (300).

But perhaps the most important effect of the carceral system and of its extension well beyond legal imprisonment is that it succeeds in making the power to punish natural and legitimate, in lowering the threshold of tolerance to penality.

(1977a: 301)

It succeeds in effacing 'what may be exhorbitant in the exercise of punishment' by 'playing the two registers in which it is deployed – the legal register of justice and the extra-legal register of discipline – against one another' (301–2).

As if this was not already more than enough food for thought, it is Foucault's guess that what he calls 'the great carceral continuum' – which connects 'the power of discipline and the power of the law, and extends without interruption from the smallest coercions to the longest penal detention' – underlies the right to punish (303). It is his guess too that it has provided the greatest support for 'the normalising power' which extends 'the activity of judging' in modern society, and that the social sciences – 'the sciences of man' – have been deeply implicated in 'a certain policy of the body, a certain way of rendering the group of men docile and useful'. They are implicated, that is, in the processes of power–knowledge which has rendered '[k]nowable man (soul, individuality, consciousness, conduct, whatever it is called)' the 'object-effect' of the 'domination-observation' which is the mode of operation of the carceral network (304–5).

But what does all this have to do with the prison movement – with political opposition to the prison? Everything. To resist we need to know exactly what it is we are resisting. As Foucault puts it, if there is 'an overall political issue around the prison', it is not the prison per se, nor even whether we should fight for 'something other than the prison'. The problem lies rather in the increasingly prevalent use of 'mechanisms of normalisation', a consequence of the proliferation of new disciplines – medicine, psychology, education, welfare – which are assuming 'an ever greater share of the powers of supervision and assessment' (306). At this point, we will leave Foucault in the midst of the 'carceral city' with its 'multiple networks' of controls and carceral mechanisms, including the prison, all of which exercise the 'power of normalisation'. For it is at this point that he ends his book, telling us now that it should be read not as a history of punishment but rather as a 'historical background to various studies of the power of normalisation and the formation of knowledge in modern society' (307–8).

Interlude (pausing for breath)

This then is the argument of *Discipline and Punish* (or some of it), as Foucault presented it in the text, and as I have re-presented it. This may have seemed like a lengthy recapitulation, but it was a necessary one given the transgressive significance of the book, which will be discussed below. At least I made it through to the end (with one small lapse), without the assistance of the secondary literature. Given that renditions of *Discipline and Punish* are in copious oversupply, such an enterprise could be read either as a feat of epic proportions or as needless repetition. But whatever the merits of this approach – one which lets the author speak, unmediated by his followers or detractors – one thing is clear: the project of *Discipline and Punish*, as annunciated there, is far from straightforward. It is therefore not surprising that its effect has been to produce a proliferation of different and frequently conflicting interpretations which might well be read as part of the 'struggle for Foucault' – that struggle to determine the 'dominant interpretation of his works' (Pearce 1988: 258). To gain a sense of the Foucault effect in the analytical field which he redesignated 'penality', we need to outline at least some of the contours of the specific struggle which is our concern – the struggle for *Discipline and Punish*. But before we turn to consider a few of the authoritative voices in the interpretative battles over Foucault's thesis about the power to punish, let us continue to privilege the author by turning to those interviews and carefully edited discussions where he sought to clarify and elaborate upon the analytical framework in which he located penality.

Foucault on *Discipline and Punish*

The first place in which Foucault elaborated on the meaning of *Discipline and Punish* was in the interview 'Prison talk' in June 1975. Here he makes clear his commitment to a new form of history – that of 'rendering apparent the point at which a certain type of discourse is produced and formed' (Foucault 1980a: 37). In the case of the prison, the aim is to analyse how it emerged 'in the movement of its formation as a discourse in the process of constituting itself'. More specifically, the analytical aim is to pinpoint the moment when it became understood that it was more efficient and profitable in terms of the economy of power to place people under surveillance than to subject them to some exemplary penalty.

(1980a: 38)

This 'moment', loosely pinpointed as the late eighteenth and early nineteenth centuries, corresponded to the formation of a new mode of exercising power, a 'local, capillary form of power', which reaches 'into the very grain of individuals', inserting itself into 'their actions and attitudes, their discourses, learning processes and everyday lives'. This led Foucault to hypothesise that 'the prison was linked from its beginning to a project for the transformation of individuals'. Moreover, its manifest failure to transform them, evident in its manufacture of new criminals, was strategically useful, both economically and politically (1980a: 39–40). This argument is by now familiar to us from *Discipline and Punish*, which he modestly describes as an attempt 'to mark out a few paths'. In particular, he wanted to emphasise the utility of the prison's production of delinquency for the bourgeoisie and the utility today of criminological discourses on the transformative impact of the prison. Such discourses, he claims, serve to justify penal measures. More broadly, they are manifestations of 'the relation between power and knowledge, the articulation of each on the other' which, he insists, is his object of analysis (1980a: 45 and 51).

Punishment then, fades from view in this interview, as in others where he begins by discussing *Discipline and Punish* but branches out into a discussion of his relationship to what he calls the 'Marx effect' (1980b: 57), or when he elaborates his analysis of power, rather than penality. For example, he maintains that what he wanted to show in *Discipline and Punish* was how from the seventeenth century 'there was a veritable technological take-off in the productivity of power' (1980c: 119). Punishment is barely mentioned in this 1977 interview, and the prison not at all. However, when questioned about *Discipline and Punish* the following year, he described it as an attempt to 'reinsert the prison within a technology which is the technology of power'. Once again then, the prison is located historically within a changing 'economy of power relationships'. It is also located analytically within Foucault's self-defined problematic: 'to work out an interpretation, a reading of a certain reality' which could be utilised 'within possible struggles'. In short, it is 'the reality of possible struggles' which Foucault wishes to 'bring to light' (1989a: 187–9). Applied to the prison, the 'effect of truth' which he wishes to produce is one which will be of assistance to the movement against penal regimes. But he rejects all the reviews which claimed that *Discipline and Punish* was about the current situation. Rather, it was 'an interpretation of history'. The unresolved problem, however, was to work out how such an analysis can be 'utilised in the current situation'. Whatever the outcome, his goal, one which could not be guaranteed in advance, was to

> produce some effects of truth which might be used for a possible battle, to be waged by those who wish to wage it, in forms yet to be found and in organisations yet to be defined.
>
> (1989a: 190–1)

So when pressed about the contemporary relevance of his book, Foucault becomes concerned to clarify the relationship between his history and the present, or, better still, between his theoretical practice and contemporary prison struggles. On several occasions he emphasised his commitment to making this connection.

> my idea was to write a book that was directly connected with a concrete activity that was taking place on the matter of the prisons. At the time a whole movement had grown up that challenged the prison system and questioned the practices involved in confining offenders. I found myself caught up in this movement, working, for example, with former prisoners, and that is why I wanted to write a history about prisons. What I wanted to do was not to tell a story, or even to analyse the contemporary situation, because that would have needed much greater experience than I had and a connection with penitential institutions much deeper than I had. No, what I wanted to write was a history book that would make the present situation comprehensible and, possibly, lead to action. If you like, I tried to write a 'treatise of intelligibility' about the penitentiary situation, I wanted to make it intelligible, and, therefore, criticisable.
>
> (1988a: 101)

Making the prison system open to criticism by writing a particular kind of history was, then, his main concern. But such was the complexity of his thesis that he found it necessary to respond to more general questions about his analysis of power. Did he see power everywhere and reduce everything to power? No, but the decision in the late eighteenth century to choose imprisonment as 'the essential mode of punishment' must be understood in the context of the development of

> a whole technique of human dressage by location, confinement, surveillance, the perpetual supervision of behaviour and tasks, in short, a whole technique of 'management' of which the prison was merely one manifestation. . .
>
> (1988a: 105)

Represented as a mere manifestation of a much broader technique of management, imprisonment appears to get lost in this more generalised thesis about power. Nevertheless, despite his interest in exposing the spread of carceral power throughout society, the desire to make punishment regimes, especially the prison, vulnerable to critique, emerges as the dominant theme in his explications of the project of *Discipline and Punish*.

Nowhere is this more apparent than in his carefully edited interview 'Questions of method', where he responds to questions about why he saw the birth of the prison as so important. Hadn't he overstated the importance of the prison in penal history, given that other modes of punishment, notably the death penalty and deportation, had remained in effect? No, he had not meant to suggest that the prison was 'the essential core of the entire penal system', but it seemed 'legitimate' to take the prison as his object of analysis, for two reasons. First, it had been neglected in previous studies of 'the problems of "the penal order" [penalité] – a confused enough term in any case'. These studies had prioritised either 'the sociological problem of the criminal population, or the juridical problem of the penal system and its basis'. With few exceptions – notably that of Rusche and Kirchheimer – they ignored the 'actual practice of punishment'. The second reason (which seems to be the same as the first), is that he wanted to address the question: '*how* does one punish?' In short, his aim was 'to write a history, not of the prison as an institution, but of the *practice of imprisonment*', but to do so for a precise political purpose – to explode the 'self-evident character' that 'prison punishment' or imprisonment acquired soon after the establishment of the penitentiaries. His role was to show how 'this way of doing things' was accepted 'at a certain moment as a principal component of the penal system, thus coming to seem an altogether natural, self-evident and in-dispensable part of it' (1981: 3–5; his emphasis).

If, as we shall see, breaching self-evidences was how Foucault came to characterise all his work, the specific task of 'shaking this false self-evidence' of the prison was, in his view, easily accomplished. Early nineteenth-century texts testified to 'the astonishment at finding the prison being used as a general means of punishment – something which had not at all been what the eighteenth-century reformers had in mind'. His research on penal imprisonment thus exceeded his 'wildest hopes' – that of achiev-ing 'a breach of self-evidence', one which makes visible 'a *singularity* at places where there is a temptation to invoke a historical constant'; one which shows that 'things weren't as necessary as all that', and that, in particular, 'it wasn't self-evident that the only thing to be done with a criminal was to lock him up' (1981: 5–6; his emphasis).

Postscripts: the author's privilege – re-imagining one's self

So much then for attempting to get away with a simplistic return to the master in order to reclaim a sense of the paradigm-shifting import of his ideas about punishment – as if we could. As one commentator has said, 'nothing could be less appropriate than to treat Foucault, as others have done, as the highest authority on the meaning and use of his own work' (Minson 1985: ix). If the goal is to measure the Foucault effect, it is obviously counter-productive to ignore the interpretative secondary literature which has mounted over the two decades since the publication in 1975 of *Surveiller et punir*. Indeed, such is the impact of his work that it cannot be contained, even in the briefest of summaries, in one chapter: it has already spilled out into the first two chapters, and will do so again in chapter 5. Compounding the difficulty of gauging the interpretative fallout of the replacement of punishment with penality, Foucault constantly revised his views about the projects and goals of his earlier work, including *Discipline and Punish*. In several such revisions, he claimed that his whole life's work was devoted to a study of power. For example, he claimed that 'the mechanisms of power, the effects of truth or if you like, the rules of power and the powers of true discourses' could be said to have been his focal concern, even though he had traversed this terrain 'in a very zig-zag fashion' (1980d: 94). These 'powers of true discourses' later became 'games of truth', including those 'found in institutions or practices of control'. Sometimes he sought to provide a sense of continuity in his work, agreeing with an interviewer that 'these games of truth no longer are concerned with coercive practices but with the pratices of self-formation of the subject' and insisting that all his analyses 'have to do essentially with the relationships of power' (1988b: 1–3).

At other times, however, Foucault drops power as a central issue, insisting rather that: 'the goal of my work during the last twenty years . . . has been to create a history of the different modes by which, in our culture, human beings are made subjects' (Foucault 1983a: 208). Certainly, one of the three 'modes of objectification which transform human beings into subjects' – 'the objectivising' of the subject in 'dividing practices' which separates the subject from others – is reminiscent of themes in *Discipline and Punish*. In fact, he gives the example of the division between criminals and the 'good boys'. But he is now adamant that 'it is not power, but the subject, which is the general theme' of his research, although he is prepared to concede that he did become 'quite involved with the question of power'. However, the power to punish seems to have faded from view. Significantly, resistance to that power does not figure in his list of the 'series of oppositions which have developed over the last few years'. His examples of these 'antiauthority struggles' includes opposition to the power of men over women and of administration over the ways people live, but not the prison struggles which had informed the writing of *Discipline and Punish* (1983a: 208–11).

It would seem from these utterances that punishment, or even penality, was never one of Foucault's central concerns. Whatever his intention, the effect of these authorial re-imaginings of his earlier projects is to undermine attempts at critical assessment – to derail the critical bandwagon with disclaimers to the effect that *Discipline and Punish* was not intended to be read as historical truth, as 'a truth-claiming discourse'. In this reshuffled scenario, genealogies – histories of the present – are not 'true' histories but rather 'fictions', or at least, more like fiction than 'true discourse'.

> I have never written anything but fictions. I do not mean to say, however, that truth is therefore absent. It seems to me that the possibility exists . . . for a fictional discourse to induce effects of truth. . . . One 'fictions' history on the basis of a political reality that makes it true, one 'fictions' a politics not yet in existence on the basis of a historical truth.
>
> (Foucault 1980e: 193)[8]

Fictioning history? A politics not yet in existence? Can Foucault get away with all this? Can he escape trial and condemnation by incessantly restating the project of *Discipline and Punish* or by strategically playing with questions of truth and fiction? Can he elude criticism by asserting that his work 'takes place between unfinished abutments and lines of dots'? Can he ward off attack by saying:

> I like to open up a space of research, try it out, and then if it doesn't work, try again somewhere else. . . . What I say ought to be taken as 'propositions', 'game openings' where those who may be interested are invited to join in; they are not meant as dogmatic assertions that have to be taken or left en bloc. My books aren't treatises in philosophy or studies of history: at most, they are philosophical fragments put to work in a historical field of problems.
>
> (1981: 4)

The answer is no, if his critics are given any say in it.

PART TWO – RECEPTIONS: READING FOUCAULT

We have arrived at last at the most difficult moment, the one when we search for ways of registering the Foucault effect without simplistically regurgitating what has been said, refuted and reiterated in countless texts. For such is the power of his work that it has generated not only a secondary literature – which has been defined as 'the academic effort to appropriate, correct, or dismiss Foucault . . . sometimes brilliantly, sometimes stupidly' – but also an identifiable 'tertiary literature commenting on the pro-liferation of "Foucaults"' (Bové 1988: viii and xxxvi). The question is: how to proceed without getting lost in this sea of Foucaults, without succumbing to the temptation to marshal all the arguments for and against Foucault? Let us attempt to negotiate all the waves which followed in the wake of the appearance of *Discipline and Punish* – the waves of discontent as well as of adulation – by selectively sampling from the authoritative commentaries, ranging from the violently hostile to the more slavish forms of worship. The underlying aim, remember, is not to try to conflate all that has been said – all those words poured on top of his own. Nor is it to resolve any of the exegetical disputes which his work has engendered. The aim is to capture the Foucault effect, utilising examples of the reception of his work,[9] in order to assess its transgressive potentiality: its potentiality to break out of conventional conceptualisations of punishment.

Against Foucault – historical irritations

'I'm delighted that historians found no major error in *Surveiller et punir*' (1988a: 101) – Foucault triumphant, in 1978, just a year after the publi-cation of the English translation of this text. He spoke too soon. Historians have been foremost amongst the critics of *Discipline and Punish*. The critiques have come thick and fast, not only from expected quarters – that of administrative historians and, at the other end of the political spectrum, Marxist historians – but also from 'fellow' exponents of the social history of punishment. The book may have appeared too late for Ignatieff to do much more than note its existence in *A Just Measure of Pain*, but as we saw in chapter 2, he distanced his work from Foucault's prison history in subsequent critical reviews of the project of the new social history of the 1970s. To reiterate, the main problem with Foucault's approach, in Ignatieff's revised or 'counter' revisionist view, is that it concentrated too much on the control aspects of punishment at the expense of the role played by consensus and informal sanctioning mechanisms (Ignatieff 1983a). Reflecting on the question of social history – the question, which he put more specifically as: 'What is it a history *of*?' – Ignatieff came to concede that while Foucault's work 'irritates historians', it at least 'dared to treat the prison and the asylums, not in and for themselves, but as sites for the study of the knowledge–power relation'. In this sense at least, Foucault remained faithful to the 'true subject' of the new social history of institutions, namely, 'the historical relation between the inside and the outside'. Yet on other issues, especially the question of agency, the question of who is doing what to whom, and, especially, the question of resistance on the part of the dominated to 'administrative logistics' (Ignatieff 1983b: 169), it is Foucault's account, above all others, which is singled out as the interpretative punching bag by social (and other) historians of punishment.

An irritation – that would seem the best way to encapsulate the effect of *Discipline and Punish* on historians. The most-cited of these irritations, or reactions to the book's 'serious errors', have been summarised in various texts, most usefully by David Garland (1990a). Blitzing through his list, we find, first, the thorny question of periodisation. Foucault's thesis that the crucial penal transformation from torture to imprisonment occurred between 1750 and 1820, culminating in 1840, has been challenged by several historians. Pieter Spierenburg dates the beginning of the decline of the European scaffold much earlier, around 1600, and its final demise much later, at the end of the nineteenth century; John Beattie argues that imprisonment was widely used as a punishment for minor offenders in early eighteenth-century England, and Garland in his book *Punishment and Welfare* dates the introduction of Foucault's individualising disciplinary techniques into British prisons at the end of the nineteenth century – a hundred years after the master's chosen 'moment' (Garland 1985: 31). Moving on, Foucault's explanation of the penal change in terms of strategic shifts in modes of exercising power also appears to be faulty. Historical research has unearthed other critical processes such as changing sensibilities about violent punishment, legal developments, especially changes in the law of evidence, changes in religious beliefs, especially those pertaining to the confessional system. Next, while he downplays the role of penal reformers, the evidence suggests that many were actively involved in shaping prison regimes. Moreover, their advocacy of more lenient punishments was not a ploy to extend control; they were genuinely committed to such reforms (Garland 1990a: 157–9).[10]

Another frequently-cited fault of *Discipline and Punish* duly listed by Garland is its failure to provide the sort of evidence required of a properly constituted historical analysis. In particular, Foucault does not document how 'the prison form' which became generalised in Western Europe in the early nineteenth century 'found its way into legislation as a result of a society-wide disciplinary strategy, rather than as an outcome of particular penal theories'. Nor does he document the 'unspecified point' later in the century when he alleges that the production of delinquency became a deliberate penal strategy. The claim that there was a 'strategic calculation' clearly requires evidentiary support as does the argument that such a covert strategy explains why the prison has survived, despite its failures, well into the twentieth century. And finally, on the question of evidence, where is the documentary basis for the key argument in *Discipline and Punish* that 'a new, normalising, disciplinary approach became dominant in the penal system with the emergence of generalised imprisonment' in the nineteenth century? On the contrary, the evidence is against such a thesis – the individualising, normalising penal methods which Foucault speaks of were not widely introduced (at least in the United Kingdom) until the end of the nineteenth century; non-disciplinary sanctions such as the fine retain a central place in penal practice, and the punitive nature of the penal process has not yet been displaced by 'the trend towards normalising disciplinary sanctions and an administrative mode of dispersing them'. As for the claim that modern society has become a 'disciplinary society', this appears to be nothing more than an unsubstantiated assertion (Garland 1990a: 160–1).[11]

There are other lists of Foucault's historical sins and transgressions.[12] For example, J. G. Merquior, one of the master's most hostile critics, features what he presents as 'the historians' judgement' – that *Discipline and Punish* is severely flawed – in his own compendium of Foucauldian faults. In particular, he happily translates and records the criticisms of the French historian Jacques Léonard – that Foucault left out the whole of the crucially significant French revolutionary period; that he therefore over-looked the penal implications of the revulsion against the bloodshed of the Terror and that, on the other hand, Napoleon's penal code of 1810 re-introduced corporal punishments, including torture, which Foucault claims disappeared with the coming of disciplinary techniques.[13] Leonard also noted that Foucault did not distinguish between different categories of prisoners (political prisoners, murderers, workers, prostitutes). Moreover, by ignoring the evidence of the persistence of old economic and religious customs, he overstated the pervasiveness and effectiveness of 'normal-isation' and other disciplinary practices in French society in the first half of the nineteenth century. Crucially too, Léonard pinpoints the key failing in Foucault's form of 'historical' explanation – it omits questions of agency. Who, if anyone or any group, was behind the penal transformations? Who benefited from them, and who lost out? For Merquior as for other critics, Léonard 'hits the nail on the head' when he says: 'One does not know for certain whether M. Foucault describes a machinery or a machination' (Merquior 1985: 101–7).

Obviously relishing the job of adding the historians' queries to his own pastiche of Foucault's *faux pas*, Merquior passes his own judgement: 'the historian of the present bungled his project'. As for Foucault's sympathetic interpreters, Merquior accuses them of failing to respond to the criticism levelled at their hero (1985: 152–3). But if Merquior overstates his case, it should be said that historians have registered a lot of complaints against *Discipline and Punish*. To sum up their irritation: Foucault's history is not 'truly historical' (Spierenburg 1984: x). And yet, notwithstanding the critiques, *Discipline and Punish* has served social historians well: it is the necessary backdrop against which they rewrite penal history. Could Spierenburg have written *The Spectacle of Suffering* if he had not been provoked 'to construct a "counter-paradigm" to Foucault's in order to get closer to the 'historical reality' he claims is missing from Foucault's account (1984: viii–ix)? Would other anti-Foucauldian histories have taken the form that they did in the absence of the irritation of *Discipline and Punish*? Unquestionably, this text has had a formative influence and some critics are prepared to concede as much. Thus, for example, in *The Promise of Punishment*, an innovative study of nineteenth-century French prisons, Patricia O'Brien declares that Foucault 'is not a social historian at all', yet she acknowledges the pivotal influence of his 'brilliant, if elusive, instititutional analyses' which, in her view, have had 'the most significant influence on the practice of the new social history of institutions' (O'Brien 1982: 7–8).

Admittedly, we have not by any means exhausted the list of historians' complaints against *Discipline and Punish*. Yet what is notable is that the critics rarely display unmitigated hostility.[14] They always seem to find at least one fruitful counterpoint in his work from which to launch their own inquiries.[15] Such is the Foucault effect. As for the master himself, what did he make of all the fuss? Seemingly, not much. Consider, for example, his bemusement at Léonard's critique. Declining to make substantive rebuttals, he contently sits back, chuckling at Léonard's satiric imaginary historian – 'the virtuous knight of exactitude . . . the doctor of inexhaustable knowledges . . . the great witness of the Real'. Furthermore, the dominant tone of his response is one of aloofness from the historians' objections, as if he were saying, with a shrug of his shoulders: 'what matter who's criticising?'. Indeed he advocates in the end an attitude of 'indifference to the obligation of saying everything, even to satisfy the jury of assembled specialists' (Foucault 1980f: 29–32).[16]

Foucault was also not averse to evading substantive criticism of his work by taking refuge in disclaimers to the effect that, as he was not an historian, his work should not be read as history (1987: 9). Concurring on this point, Garland maintains that 'it is arguable that *Discipline and Punish* is not primarily a historical text' but rather a work of social theory. In Garland's view, the 'real core' of *Discipline and Punish* is what he calls its 'power perspective' – its interpretation of punishment exclusively in terms of power, indeed as a form of power in itself (a 'political technology' no less) (Garland 1990a: 162). We shall return to Garland's critique of the 'power perspective', but for now let us take another path which is opened up by a reading of *Discipline and Punish* as social theory – that of Marxist and feminist reactions to the text. Of course, in some quarters it would be simply unacceptable to lump feminists and Marxists together, and in most circumstances I would agree. Certainly, it would be highly problematic to suggest that Marxist or feminist analysts have been uniformly for or against Foucault, for their responses have been quite diverse. But providing a sense of the divergent reactions provoked by *Discipline and Punish* is precisely our concern here.

Marxist and feminist receptions

First, let us consider Marxist receptions of Foucault's work. Even if we limit our focus to what he had to say about punishment, a wide range of options have been taken. At one extreme are those who dismiss the work because it transgresses the foundational tenets of Marxist analysis. Bob Fine, for example, condemns Foucault's account of the effects of the prison as functionalist and refuses its association of the prison with industrial society rather than capital (1979 and 1980), while John Lea challenges the idea that factory discipline was 'simply identical with the subordination of labour to capital' (1979: 77). Others, as we saw in chapter 2, draw on *Discipline and Punish* for insights into the operation of disciplinary power in modern capitalist societies. Melossi and Pavarini's study, which argues for the compatibility of Foucault's disciplinary thesis and the Marxist project, is a case in point. Heinz Steinert, who criticises Foucault for failing to see that discipline can be derived from the capitalist mode of extraction of surplus value, but who nevertheless acknowledges that 'discipline' is a useful category, could also be placed in this camp (Steinert 1983). At the other end of the spectrum are those who read *Discipline and Punish* as 'a new mode of analysis' carrying them 'beyond Marxism' (Smart 1986: 157–8).[17] Mark Poster exemplifies this last approach, arguing that, by writing a history in which the mode of production is not privileged as 'the totalising centre of history', *Discipline and Punish* goes 'a long way toward overcoming the customary limitations' of the Marxist problematic (Poster 1984: 95 and 1989: 71). Thus inspired, Poster suggests that the primacy of the mode of economic production be replaced by a 'mode of information' which, however, is never clearly defined. Taking another tack altogether, Jeff Minson rejects the notion that Foucault's work can be placed in theoretical competition with Marxism inasmuch as 'the Marxist tradition is far too big and variegated, and Michel Foucault far too inconsiderable a fish, to place them in the same balance' (1985: 11). At the same time, however, he argues that notwithstanding his 'flaws', Foucault presented Marxist-orientated socialist theories and politics with 'some inescapable challenges' – including the challenge of coming to grips with his work on penality (Minson 1986: 107).

It is beyond the scope of this book to enter into the debate about how best to represent the relationship between Marxist and Foucauldian analytical frameworks. Nor is this the place to arbitrate between the various Marxist readings of *Discipline and Punish*. Suffice it to note that the fact that Marxist responses cannot be easily categorised as for or against *Discipline and Punish* is hardly surprising: Foucault was never systematic about Marxism, so why should their response be univocal? The crucial point is that in the process of critiquing and coming to grips with his theses about disciplinary power and the operation of modern law – the juridical sphere – Marxists have provided more sophisticated understandings of penality. Steven Spitzer's analysis of the rationalisation of crime control in Western capitalist societies, referred to in chapter 2, is a case in point (1983). Barry Smart's effort to sketch the lines of a productive meeting between Foucault and Marxism on the question the state, power and social regulation is another (1983a and 1983b).

As for feminist receptions of *Discipline and Punish*, those reacting to his ideas about punishment will be considered in chapter 4 while those extending his ideas about discipline will be considered in chapter 5, where we will see them taking disciplined and docile bodies to places Foucault would never have dreamed of. As we shall see, feminists have been more predisposed to engage with his disciplinary thesis than with his ideas about penal practices, leaving something of a lacuna in feminist analyses of penality per se. Still, their extensions of the disciplinary thesis are very suggestive about the directions which a more deeply reflective – that is, feminist – Foucauldian analysis of penality should take. Here it suffices to note that their engagments with *Discipline and Punish* can be read as regional instances of a fairly widespread recognition by feminists of the potentiality of the work of this 'profoundly androcentric writer', notwithstanding the fact that, as Meaghan Morris put it, 'any feminists drawn into sending Love Letters to Foucault would be in no danger of reciprocity' (Morris 1988: 55). Some don't care. As Nancy Fraser has said, Foucault may not be 'much good as a husband' and 'one wouldn't want, politically speaking, to cohabit with him indefinitely'. And yet:

> he makes a very interesting lover indeed. His very outrageousness in refusing standard humanist virtues, narrative conventions, and political categories provides just the jolt we occasionally need to dereify our usual patterns of self-interpretation and renew our sense that, just possibly, they may not tell the whole story.
>
> (Fraser 1989: 65–6)

Fraser's point is well taken. The fact that Foucault himself does not come close to telling the whole story or to being a fully satisfying object of desire is of little consequence: feminists have their own political and analytical agendas and are free to use him or not as they please.

There are of course more specific critical observations which have not been considered here. In particular, Foucault's notion of the body has been widely critiqued from Marxist and socialist feminist perspectives (e.g. Dews 1987; Minson 1985; Fraser 1989) as well as from poststructuralist feminist perspectives (e.g. Butler 1990). His analysis of sovereign or 'juridical' power and legalism has also received considerable critical attention from Marxist quarters (e.g. Palmer and Pearce 1983) as has his analysis of the role of the state in the development of the disciplinary society. While sympathetic Marxists attempt to synthesise Foucault's analysis of power relations with Marxism, others insist that he has set up an untenable opposition between state power and an all-pervading discipline, thereby overstating the incompatibility of juridical power and disciplinary power (e.g. Steinert 1983; Minson 1985). Yet no matter how devastating or dismissive these critiques are, they all serve to confirm the Foucault effect. The most savaged of the new social historians of punishment and yet the most influential, Foucault survives the barbs of the Marxist Pharisees and lives on secure in the role of the quintessential Messiah of penality – sacrificed for his excesses, bearing the cross of the attack of lesser lights, but liberating all who would follow the Foucauldian light out of dungeon darkness.

For Foucault – the Foucauldians

The term 'Foucauldian' is deployed here loosely, and perhaps to some unforgivably: no doubt many would protest at being labelled a Foucauldian, let alone a 'guardian of the temple'. Other commentators, Foucault's English translators for example, would be quite content. After all, their exegetical contributions amount to little more than translation and exposition, so keen are they to allow His Master's Voice to be heard, unbroken by the din of their own ecstatic interruptions, much less by that of the madding crowd of critics.[18] At any rate, I have here deposited indiscriminately a host of texts into the Foucauldian basket. They range from the sycophantic to stinging yet ultimately sympathetic critiques. Yet diverse as these receptions are, and strident though the protests may be that it is a travesty to categorise some and not other commentators as Foucauldian, or even to categorise them at all, those labelled 'Foucauldian' here have one thing in common: they have all followed the master's direction to use his books as 'little tool boxes' (quoted in Patton 1979: 115). By developing his new instruments for understanding punishment – notably, power, micro-power, discipline, technology and strategy – they provide clear examples of the effectivity of *Discipline and Punish* in producing transgressive interpretative breakthroughs in the analysis of punishment.

Perhaps the most useful Foucauldian glosses on *Discipline and Punish* are those which provide reading strategies – that is, different ways of receiving the text. Here Foucault set an example, declaring that his work should be read not as history but as 'a philosophical exercise' in which the aim is to learn 'to what extent the effort to think one's own history can free thought from what it silently thinks, and so enable it to think differently' (Foucault 1987: 9). Thus Hubert Dreyfus and Paul Rabinow are simply following the master's example in dismissing historical objections to the book. Undoubtedly he would approve their giving historians short shrift, as they do in a footnote:

> There is obviously no simple appeal to the facts involved in evaluating Foucault's historical theses . . . most of these historians have mis-understood his argument and hence even their minor factual corrections are simply beside the point.
>
> (Dreyfus and Rabinow 1983: 126)

Their strategy is to read *Discipline and Punish* not as history but as 'a geneaology of structuralist discourse and associated practices' (1983: 155). The French philosopher Gilles Deleuze, on the other hand, reads it as a map – a cartography of the 'Divine Comedy of punishment' – in his homage to Foucault, the self-defined 'cartographer' (Deleuze 1988: 23 and 44). Still another tactic has been to carefully distinguish standard histories from Foucault's 'genealogical' quest to discover the conditions of emergence of the carceral power to punish, and, more particularly, to determine why the penitentiary reform proposals were 'so readily acceptable'. In this way, *Discipline and Punish* is still read as history – it is asking 'historical questions concerning the acceptability and perpetuation of generalised imprisonment' – but it is a different kind of history, one which is concerned not with a history of institutions or of ideas but rather with the form of the exercise of power which characterises the modern prison (Minson 1985: 20–3).

By contrast, Paul Patton refuses the idea of reading *Discipline and Punish* as history. Given that the object of analysis is 'the carceral' rather than the institution of the prison and that the book's central concern is to define 'the specificity of discipline as a form of exercise of power on the body', he argues that it should not be received as a 'kind of "genetic" history of the evolution of the penal apparatus'. Instead, he interprets the project of *Discipline and Punish* as 'morphological rather than genetic, or, if you like, diachronic rather than synchronic' (Patton 1979: 114, 128–30). That is:

> It is less a matter of tracing the historical thread of the apparatus of punishment, than of characterising the kind of power exercised in the

prison, and of defining the nature of the general system of power within which the prison functions.

(Patton 1979: 130)

Imprisonment as a generalised form of punishment belongs in a 'non-discursive historical series' – that of the relations between power and the body. Patton concedes that Foucault's explanation of the emergence of the prison as the predominant mode of judicial punishment – 'the final figure of the age of disciplines' – is unsatisfactory in that 'next to nothing is said about the actual historical circumstances of the introduction of the prison'. But in his view, the objections of historians like Leonard miss the mark.

> Foucault's explanation of the birth of the prison needs to be situated not in the field of an analysis of the political and social events surrounding the introduction of the prison, but in the field of an analysis of the forms of (micro-) power in society.

(1979: 135–7)

From this standpoint, the historians' objections are 'based on the illusion that Foucault is talking at the level of the *history* of the mechanisms of disciplinary power, in the sense in which historians understand that term'. At this level, innumerable objections can be raised to the idea that there was 'a uniform and massive disciplinarisation of society' in the eighteenth and nineteenth centuries or to Foucault's neglect of the resistance of workers and prisoners. But 'such "historian's history"' was not Foucault's primary concern. Rather:

> His analysis of discipline forms part of a morphology of the will to power, that is, the characterisation of the forms of exercise of power, rather than a history of their social implantation.

(1979: 137–9)

Such a morphology of the programme of disciplinary power must be separated from 'the real, historical progress of its techniques'. Furthermore, the history of the emergence of the prison is dependent on 'the morphological question' – the question of the form of power which the prison represents (1979: 137–9).[19]

There have been other moves made by Foucauldians to defend Foucault, for example by explaining what he meant by 'the disciplinary society' (e.g. Ewald 1992) or by rejecting 'literalistic' objections to his work on the ground that he is 'engaging in a legitimate rhetorical tactic, telling us lies about the past in order to open our eyes to the reality of the present'. In this reading, Foucault's enterprise is 'a prophetic one': his interest is in 'changing the way things are', not in 'logical or historical correctness for its own sake'. Such a reading purports to save *Discipline and Punish* from those 'naive readings' which seek to find 'true propositions regarding the actual institution' of the prison (Megill 1985: 244–6). Still another move has been to read his work as having the impact of 'a force of flight' from our entrapment in modern systems of thought, one which teaches us 'how to doubt the order of things' (Bernauer 1990: 184). Yet for all the diversity of these interpretations, they have one thing in common: they are profoundly masculinist and, in this significant respect, blindly accepting of the order of things. The question of the absence of gender, let alone of women, in Foucault's work completely passes them by.[20]

From penology to a 'social' analysis of penality

On a happier note, it should be recalled that it was *Discipline and Punish* which provided the spark which ignited the movement from penology to 'the social analysis of penality' (Garland and Young 1983) or, alternatively, to 'the sociology of penal policies' (Faugeron and Houchon 1987) – a movement led by progressive sociologists interested in charting changing penal configurations in late twentieth-century Western societies. In this task they were more than ably assisted by Foucault's methodological directives to study power 'at its extremities' or in its more 'local' forms where it becomes 'less legal'; to focus less on conscious intention than on 'the point of application of power'; to ask 'how things work at the level of ongoing subjection, at the level of those continuous and uninterrupted processes which subject our bodies', and to reconceptualise 'mechanisms of exclusion' as including 'apparatuses of surveillance, the medicalisation of sexuality, of madness, of delinquency, all the micro-mechanisms of power' (Foucault 1980d: 96–102). By providing such a smorgasbord of analytical possibilities, Foucault played a pivotal role in freeing penality from the confines of traditional penology's narrow, empiricist obsession with issues of technical efficiency. It was his ideas about the 'carceral city' and the dispersal of social control throughout the disciplinary society which opened up the penal field to studies of decarceration and even 'trans-carceration' (e.g. Lowman *et al.* 1987).

Once again, this is not to suggest that the proliferation of Foucauldian critiques of decarceration policies in the late 1970s and early 1980s should be counted as an unqualified analytical success or that these studies came close to specifying 'the social' in ways which would have purchase with feminist theorists. The so-called 'dispersal of discipline thesis' (Bottoms 1983), based on Foucault's notion of 'indefinite discipline', may have contributed to an understanding of the ways in which penal institutions are extended into the community via the blurring of the boundaries between the institution and the community, the widening of the social control mesh and the 'penetration' of the state into the community. However, this last idea – that the 'blurring of social control implies the deeper penetration of social control into the social body' (Cohen 1979: 356) – cannot go unchallenged.[21] Feminist analysts may have been bemused that 'penetration' was the operative word in this form of Foucauldian social control theorisation, but what were they to make of the alarmist visions conjured up by all the 'social control talk' (Cohen 1983) in these penetrating – more phallic than penal – masculinist analyses?[22] Surely they could only gasp with incredulity at the futuristic scenarios conjured up by masculinist Foucauldian discourse – 'the spectre of expanded state control' or 'the nightmare of the benevolent state gone haywire' (Austin and Krisberg 1981: 183 and 188) and the emergence of a 'carceral archipelago' characterised by 'an intensity of intervention at least as great as that in most maximum security prisons' (Cohen 1979: 352). For women have always been controlled and disciplined, if not in the state-controlled ways anticipated by the Foucauldian social control theorists at least by other state control systems, notably social security, and, more broadly, within 'civil society'. On the other hand, the 'spectre' of expanding state control is not self-evidently regressive for women. Their experience in the family, a site of oppression and control for many women, has demonstrated that there is nothing inherently progressive about the defence of 'a sphere of private, indvidual relations, autonomous of regulation' (Brown and Hogg 1985a: 409).

To be sure, masculinist Foucauldian sociologists of social control have withdrawn from some of their more alarmist, state-focused 'dispersal of discipline' notions and, in the process, have provided more useful points of departure for a clarification of the complex nature of the interplay of social and legal controls in modern Western societies. But most of them still suffer from a form of 'sanction myopia' (Freiberg 1987: 243) which precludes them from extending their masculinist gaze beyond criminal or civil penalties to the question of gendered sanctions. However, studies exploring the dispersal of non-disciplinary as well as disciplinary forms of punishment have relevance for a feminist analysis of penality (Bottoms 1983). So too do studies calling for an examination of the internal differentiation of the penal realm and, more broadly, for a 'social' analysis which explores the 'social foundations of penality' (Garland and Young 1983: 4–5). Furthermore, *Discipline and Punish* is open to less alarmist, perhaps less phallic and more feminist, readings. In particular, Foucault's ideas about the establishment of a 'carceral network', understood as an extension of surveillance and normalisation throughout society (Foucault 1977a: 300–8), connect in self-evident ways to feminist sociologies of the social control of women, thereby providing an analytical space in which women can be included in any properly-constituted 'social' analysis of penality.

BEYOND FOUCAULT?

There is today what could be categorised as a third response to Foucault's analysis of punishment, one which claims to move beyond the stances taken by those who are for as well as those against *Discipline and Punish*.[23] The leading exponent of this position is David Garland, an erstwhile Foucauldian who acknowledges Foucault's influence on his historical analysis of punishment regimes in late nineteenth-century England, but who has now arrived at a post-Foucauldian analytical stage.[24] The drift of Garland's argument is that it is time to move beyond the social control framework which dominated the sociology of punishment in the 1980s. What is required is 'a wider, more flexible and more multi-dimensional framework' which allows for the impact of 'cultural sensibilities' on the punishment process. Punishment is not simply an exercise of power; it expresses 'social sentiments', notably passion. Indeed, 'the essence of punishment is irrational, unthinking emotion'. Thus punishment must be conceptualised not only in terms of the power to punish, but also as an 'urge to punish' – as 'an emotional reaction which flares up at the violation of cherished social sentiments'. We need to focus on the '*tragic* aspects of punishment' (Garland 1983b: 3–7; his emphasis). In this Durkheimian-influenced framework, attention is drawn to

the non-instrumental aspects of punishment – its emotional aspect, its social origins, its expression of values and culture and its effect *beyond* the relationship of controlled and controlling.

(1990b: 9; my emphasis)

Crucially, it was Foucault, according to Garland, who led us down this treacherous 'control' path and a 'Foucault-derived "sociology of control" which reduced the sociology of punishment to 'a sociology of control and domination', thereby closing off important questions about punishment. By over-emphasising power and control issues, by offering an interpretation of punishment as a 'political technology', *Discipline and Punish* led us to overlook the fact that punishment is a 'social institution'. More particularly, punishment is 'a symbolically deep event . . . an event which has a profound cultural resonance' with the public, and it cannot be understood 'within a purely instrumental framework' (1990b: 10–12).

This critique of Foucault's so-called 'power perspective' is the central plank in Garland's bid to transcend sociological disagreements about how to theorise punishment (1990a: 162). He claims that it is time for the

sociology of punishment to strive for an 'integrated, pluralistic interpretation', a 'balanced synopsis' – a 'synthesis', no less – of the range of
perspectives available. Interestingly, punishment is understood here as a
complex legal process which Garland proposes to 'capture' with the concept of 'penality' – a concept which he not only borrows from Foucault but
unashamedly appropriates as his own, defining it as 'the network of laws,
processes, discourses, representations and institutions which make up the
penal realm'. While Foucault's analytical interests extended to non-legal
forms of punishment, Garland's narrower goal is to understand 'legal
punishment and its social foundations'. He therefore focuses on those
punishments which are 'authorised by law' – the 'non-legal but often
routine forms of punishment which occur in modern criminal justice', such
as the 'implicit penalties' found in police and prosecution practices, are not
his concern (1990a: 15–18). Punishment might be a social institution, but
Garland is concerned only with the its legal or 'authorised' manifestations
in the criminal justice system. Returning to his critique of Foucault, we find
Garland accounting for the inadequacies in the argument of *Discipline and
Punish* – for example, the account of the prison's survival – in terms of
Foucault's failure to acknowledge 'the role of any values other than power
and control' in the history of punishment. This also led Foucault to neglect
those ideological and political forces which opposed the introduction and
extension of disciplinary power. As a result, *Discipline and Punish* tells a
story of 'meticulous domination and thoroughgoing control' which gives
the impression that 'society's practices of normalisation – its imposition of
standards upon conduct – are oppressive in all their aspects' (1990a:
166–9).

But is this impression so wrong? Is it really time to revise it? Is the
critical project to which Foucault contributed so much, now exhausted,
such that we need a synthesis of Foucauldian, Weberian and Durkheimian
themes to understand the 'social' institution of punishment? The answers
to these questions depend on one's social position and theoretical
standpoint. Those at the bottom, those more likely to be on the receiving
end of legal punishment, might not be as sanguine as Garland about the
'cultural' values and 'social sentiments' which are enshrined in his new
synthesis. Those on the receiving end of disciplinary practices, whether
these occur within or without the criminal justice system, might be less
inclined than Garland to narrow the analytical parameters of 'penality' to
'authorised' punishments. Indeed, studies of women offenders as well as
women victims who undergo Western criminal justice processes indicate
that it is precisely the non-legal forms of punishment – the 'implicit
penalties' – which punish women most (e.g. Eaton 1986). And studies of
disciplinary regimes imposed on the lived female body in Western societies

come to similar conclusions, as we shall see in chapter 5. The evidence of these studies suggests strongly that Foucault's disciplinary thesis still has a purchase and that the critical project highlighting the control aspects of punishment is far from exhausted. However, if this evidence is not convincing for those like Garland who are determined to move beyond Foucault, they could at least acknowledge that it was not they, but rather Foucault, who proposed the concept of 'penality' in order to take it beyond the narrow parameters of conventional understandings of punishment. We can hope too that, as they develop their 'new' pluralistic conceptualisations of punishment, post-critical scholars on a synthesing mission will take into account that the 'social' is profoundly gendered and that a masculinist perspective on punishment regimes is just as profoundly limited.[25]

RECLAIMING FOUCAULT: THE POLITICALITY OF THE POWER TO PUNISH

By now it must be obvious that I have succumbed to the temptation which the chapter set out to avoid: that of providing a kind of rough taxonomy of interpretative inclinations provoked by *Discipline and Punish*. But what to do with it? While I have no intention of entering the fraught minefield of interpretative battles for or against Foucault, I do want to suggest that two recent interpretative trends have worked to camouflage or at least diminish the significance of his analysis of the power to punish. First, the attempt to move beyond Foucault seems premature in that it blocks off bids to develop *Discipline and Punish* in still more analytically useful – that is, transgressive – ways, some of which will be explored in chapters 4 and 5. Second and related, the dominant interpretative tendency, that of emphasising the discipline of *Discipline and Punish* to the detriment (analytically speaking) of punishment, has had deleterious effects. It overpowers the analysis of punishment, such that it is customary in some circles today to go so far as to say, or at least imply, that Foucault was not interested in punishment. According to Pasquale Pasquino, for example, the sub-title 'birth of the prison' displays 'a concern somewhat different from the true object of the book'. It is little more than a 'pretext' for the study of a problem which Foucault defines at the end of the book – 'the power of normalisation and the formation of knowledge in modern society'. Thus it is 'the disciplines' or rather 'the conditions of possibility of modern society' which constitute 'the real theme' of the book. In brief, 'Foucault's problem is that of interrogating modernity around the very construction of the subject' (Pasquino 1986: 97–8).[26] Yet while it is well to be reminded of the diverse range of issues which *Discipline and Punish* throws into relief, a reading of Foucault's texts indicates that he emphatically *was* interested in the penal question. Indeed, the elision of this interest in the secondary literature betrays his active involvement in prison politics.

Now that Foucault's biography has detailed his involvement in the prison movement in France in the early 1970s (Eribon 1991), there is no longer an excuse for ignoring or underplaying the political connectedness of *Discipline and Punish* to the prison struggle. But it should have been apparent much earlier, if not in *Discipline and Punish* where he makes the prison riots of the early 1970s one of his key reference points, then in his interviews where he elaborated on his objectives. In 'Questions of method' for example, when pressed about the allegedly 'anaesthetic' or deleterious effect of his thesis about disciplinary power on prison struggles and resistance generally, he replies that his 'project', far from being comparable with revolutionary programmes designed to overturn society, is more modest in scope. It is simply this:

> To give some assistance in wearing away certain self-evidences and commonplaces about madness, normality, illness, crime and punishment; to bring it about, together with many others, that certain phrases can no longer be spoken so lightly, certain acts no longer, or at least no longer so unhesitatingly performed, to contribute to changing certain things in people's ways of perceiving and doing things, to participate in this difficult displacement of forms of sensibility and thresholds of tolerance . . .
>
> (Foucault 1981: 11–12)

Importantly, one of the principal sites selected by Foucault for wearing away self-evidences, for altering people's perceptions of the intolerable, was the prison system in France.[27] Moreover, he became aware of that 'extremely strange reality that we call confinement' years before he wrote *Discipline and Punish*. What struck him about this practice of confinement was that while it was 'accepted by both sides as absolutely self-evident', it was 'far from being self-evident' (Foucault 1988a: 96–7). The clearly-defined goal of *Discipline and Punish*, as well as of the Prison Information Group (GIP) he helped establish in France, was precisely to breach this false self-evidence of the prison.

Foucault's specific concern with the question of penality re-emerged yet again in an interview given shortly before his death. Here he explains one last time precisely what he had intended to do in this book. It was not to write a critical work which took the form of a denunciation of the penal system today. Nor was he interested in writing an historical account explaining how penal institutions functioned in the nineteenth century. Rather, he had 'tried to pose another problem' – that of discovering 'the system of thought, the form of rationality' which since the late eighteenth century had produced the idea that the prison was the best means to punish. To 'give oneself the means to think what could yield to a real, profound and radical transformation' was only possible if we isolated 'the system of rationality underlying punitive practices' (1989b: 280). That is, to transform the penal system it is necessary to examine the thought structures which sustain it. In this final reformulation of his project, Foucault provides an important connecting point to his earlier declarations about the meaning of his work. This connecting point is the 'specific intellectual', a figure which appeared in his work in the 1970s. The function of the specific intellectual, as described then, was to become involved in local political struggles by deciphering specific regimes of truth (1980c: 126–33). Now, finally, it is to isolate 'systems of thought that have now become familiar to us, that appear evident to us, and that have become part of our perceptions, attitudes and behaviour' (1989b: 282).

Here the labyrinthine path along which Foucault stages and restages his overall project returns to a familiar theme, that of the all-important imperative to breach self-evidences. We may not yet have encountered 'problematisation', the notion which finally announces itself, in his last interviews, as underlying all his work: after all, Foucault concedes that he never 'isolated this notion sufficiently'. But it does not come as a surprise to find him reformulating the goal of *Discipline and Punish* again, this time as a 'problematisation' – apparently, he was 'trying to analyse the changes in the problematisation of the relations between crime and punishment through penal practices and penitentiary institutions' in the late eighteenth and early nineteenth centuries (1988c: 257). Yet if this does seem new, he reiterates the by now familiar theme of the role of the intellectual, themes which highlight the politicality of all his work.

> The work of an intellectual is not to shape others' political will; it is, through the analyses that he carries out in his own field, to question over and over again what is postulated as self-evident, to disturb other people's mental habits, the way they do and think things, to dissipate what is familiar and accepted, to re-examine rules and institutions on the basis of this re-problematisation (in which he carries out his specific task as an intellectual) to participate in the formation of a political will (in which he has his role as a citizen to play).
>
> (1988c: 265)

Here, perhaps, is the essential Foucault, happily disrupting other people's modes of thought and behaviours; breaching the self-evidence of the familiar, including especially the self-evidence of oppressive institutions; labouring hard over the relationship between the theoretical work of the intellectual dissident and political practice, and yet, at the same time, abjectly failing to problematise the most familiar relationship of all, that of gender, thereby failing, from beginning to end, to breach the self-evidence of the thoroughly masculinist paradigms which have imprisoned the theorisation of penality all along. Surely in formulating what was required in terms of 'a ramified, penetrative perception of the present' (1980b: 62), and in contemplating the role of the intellectual exclusively in male terms, Foucault destined that his androcentric gaze would continue to focus unblinkingly on the punishment of men.[28] On the one hand, then, he dissipates the familiar in an explosively powerful way, insisting that historical analysis be part of political struggle: 'The point is not to give to the movement a direction or a theoretical apparatus, but to set up possible strategies' (Foucault in Gandal 1986: 123). On the other hand, he has insufficiently specified the form of both the analysis and of the struggle required to transform penal regimes. As a consequence, the political effectivity of his efforts to breach the self-evidence of oppressive institutions and practices is not as straightforward or, indeed, self-evident as he might have hoped.[29]

Concluding note

In the same 1977 interview where Foucault expressed misguided or premature delight that historians had found no major faults with *Discipline and Punish*, he also expressed his satisfaction that prisoners read it in their cells (1988a: 101). It is impossible to know whether this is true or how many prisoners have read the book, let alone what they made of it. We do know, or at least we are told by his friend Gilles Deleuze, that he felt that his Prison Information Group was a failure (Eribon 1991: 234). What then, are we to make of the possibility of bridging the gap between theoretical texts and incarcerated populations, between theory and activism and of the possibility of wearing away the self-evidence of punitive responses to crime? Would Foucault believe that the conditions of emergence of a progressive, theoretically-informed strategy around, or rather against, penality have now dissipated? Would he despair that today, two decades after the publication of *Surveiller et punir*, the self-evidence of the prison appears to be secure against both theoretical and activist transgressions? How can we know, and, anyway, what does it matter? What matters, in Foucault's view, is the speech and resistance of the imprisoned:

> when the prisoners began to speak, they possessed an individual theory of prisons, the penal system, and justice. It is this form of discourse which ultimately matters, a discourse against power, the counter-discourse of prisoners and those we call delinquents – and not a theory *about* delinquents.

> (Foucault 1977c: 209; his emphasis)

This then is what ultimately matters, according to the theorist who declared that theory is itself practice, that theory is 'the regional system' of the 'struggle against power' and who, we are informed by a temple guardian, taught us 'the indignity of speaking for others' (1977c: 208–9). As such claims surely require further scrutiny, we will return to the crucial question – that of merging theory with activism in the prison movement – in the last chapter. There we will ponder Paul Sedgwick's observation that Foucault's work – and by extension, any transgressive analysis of penality – will ultimately be assessed by its capacity to 'aid in the formation of an informed political practice' (1982: 148). But first, let us consider another question, one which seemed to be beyond Foucault's intellectual horizon – that of the lonely, yet-to-be-adequately-theorised figure of the woman inmate. More broadly, let us turn to the question of the disciplining and punishment of women.[30]

4   Feminist analytical approaches to women's imprisonment

> The female prison community has been overlooked: it merits study as does any other complex organisation, in order to add to the growing body of theory on group behaviour.
>
> (Giallombardo 1966: 1)

Critical feminist approaches to penality have really only begun to emerge over the past decade, and even then they have focused almost exclusively on women's imprisonment. British sociological studies, in particular the work of Pat Carlen, and revisionist histories of women's imprisonment have commenced a process which will eventually fundamentally transform critical analyses of punishment regimes. Progress in this direction, however, has been slow. On the one hand, critical masculinist analysts of penality, having only recently constructed their own subversive paradigms, appear to be incapable of registering the import of the new scholarship on women offenders. On the other hand, feminist research initiatives have remained precisely that: disparate empirical studies which are still today missing the benefit of a sustained critical dialogue, let alone an active theoretical engagement with issues raised by critical but non-feminist analysts. The purpose of this chapter is to explore these emergent feminist approaches to the question of the punishment of women with a view to suggesting ways in which they can be made to impact in a transformative way on the study of penality.

A point of clarification, one which goes to the heart of the theoretical quandary besetting the field of women and penality, is in order before we start. As Pat Carlen, arguably the most theoretically rigorous analyst of lawbreaking women, has pointed out, not all the authors of the new revisionist accounts of women's encounters with the criminal justice and penal systems which have appeared over the past decade claim a feminist perspective. Carlen, who is herself ambivalent about making such a claim, resolves this problem in the following way:

because they have collectively contributed to a demolition of certain sexist myths concerning women's lawbreaking and have called into question the more discriminatory and oppressive forms of the social control and regulation of women, I shall . . . use 'feminist' very loosely to refer to all those who, in writing of women lawbreakers, have been concerned to remedy the wrongs done to *women* criminals by criminologists, police, courts, and prisons.

(Carlen 1990a: 107; her emphasis)

We shall have occasion to return to the question of feminism in relation to critical approaches to penality, but for now it is appropriate to begin with an overview of the diverse work being done in the broad area of women offenders in Western criminal justice and penal systems.

SENTENCING WOMEN TO PRISON

New sentencing studies

First, we should consider the new directions taken by recent research on the sentencing of women. Research in this area currently takes two broad forms. The first and still dominant form of analysis, especially in the United States, is a hypothesis-testing mode of inquiry which remains preoccupied with now antiquated questions about the alleged impact of 'chivalry' and 'women's liberation' on the sentencing process. These statistically-based, quantitative studies deploy multiple regression, multivariate logistic analysis and loglinear modelling to test endlessly whether chivalrous magistrates sentence women more leniently than men, or whether women's liberation leads to crime. Such studies, which produce what they call 'descriptive data on females', leave much to be desired. Their questions and conclusions are frequently misinformed by simplistic, masculinist constructions of gender, including the assumption that women – the female data – constitute an undifferentiated unity which is advantaged or disadvantaged at different decision points: arrests, committal or sentencing. Furthermore, even when the data are controlled for offence type and prior convictions, the results are unclear (Parisi 1982; Gelsthorpe 1987). Some studies find that women are treated preferentially in court (Steffensmeier 1980) others that they are treated more harshly (Smart 1976; Dominelli 1984; Chesney-Lind 1978); still others that they receive equal treatment; or that disparities in sentencing are diminishing (Douglas 1987; Kempinen 1983), or that differential sentencing occurs for felonies but not misdemeanours (Zingraff and Thomson 1984). Overall, however, the more rigorous of these studies find that when legally relevant considerations are taken into account – such as the fact that women commit less serious offences and are less likely to have prior convictions – sex differences in sentencing disappear, although domestic circumstances, in particular marital status, have been found to be more important in the sentencing of women (Farrington and Morris 1983: 247).

Over the past decade, several British feminist sociologists have initiated and developed a more sophisticated form of research on women offenders. Breaking out from the limitations imposed by empiricist, masculinist paradigms, they have shown that gender-differentiating processes operate in far more complex ways than hypothesis-testing models allow, and may not in fact be exposed by statistical correlations which purport to demonstrate a direct and quantifiable empirical association between gender and law enforcement processes.[1] These analysts have made a convincing case for developing a more theoretically-informed approach to sex/gender questions in the criminal justice system, one which recognises that the key issue is not whether women are treated differently from men but how different categories of women are treated by the courts (e.g. Smart 1976). They argue that it is not women per se who receive different sentences but women in their gender roles as women and mothers. Thus, women who display appropriate feminine and middle-class characteristics are more likely to be treated more leniently than those who are working-class, black, unmarried or in any other way perceived as 'deviant' (e.g. Hudson 1987: 119–21). More broadly, these new research initiatives have displayed a more sophisticated understanding of the social constructions of sex, sexuality and gender which inform criminal justice agents' perceptions of normal and criminal women (e.g. Worrall 1990), or of good or wayward girls negotiating the enormously difficult task of 'growing up good' in Western societies (Cain 1989).

These new studies of the ideologically-based constructions of sex and gender and their deconstructions of the discourses of sexuality, domesticity and pathology which colour magistrates' and judges' perceptions of women offenders have transformed the nature of research in the field.[2] It is now clear that we need to abandon simplistic theorisations of lenient-versus-severe treatment of women in courts. Far more interesting questions arise from an exploration of the impact of the ideology of 'familialism' on the expectations which magistrates, probation officers and social workers have of women offenders' capabilities. An overriding concern with women's domestic responsibilities, as Lena Dominelli has argued, does not necessarily translate into leniency for them. Familial ideology can operate instead to give male offenders involved in domestic duties such as child care a source of leniency not available to women (Dominelli 1984: 101). Mary Eaton came to similar conclusions in her pathbreaking study of the of familial ideology in sentencing practices in London magistrates' courts. Eaton rejects as too limited the approach which studies differential sentencing by comparing court disposals of cases involving women with those involving men. Sentencing, the end point of the criminal justice process, is the wrong starting point because very few women appear in court under the same circumstances as men do, or for the same offences. Women are disadvantaged in court, 'not specifically in relation to men defendants, but more generally in relation to men within the family and consequently throughout society'. Eaton argues, convincingly, that it is more fruitful to understand the processes involved in sentencing – the pleas of mitigation, social work reports, magistrates' assumptions – within a broader social context. Focusing on the way courts make use of gender roles within the family, she demonstrates how the courts judge male and female defendants in the context of their families, thereby preserving differences based on sexual inequality (Eaton 1986: 12–31 and 87–98).

Eaton's work typifies the new mode of British sentencing research which focuses on the entire criminalisation process, starting with women's lives and then moving on to examine how 'the social control of women leads to state control' (Chadwick and Little 1987: 255). The wide-ranging approach of this work has provided important guidelines for research on women prisoners, who rarely constitute more than 5 per cent of any Western prison population and who, consequently, continue to be ignored even by otherwise progressive analysts. For example, as we have seen, Garland and Young may have been strong advocates of a move from traditional penology to 'a social analysis of penality', but the 'social' does not appear to include women in their masculinist analytical framework.[3] While it is all very well to assert the importance of recognising internal differentiations within the prison system, it is another matter altogether to classify, without further elaboration, women prisoners with sex offenders as objects of different internal practices. Surely analysts who purport to be 'progressive', as Garland and Young do, must take pains to distinguish women prisoners from sex offenders (1983: 23). The same point holds for the recent prison study which, while proclaiming the need to move from penology to a sociology of penal policies, relegated women prisoners to a footnote in apparent oblivion of the trivialising effect of such a discursive manoeuvre (Faugeron and Houchon 1987). Certainly, the failure of masculinist sociologists and social historians to address the question of women's imprisonment, let alone the question of how an analysis of the punishment of women might impact on their theories of penality – theories based on studies of the punishment of men – is a clear sign that their critical analytical frameworks require a major overhaul. In the meantime, in the face of such relentless masculinist blindness to the necessity of including women prisoners in any progressive examination of penality, feminist researchers have insisted that women prisoners be treated as a subject worthy of progressive, theoretical study in their own right. Here the work of the British criminologist Pat Carlen is exemplary.

Pat Carlen

Carlen's work – in particular, her definitive sociological study of women's imprisonment in Scotland (1983a), her autobiography-facilitating text which allowed British women ex-prisoners to speak for themselves (1985), her ethnography of the socio-biographies of thirty-nine women with criminal convictions (1988) and her suggestions for alternatives to women's imprisonment (1990a and 1990b) – have had a transforming effect on Western research on women prisoners. While some of the policy implications which she draws from her work on lawbreaking women will be explored later, it is essential to begin with a consideration of her now classic *Women's Imprisonment: A Study in Social Control* (1983a), the text which focuses on the 'moment' of imprisonment for women and which placed the analysis of 'female' imprisonment firmly and irrevocably in the broader context of the social control of women.

Briefly, Carlen's *Women's Imprisonment* is a field-work study of Scotland's only women's prison, Cornton Vale. But it is much more than that, for Carlen's analytical concerns cannot be confined to one particular prison. While she retains her focus on Cornton Vale, her project is more ambitious: it is to locate 'the wider meanings of the moment of prison', meanings which cannot be contained within one particular institution, nor within what she calls 'the female subject of penology'. Rather, the meanings of women's imprisonment 'must be constantly open to question' – that is, open to empirical and theoretical investigation not only of the women themselves, but also of men, families and the authorities, of alcoholism, 'madness', 'badness' and 'sickness' and of 'a type of dismissive society in general' (1983a: 1–2). Carlen's investigation takes the form of a case-study. She interviewed twenty women who were serving or who had served short-term sentences with a view to exploring 'the changing and various meanings of imprisonment within Great Britain' and, more broadly, 'the invisible nature of the social control of women'. Her aim was

> to assess the 'moment' of prison: in other words, to theorise about the relationships between the biographies of women prisoners, the discourses which constitute them and the politics which render them the 'female' subject (albeit denied) of penology.
>
> (1983a: 3)

Carlen's inquiry into invisible women prisoners very quickly establishes the pertinence of her initially somewhat surprising question: 'Is the modern prison necessarily about crime and punishment at all?' (1983a: 4). Having determined that, at the time of her study (1979–80), most Scottish women under sentence had been charged with very minor offences – approximately half were convicted for non-payment of fines, a third were convicted for breach of the peace, and another third were convicted for minor property crimes – Carlen sets sail on a different course, insisting that the denied meanings of women's imprisonment in Scotland are to be found neither within the walls of Cornton Vale nor within the official crime statistics. Rather, they are to be located

> within discursive forms and practices which, conventionally, are considered to be quite unrelated to penology – within, for example, the conventions of the family and the kirk; within traditional forms of public conviviality and ethics of domesticity and masculinity; within some peculiar absences in Scottish social work practice; within the ideological practices of contempt psychiatry; and within some over-determined presences (e.g. alcohol, unemployment, poverty) within Scottish culture and society.
>
> (1983a: 15)

Much of the book is concerned with tracing the impact of these over-determined presences on the lives of the women prisoners and demonstrating that the Scottish female offenders most likely to be imprisoned are those who have 'stepped outwith domestic discipline' (1983a: 16). Carlen's appropriation of this Scottish word, 'outwith', helps capture the outsider, marginal status of women prisoners inasmuch as its more subtle meaning of 'beyond (out) but not lacking (with)' helps to convey what she calls 'the contradictory states of consciousness engendered by the competing definitions of women' (1983a: 233). Applying this idea to her groups of Scottish women prisoners, she argues that:

> offending women are seen as being outwith family, sociability, femininity and adulthood. Although in penal discourse they are often seen as being outwith 'real' criminality too, they are also: rejected by hospital alcohol units as being outwith motivation; rejected by social workers as being outwith reform and beyond help; and rejected by psychiatrists as being outwith treatment and beyond cure.
>
> (1983a: 155)

In this way, Carlen captures some of the key over-determining processes which propel some women into the prison system. In a most helpful way, too, she notes that women's imprisonment in Scotland is imprisonment not only 'in the general sense in that it has all the repressive organisational features common to men's prisons'; it is also a form of imprisonment specific to women inasmuch as family life and social isolation, 'two modes for controlling many Scottish women outside prison', are also 'incorporated into the prison regime to produce a very fine disciplinary web which denies women both personality and full adult status' (1983a: 16). While this is very reminiscent of themes from *Discipline and Punish*, Carlen does not explicitly acknowledge Foucault's influence on her theoretical framework.[4] Nevertheless, her approach could fairly be described as Foucauldian, especially in those sections where she describes disciplinary regimes within and without the prison. But however one characterises Carlen's approach, it is certainly very useful for understanding the specific ways in which penal and non-penal control mechanisms intersect in the lives of Scottish women prisoners who, as she argues, suffer the multiple burdens of being constructed as 'both within and without sociability, femininity and adulthood; and then defined out of existence as being beyond care, cure and recognition'. But, importantly, she notes that this situation is not specific to Scotland: invisibility as well as training for domesticity and motherhood have always been dominant features of women's prison regimes in Great Britain and the United States (1983a: 17–19).

Carlen's elucidation of the specific elements in Scottish culture which contribute to what she calls the 'non-penal disciplining of women' (1983a: 33) – notably domestic responsibilities in slum housing and men's violence in the home – is one of the strongest sections of the book. Most importantly, it opens up a much more fruitful approach to the question of women's imprisonment. As Carlen explains, the social situation of working-class women is a complex one. For example, 'the non-penal and informal disciplining of women does not usually take the form of extreme physical violence'. Nevertheless, women prisoners who had been or still were in relationships with men were 'controlled and increasingly isolated in a multitude of non-violent ways' which related to ideologies about women's place in the family (44). As for the penal control of women, this should be seen as

> a very specific form of social control especially tailored for the disciplining of women. For the majority of these imprisoned women have not merely broken the law. As women, mothers and wives they have, also, somehow stepped out of place.
>
> (1983a: 59)

Noting discriminatory sentencing practices which impact disproportionately on these women who have stepped out of place, Carlen moves on to examine the specific prison regime imposed on women in Cornton Vale. Here the training programme emphasising family and the home and the organisation of the blocks into 'family' units comprised of seven women are singled out for special criticism. Prison administrators would do well to consider Carlen's critique as it demonstrates convincingly that unit management 'results in women prisoners being rigidly disciplined in a way that further increases their isolation and dependency' (1983a: 73).[5]

As Carlen makes clear, women's imprisonment, at least in Scotland,

> is imprisonment in the general sense that it has all the repressive organ-
> isational features common to men's prisons; at the same time, it is a
> form of imprisonment specific to women in that it has repressive
> features not to be found in men's prisons.

(1983a: 76)

Crucially too, she demonstrates that these specific repressive features centre on family structure: 'the woman's place in the family is constitutive of, and conditions, the meanings of her imprisonment from the sentencing stage onwards'. Whether the woman prisoner has family or not, 'there is no judg-mental space where she, the crime and the punishment can be constituted as being family-immune'. Moreover, inasmuch as she is imprisoned 'for her own good', the prison becomes 'home'. In this way, the discourses of family life are incorporated into the state's penal institutions for women (86).

It is one of the strengths of Carlen's study that she is able to theorise the ways in which 'definitions of legitimate womanhood' saturate this women's prison and at the same time demonstrate how imprisoned women are deconstructed and reconstructed within penal discourses and practices 'to the point of debilitation'. Such is the fate of women prisoners who are 'contradictorily defined as being: both within and without sociability; both within and without femininity; and . . . both within and without adulthood'. This is especially the case for short-term prisoners, for whom the disci-plinary organisation of Cornton Vale was devised. Carlen's evidence suggests that these prisoners receive 'an even stricter and more coercive surveillance than do their counterparts in men's prisons'. This control is enhanced by the family unit system which allows for a rigid surveillance in which their every move is monitored. As Carlen starkly reminds us, this form of prison discipline ensures that the women are 'mentally and emotionally straitjacketed into the same debilitating tension and isolation which they have already experienced in nuclear family situations outside the prison' (1983a: 90–108). Overall, she found that

> the general features of the hierarchical discipline combine with the
> domestic work programme, with the denial to prisoners of sociability
> and adult womanhood and with the organisation of the women into
> small family units, to ensure a mental and bodily surveillance which
> denudes the prisoners' daily life of all dignity and independence.

(1983a: 111)

However, while it is well to be reminded that women are disciplined in constricting gender-specific ways, Carlen falls into the trap of contrasting the realm of surveillance which is the women's prison with a supposedly mutually supportive counter-culture in male prisons which mitigates against a close surveillance. While women prisoners are regulated right down to the last details of their 'self-presentation' (1983a: 113), it does not follow that they cannot, or do not, form resistant networks. Equally, the notion of a male prison 'counter-culture' elides the realities of brutality and self-destructiveness within the men's prison system. By contrast, a strength of Carlen's study is her analysis of the figure of the 'disordered' or emotionally disturbed woman prisoner. Drawing on Foucault's work on the history of the fusion of medical and penal interventions in nineteenth-century Western control systems, she notes that, at any one time, about two-thirds of the women in Cornton Vale are likely to be 'disordered offenders' with a history of mental illness (1983a: 196–7). Her incisive critique of the application of the elusive label 'personality disorder' to women offenders contributes to the clarification of the contradictory situation of women in prison:

> the women are physically located in the prison on the grounds that they are physically (and permanently) located within a psychiatric category whose pathology is always already denied. So, being seen as neither wholly mad nor wholly bad, they are treated to a disciplinary regime where they are actually infantilised at the same time as attempts are made to make them feel guilty about their double, triple, quadruple or even quintuple refusal of family, work, gender, health and reason.
>
> (1983a: 209)

In conclusion, Carlen achieves her main aim, which was to show that

> the dominant meaning of women's imprisonment in Scotland is that it is imprisonment denied: it is denied that the women's prison is a 'real prison', it is denied that the prisoners are 'real women'.
>
> (1983a: 211)

It remains only to draw out the implications of her research for penal politics. In brief, these are that a policy of shorter sentences will only be just if most present categories of short-term prisoners, especially persistent petty women offenders, are removed from prison; that imprisonment be reserved for the gravest offences, and that the small unit system be abandoned. Finally, Carlen concludes by agreeing with Rusche and Kirchheimer, Foucault and the other critics that prisons are 'used as much for storing away those deemed to be socially useless' as for punishing the deserving and dangerous or protecting society. It follows that 'the question "what are prisons for?" must be continually posed' (218). So must the more specific question – why, in the face of the huge costs involved, do we continue to imprison women charged with minor offences? The reasons, as Carlen demonstrates here, are complex, and, significantly, they are 'only obliquely connected with the punishment of crime' (115).

Carlen's 1983 study of Cornton Vale has warranted a close analysis because it remains an important role model of transgressive research on women's imprisonment – research which breaks out from the restrictions of conventional modes of analysis – and also because of all the insights it provides into a specific penal regime. Her later study, *Women, Crime and Poverty* (1988), an ethnographic analysis of women's lawbreaking and criminalisation which draws attention to the changing circumstances of women's imprisonment in the late 1980s, may be dealt with more briefly. Her main concern in this book is with formulating policy recommendations for keeping women out of prison. As she says, women may be only 3 per cent of the British prison population, but there is still 'grave cause for concern about women's imprisonment' because the proportionate use of imprisonment for women more than doubled in the United Kingdom in the 1980s. Further, women were being sent to prison for less serious offences than men (Carlen 1988: 4). Importantly, Carlen broadens the basis of the study to show how 'class-biased and racist inequities in the administration of welfare and criminal law are intertwined with discriminatory typifications of gender-competence' (1988: 74). She then proceeds to highlight major factors in the criminalisation of women – poverty, racism, being placed in care, drug addiction and the discrimination which flows from 'a judicial logic shaped by outdated typifications of both femininity and women's proper place in an idealised nuclear family' (1988: 151). She also draws out the significant policy implications of the new research, including the need to sensitise court personnel to the stereotyping that diverts attention from 'contemporary women's actual gender problems', and the need for a 'radical rethinking of the concept of culpability in terms of what a reasonable woman (often with prior experience of her relative power-lessness in face of male violence) might be justified in doing in certain circumstances' (1988: 152).

In *Women, Crime and Poverty* Carlen endorses what are now long-standing feminist proposals for reducing women's imprisonment: that women should not be imprisoned for non-violent offences or for non-payment of fines; that only exceptionally should they be remanded in prison before trial, and that community-based programmes be expanded to meet the special needs of young women at risk of state incarceration. As Carlen notes, 'all these proposals have been made before': consequently it is high time that legislative changes were made to 'effect a more rational and coherent system of sentencing' which will impact progressively on women (Carlen 1988: 157). Next, she outlines 'fundamental structural and ideological changes' which need to be made if fewer women 'are to be caught up in criminal careers'. These include changes in policies related to housing, social security, taxation, wage and pension structures, working conditions and community child care, all of which are designed to give women in poverty and with criminal convictions 'a chance of surviving without resorting to crime again.' Finally, she suggests that we need to develop 'more sophisticated models of culpability, responsibility and accountability' which can take account of women's social disadvantages. Otherwise, as Carlen says, 'in the future many more young women will be sentenced to lives of poverty', and 'many more will be outlawed by careers in crime' (Carlen 1988: 161–3).

Pat Carlen then, provides several insights into how research and political agendas are inextricably connected. Most important, she demonstrates how to explore the ways in which women's imprisonment relates to gender relations outside the criminal justice system, but without losing sight of imprisoned women. In a most useful way, her work has informed progressive research on women's imprisonment elsewhere. For example, critical analysts of prisons in the state of New South Wales in Australia have acknowledged Carlen's work in their recognition that research and political strategies centred on women's prisons have to address the diverse field of institutions and practices – refuges, domestic violence, welfare provision and housing – but somehow without consigning women in prison to invisibility again (Brown, Kramer and Quinn 1988; Brown 1989). Yet notwithstanding the importance of her work for transforming the analytical field of penality, Carlen omits to consider the centrality of an historical perspective to a critical understanding of the imprisonment of women. The question we need to address is the one raised in chapter 2: namely, how will looking at gender differentiation in the field of penality challenge the findings of the male-focused revisionist histories which emerged in the 1980s? Here recent North American studies of women's prisons provide some useful research models.

REVISIONIST HISTORIES OF WOMEN'S IMPRISONMENT

To date, relatively few historians have attempted to redress the gender imbalance which remained after 'the new social histories' of the 1970s revised the story of nineteenth- and early twentieth-century prisons systems in the Western world. But over the last decade some brave souls, notably Estelle Freedman, Nicole Rafter, Patricia O'Brien and Dobash, Dobash and Guttridge, have taken up the challenge of providing a fully 'social' or revisionist punishment history, one which includes women. At a general level, these new revisionists have sought to demonstrate how women's prisons must be understood within the different context of women's historical experience and how the unique origins and functions of women's prisons raise important questions about the received history of 'the' prison system. More specifically, they have begun the important process of closely examining historical records which provide evidence of the singular experiences of women under particular penal regimes in the United States, France and Great Britain. Inasmuch as their work has been instrumental in reconstructing the historical realities of women's imprisonment in that country, their key findings should be noted.

Freedman: *Their Sisters' Keepers*

For Freedman, women prison reformers – 'their Sisters' Keepers' – provide the focus for a study of women's prison reform in the United States between 1830 and 1930, and women's history, rather than the history of prisons, provides the 'central context' (Freedman 1981: 1–2). Freedman maintains that, in order to understand why reformers came to view women prisoners as a special group, we need to study women's place in nineteenth-century prisons. Finding that very few women entered the early North American prisons either as inmates or keepers, she explains that women 'were not at first considered a significant part of America's dangerous classes'. Further, she suggested that this 'initial infrequency of women's incarceration' could be explained in terms of 'their different historical relationship to institutions of social control' such as the family and church.

> Because women's behaviour was more closely regulated by these private institutions, they were less likely to become subjects of new public agencies of punishment, at least for the reasons that men were.
>
> (1981: 10)

In this way, Freedman's study is immediately tied to the question of women's crime patterns – patterns which changed over the nineteenth century to reflect rising conviction rates for property and public order offences. Returning to the question of penality, she claims that women who served time in penal institutions between 1820 and 1870 were not subject to the same prison regimes as male inmates. The men experienced isolation, silence and hard labour, but the dearth of accommodation for women inmates 'made isolation and silence impossible for them, and productive labor was not considered an important part of their routine'. However, the neglect of women prisoners was 'rarely benevolent'. On the contrary, 'a pattern of overcrowding, harsh treatment, and sexual abuse recurred' throughout the nineteenth-century women's prison system (1981: 11–15).

Freedman's analysis then turns to the involvement of middle-class women in prison reform in the post Civil War era. She focuses on the establishment after 1870 of separate women's prisons – the women's reformatories – the ideologies and penal practices of the reformers and the inmates themselves. She found that over time these 'feminine institutions' came to resemble traditional prisons. While they remained unique in the domestic content of their retraining programmes, women's reformatories came to rely increasingly on their control functions, creating a 'tension between domesticity and discipline' which pervaded the system (90). Freedman finds a wealth of evidence pertaining to the retraining programmes and goals of 'womanhood', but far less information about the effects of the reformatory methods on prisoners. Noting that the 'most difficult problem in prison history is reconstructing the inmate experience', she discovers very few incidents of resistance or rebellion: the bulk of the evidence suggests that 'most inmates complied with official routines'. As for the retraining programmes, they had a mixed success – the tension between teaching traditional feminine ideals of purity and submissiveness and training women to be self-sufficient was a large part of the problem (1981: 100–6).

Next, Freedman focuses on the 'new criminology' of women developed by progressive reformers between 1900 and 1920. This criminology was, she argues, partly a response to the movement known as the 'new penology' developed by male and female reformers seeking new methods to replace those used in discredited nineteenth-century prisons. Informing their ideas were new scientific investigations of the causes of crime. Freedman argues that despite the popularity of biological determinism and hereditarian theories, women researchers and reformers 'often remained more suspicious' of these theories and instead made a major contribution to the development of environmental or social and economic explanations of women's crime (1981: 109–11). In the process, she provides a rare glimpse of an important though under-researched aspect of penal research undertaken by women social scientists in the early decades of the twentieth century – research which contributed to the development of a more progressive sociological criminology. Freedman concludes her account in the 1930s, the end of the progressive era, by which time 'women's prisons were becoming a standard feature of the American criminal justice system' (1981: 143). In her assessment, the reform movement was largely a failure inasmuch as after the 1920s the separate prisons were now run by women who lacked the critical approach to men's prisons taken by earlier reformers. Moreover, these prisons no longer existed to serve women. Rather, they supported the male-dominated system and adopted its values. Thus the fate of the women's prison movement, in Freedman's reading, was to testify to the capacity of American institutions to 'accommodate reform for conservative ends'. The story ends where it began: with women's prison reformers, their legacy and the need for ongoing scrutiny of the women's prison system today (1981: 151–7).

Rafter's *Partial Justice*

In contrast to Freedman's focus on reformers, Nicole Rafter's more ambitious goal was to deal with 'an entire institutional system for women' in the United States and, in particular, with the intersections between gender, race and class (Rafter 1990: xiv). Her main concern was to correct the 'skewed picture' of the history of incarceration which emerges if we fail to notice that women as well as men inhabited the nineteenth-century penitentiaries. As she points out in *Partial Justice: Women in State Prisons, 1800-1935* (1985a), a distorted picture emerges from traditional approaches as well as from the 'new' revisionist male-focused prison histories of the 1970s – histories which continue to 'limit our access to a significant chapter in the history of women' (Rafter 1985a: xiii). Rafter thus aims to set the record straight by considering the history of the imprisonment of women in the United States from an explicitly feminist and socialist perspective. Her main points are as follows. First, although it has been long established that the reformatories established between 1870 and 1930 played a crucial role in the development of the North American women's prison system, this is only a partial picture. The 'custodial' model – which was more 'masculine' because it resembled maximum security prisons for men -- was the first of the two styles of women's prisons to emerge, and was more widely adopted in North America than the reformatory. Thus, the almost exclusive focus of traditional studies on reformatories has produced a distorted picture of the women's prison system which obscures our understanding of the origins of the problems faced by that system today. Most importantly, this focus has blinded us to the development of a 'bifurcated' women's prison system in which minor offenders, who were overwhelmingly white, were placed in reformatory institutions while felons, who were disproportionately black women, were sent to custodial institutions (Rafter 1982; 1985a). Moreover, while Rafter argues that white women were subjected to especially repressive forms of treatment in the reformatories, she notes that black women were over-represented in the custodial prisons throughout the period under review, 1865 to 1935. Surveying the evidence pertaining to regional variations in sentencing patterns, she concludes that nearly every aspect of treatment within the women's prison system was 'shaped by attitudes that devalued blacks' (1985a: 154–5). At the same time, Rafter also argues that the establishment of the women's reformatory after 1870 was a 'major development in prison history' because this new model 'broke radically with male-orientated prison traditions, creating a set of feminised penal practices' and extending state control over a population of young, mainly white, working-class women convicted of 'minor sex-related offences' (1985a: 288–90).

Consistent with a socialist–feminist approach, Rafter situates her study of the women's reformatory movement in the context of a variety of late nineteenth- and early twentieth-century social changes which have been associated with immigration, urbanisation, the development of capitalism and with changes in gender roles and the widening of class divisions in the United States. As well, she situates her prison history within the broader movement to establish institutions for 'the dependent, defective and delinquent classes'. Changes in the handling of juvenile offenders, especially girls, provided models for the new reformatory type of prison for adult women, and the so-called social feminist and social purity movements were, she claims, 'as influential as institutional developments on the evolution of women's reformatories'. It is here, in the post Civil War movement of middle-class women into public affairs concerning women and children, that class and gender factors intersect in Rafter's analysis (1983: 305–6). Writing as she does from a 'social control' perspective, Rafter questions Freedman's emphasis on sisterliness between reformers and prisoners. While Freedman emphasises the humanitarianism of the reformers, Rafter claims that the key factors are 'the solidification of gender roles' in nineteenth-century North America, as well as 'the hardening of division between social classes'. As she sees it, these factors met head on in the bodies of the working-class offender and the middle-class reformer.

> Two groups of women – the working-class offenders and the middle-class reformers – met, so to speak, at the gate of the women's reformatory. The struggle between them was economically functional in some ways to the reformers: it helped maintain a pool of cheap domestic labour for women like themselves, and, by keeping women in the surplus labour force, it undergirded the economic system to which they owed their privileged position. But such purely economic explanations do not account adequately for the dedication with which the reformers went about their tasks of rescue and reform. The struggle also involved the definition of gender. Reformers hoped to recast offenders in their own image, to have them embrace the values . . . of the lady.
>
> (1985a: 175)

Moreover, Rafter argues that this control strategy worked: the working-class offenders 'were, in fact, reformed'. More broadly, she argues that the women's reformatory movement was an attempt to 'increase middle-class control over white working-class women' rather than a humanitarian effort, as Freedman's interpretation had suggested (1990: xiii). To support her case, Rafter provides a close analysis – one informed by feminist theorists who have explored 'the ways in which social controls are exercised on women *as women*' – of the 'techniques of social control' deployed in the women's reformatory at Albion, New York (1985a: 158; her emphasis).

Rafter has contributed in significant ways to the process of producing the histories of women's imprisonment which she predicted would be written over the decade spanning 1980 to 1990. Indeed, it is instructive to note that in 1980 she anticipated that over the next decade feminist scholars would establish 'an empirical foundation for theory about the punishment of women'. Furthermore, she hoped that this new research would 'clarify the role played by female institutions' in the development of the whole prison system and, in the process, 'force us to rethink some of our assumptions about the incarceration process' (Rafter 1980: 263, 267). While research on women's prison history has not expanded as rapidly as Rafter may have hoped, she herself has continued to contribute to the project. Her revised edition of *Partial Justice*, which extends the analysis beyond 1935 to the late 1980s, continues the challenge to hegemonic masculinist accounts of the prison system. For example, she singles out the 'gender bias' of David Rothman's revisionist social history of changing penal patterns, a bias which she argues leads him to misread 'the evolution of state control' in the early twentieth century. Specifically, she claims that his thesis about the significance of a movement for alternatives to incarceration in the early twentieth century is contradicted by 'the reality' that the women's prison system greatly expanded during the progressive period, a time in which institutions for women were established 'at a faster rate than in any period until the 1970s' (1990: xiii). In the light of such findings about 'the reality' of penal changes taking place in women's prisons, it would seem that 'social' historians like Rothman have two choices: either they have to specify that their accounts are limited to changes taking place in men's prisons, or they will have to revise substantially their historical explanations and theories about supposedly universal, non-gendered penal transformations.

Several observations are salient here. On the positive side, Rafter does provide a lot of the goods. Most important, she forces us to revise the revisionists' account of the history of imprisonment. For while she concedes to the revisionists that the emergence of the penitentiary was indeed 'one of the most dramatic innovations in the history of punishment', she insists that we note that it was inhabited by women as well as men (Rafter 1985a: 3). She also forces us to rethink periodisation. For example, the 1870s, a time when the penal treatment of women began to undergo a 'revolutionary change' by breaking with custodialism to produce a unique model of prison – the reformatory – must now loom large in any history of women's imprisonment, at least in the United States. Again, the year 1933, when the two types of women's prison merged on one site, at least in New York, provides us with a date for the end of the bifurcated system and the beginning of the process which produced the 'mixed code of custodialism and nurturance' which is the women's prison system today (Rafter 1983: 255–6).

Rafter's work on the North American women's prison system thus provides some useful points for comparison with historical research on women's imprisonment elsewhere, some of which have already been taken up by critical scholars elsewhere, as we will see. For now, we need to note the shortcomings of Rafter's approach. First, she fails to provide methodological directives beyond a comparative analysis which privileges men and their prisons. Rafter's modus operandi is to compare historical differences between the incarceration of men and women – a comparative project which for her '*necessarily* starts with prisons that mainly held men' (Rafter 1990: xxv, emphasis added). In this paradigm, men and male prisons necessarily remain the norms from which women and women's prisons deviate. Second, the 'theory' about the punishment of women which was supposed to materialise from Rafter's study leaves something to be desired. Her theoretical conclusions appear to be that changes in gender roles and class relationships influenced the women's reformatory movement which, interestingly, is presented as a struggle between two groups of women. On one side are middle-class women, who needed to maintain a cheap pool of domestic labour; on the other side are working-class women who needed to be taught 'a new concept of womanhood' (1985a: 175). Strangely, neither working-class women nor middle-class men have agency here. Surely this is a double falsification of women's relative power: on the one hand, working-class women resisted the imposition of middle-class norms of womanhood; on the other hand, middle-class women did not control the domestic labour market. Rafter's only other theoretical conclusion appears to be that we should pay attention to 'variations' within the prison system – variations such as 'period, region and inmates' sex, race and age' (1985a: 180). Thus, women finally emerge from this feminist and socialist prison history as a 'variation': they are not a subject in their own right.

There are then, limits to the transformative power of this kind of feminist prison history. By including women, Rafter has revised the masculinist, revisionist picture of the evolution of the prison system. But adding women to revisionist prison history – women, moreover, who are represented as struggling primarily against each other – does not fundamentally challenge the androcentric nature of the revisionist theoretical framework. It does not disturb the newly laid down 'master patterns' of nineteenth-century penality in Western Europe. Nor does Rafter's feminist history accomplish a paradigm shift such as that achieved by the revisionists themselves when they set about exposing traditional prison history as hopelessly teleologically biased and thus, effectively, 'ahistorical history' (Cohen and Scull 1983; Mayer 1983: 22). Furthermore, her either-or model of historical explanation, which assumes that the prison reform movement was either humanitarian or control orientated, sets up a false binary opposition which fails to convey the complexity of discursive and non-discursive penal practices in nineteenth-century North America. Ultimately, Rafter's women's prison history takes the form of an auxiliary history – a 'variation' on the male-focused historiography of the masculinist revisionists. The methodological implications are limited to the application of a revised ('add-in-women') revisionist framework to any particular set of historical records pertaining to imprisonment. In effect, this amounts to a call for a gender-sensitive revisionist prison history rather than a transformation of the masculinist framework of the new social history. Women prisoners who lived and died under past penal regimes surely deserve more.

TOWARDS A FOUCAULDIAN HISTORY OF WOMEN'S IMPRISONMENT

Dobash, Dobash and Gutteridge

For all its methodological limitations, Rafter's work stands out as an important, and still rare, feminist foray into research on the history of women's imprisonment. As such, it provides a useful research model for other work in this field. For example, in the briefly-titled *The Imprisonment of Women* (1986), which is in fact a history of women's imprisonment in Great Britain, Dobash, Dobash and Gutteridge have built on Rafter's, and also Estelle Freedman's, work in order to draw a comparative picture of conditions in the two countries. This British study warrants a close analysis, not simply because of the points of comparison made with the North American penal establishments for women but, more crucially, because it offers the beginnings of a comparative analytical and theoretical framework focusing on women in prison. Furthermore, this study not only commences the important process of drawing together the different threads of critical approaches to women's imprisonment, its authors go so far as to pay a debt to Foucault for the 'many theoretical ideas' they got from his work and, interestingly, also from discussions with him (1986: vii). The stage is thus set for the writing of a genealogy of women's imprisonment, blessed by the master theorist of penality himself. At the very least, *The*

Imprisonment of Women holds out the promise of a theoretical engagement with the issues which have concerned those critical but non-feminist analysts of men's prisons who paved the way for the establishment of a 'social' analysis of penality.

Dobash, Dobash and Guttridge commence with an informative overview of the state of research in the field at the time of writing The Imprisonment of Women. They note that, until the early 1980s, most research on women's experience of confinement was carried out in North America. They note too that much of this research was conducted in the 1960s and took the form of studies of prisoners' coping mechanisms. The dominant and still commonplace view was that men cope in prison by adopting 'a virulent anti-social, anti-staff subculture' which 'was seen as an impediment to rehabilitation'. Similar assumptions, 'although often not articulated, underpinned the research on women in prison'. Women prisoners, according to the received accounts, may not have developed 'virulent anti-staff norms' like the men, but they did establish various forms of family and 'homosexual' relationships as coping mechanisms. Rose Giallombardo's now classic *Society of Women: A Study of a Women's Prison* (1966) typifies this approach, focusing as it did on the ways in which women adapted to life in a North American prison. Dobash, Dobash and Guttridge surmise that this focus in the North American studies on the sexual orientations of women prisoners may have reflected 'prevalent theories about women's crime which stressed its bio-psychological and sexual basis'. But whatever the explanation, the important point to note is that subsequent research has focused on the sexual and familial behavioural patterns amongst women prisoners 'to the neglect of a great many issues about the prison itself, its regimes, policies, practices and orientations to those confined'. Furthermore, as late as the 1970s, British research on women in prison was 'dominated by bio-psychological perspectives about women and girls' who were 'more likely than male prisoners to be seen as low in intelligence, maladjusted, emotionally disturbed and in need of psychological and psychiatric intervention' (1986: 5–6).

Dobash, Dobash and Guttridge acknowledge that recent critical research on the imprisonment of women in Britain, such as that of Pat Carlen, has moved away from this preoccupation with the bio-psychological nature of women in confinement. But they claim that the biographical mode of analysis which Carlen has deployed necessitates a concentration on the nature of individual prison experiences which in turn entails a continual neglect of 'wider' but unspecified issues. As Carlen is very much concerned with a range of wider penal issues, especially policy issues, she would have good cause to dispute this criticism. But rather than enter into the debate, let us keep the focus on *The Imprisonment of Women*, which moves on to critique the conventional account of the creation of the nineteenth-century prison as 'an exceptional, unique and progressive development'. Here Ann Smith's account of the incarceration of women (1962) as a history of 'steady progress reaching its pinnacle in the thera-peutic ideals of the present era' provides the perfect example of the kind of conventional, administrative history which Dobash, Dobash and Guttridge intend to replace with a fully-informed critical approach. This desire to write a new kind of women's prison history leads inexorably to an appre-ciation of the work of feminist historians and other critical scholars who moved beyond the 'conventional, reductionist and individual approaches' of 'conventional histories emphasising administration and progressive development'. Rusche and Kirchheimer and the revisionist historians of the 1970s are mentioned, but it is Foucault's analysis of the penitentiary as a new strategy of power, 'the apex of the carceral society', which is presented as the most significant of the new critical paradigms (1986: 7–8). However, Foucault, along with the other revisionist masculinist historians, is criticised for failing to consider that 'patriarchal and gender-based assumptions' might have played a role in the development of the prison. Questions omitted in conventional social histories need to be asked:

> Were women sent to prison during the nineteenth century also seen as potential labour power to be transformed into disciplined workers, or did other sorts of assumptions dictate penal responses? If patriarchal assumptions were apparent, did they result in the creation of unique institutions for the punishment and reform of women and did prisons for women become the sites for the generation of new theories of the criminality of women?
>
> (1986: 9)

Here Freedman's and Rafter's prison studies are held up as models of the kind of enquiry into the impact of patriarchal assumptions on the develop-ment of forms of confinement for women in the nineteenth and twentieth centuries. Freedman may have overstated the case for the supposedly 'sisterly' relationship between prison staff and prisoner, but Rafter is seen to have demonstrated convincingly that the degrading penal regimes suffered by black and poor white women in the prisons and jails were not informed by the benevolent, sisterly and therapeutic ideals of the reforma-tories in late nineteenth-century North America. Dobash, Dobash and Guttridge point out that in Great Britain, on the other hand, there has been no comparable work on what they call the 'critical history of women in prison'. Further, they claim that the problem created by the dearth of a critical British historical analysis has been compounded by a failure to investigate conditions inside contemporary British prisons for women.

They therefore set out to provide a critical account of past and present penal regimes for women in Britain, paying particular attention to

> how class and gender assumptions have shaped the imprisonment of women over time; the operation of regimes of punishment and discipline; the content of authoritative, official discourses on the criminality and imprisonment of women, and the way official conceptions and government policies have been translated into prison practices.
>
> (1986: 10–11)

Elaborating on their project, Dobash, Dobash and Guttridge insist that the study of women's imprisonment must be situated 'in the overall context of women in society and relative to the criminality of women'. Indeed, they hope to 'contribute to an understanding of the criminality of women' by placing it in a changing socioeconomic context. Evidently then, there will be no attempt here to break the bond between crime and punishment, an analytical move which critical analysts have been calling for since Rusche and Kirchheimer; on the contrary, changing patterns of criminality are seen to be inextricably connected to the question of punishment in *The Imprisonment of Women*. Importantly too, the authors claim a commitment to examining the ways in which women have reacted to and struggled against past and present penal regimes, thereby promising to tell a story neglected by administrative and social histories alike – the story of the prison from the bottom up. Interestingly, they claim to have 'good historical evidence' of the ways in which women struggled against 'the new technology of imprisonment'. Finally, their aim is to provide a historical background for understanding current penal developments, including especially the impact of medical discourses on penal policies for women. To that end, the historical analysis is to be supplemented with a field-work study at the Scottish women's prison, Cornton Vale (1986: 11).

So much for the proposed project of Dobash, Dobash and Guttridge. I have considered it at some length because it affords such a wide-ranging overview of old and relatively new research directions on the imprisonment of women. Turning to their own research, we find that most of their 'good historical evidence' has been drawn from the secondary literature and amounts to little more than a summary of previous research findings. They begin with pre-industrial punishments for women, noting that the fourteenth- to seventeenth-century witchcraft executions 'represented only the most dramatic of a number of unique offences and punishments for which women were the primary targets' and that community chastisements of women were 'likely to be more physical, direct and serious' than those directed at men. In good Foucauldian style, they note that these physical and symbolic punishments, such as the ducking and bridling of women, focused on the body, that indeed the body was the 'point for the manifestation of power'. Moreover, they highlight other important research findings which do not figure in masculinist accounts of the origins of the prison. For example, long-term confinement in convents, which were effectively prisons for the many involuntary entrants, pre-dated by centuries the development of systematic confinement in the late 1500s and early 1600s; the Dutch established the first distinct penal establishment for women in 1597, and the mid-seventeenth-century *Spinhuis*, 'probably the first truly purpose-built penal institution for women', was the precursor of penal developments in nineteenth-century Europe (1986: 20–4).

These points have been made before, as have those about economic changes in the eighteenth century and the coming of the penitentiary in the nineteenth century. Points about the role of reformers have been well rehearsed before too, although the authors offer an interesting interpretation of Elizabeth Fry's work, particularly her later penal work as involving 'new forms of discipline and technologies of correction'. They also trace the prison careers of women sentenced to penal servitude in British penitentiaries, commenting that the Penal Servitude Acts of the 1850s 'marked the beginning of distinct official differences in the treatment of women offenders' who were 'subjected to a tighter regime' than male inmates. Crucially, and this is a point to which we will return, they argue that women were 'more closely confined in this new regime created specifically for them'. Here then, is important evidence that criminalised women, ignored in masculinist accounts of penality, may have had a closer association with the development of the disciplinary regimes of the nineteenth century than male prisoners. For while these regimes were in some ways similar for men and women, the evidence suggests strongly that surveillance and regulation were 'always closer and more omnipresent than that usually directed at men' (1986: 51–61).[6]

The section on penal regimes in Britain during the period from 1840 to 1870 – the age of the 'great confinement' – is one of the strongest in the book. Based on primary evidence, it focuses on the nature of the regimes for women in the new and reconstituted prisons and, to a much lesser extent, women's reactions to this confinement. Their claim that women were subjected to a tighter disciplinary regime is supported by evidence pertaining to the establishment by the 1860s of what they call a 'wide interlocking carceral network' of refuges, asylums, reformatories, shelters. While these institutions were 'not necessarily penal', women could be sent to them for an indeterminate period after they had completed their sentence in a convict prison such as Millbank or Brixton. Other institutions were created at this time to confine and train working-class women:

reformatories and refuges to save and reform young women and inter-mediate prisons for the reception of women released from convict prisons. As well, the ancient Magdalen Houses of asylum for prostitutes were resurrected in order to transform the nineteenth-century prostitute into 'a new reformed woman'. Clearly, all these institutions 'constituted signi-ficant developments in the extension of a carceral net of supervision and correction for women' (1986: 72–6). On the important question of women prisoners' reactions to the imposition of these disciplinary regimes, Dobash, Dobash and Guttridge repeat their claim that there are 'some good and surprising sources of information about women's responses to prison', notably official reports and, very occasionally, a first-hand account inform-ing us of the resistances and struggles of 'bold and strategic' women prisoners. But, in fact, they unearth very few episodes involving women in revolt or protest. What they do find is that, then as now, self-mutilation and other forms of self-destructive or inward-focused individual actions such as wrecking cells were more common responses by women to imprisonment (77–84). The point is not made clearly, but the evidence of contemporary observers suggests that the refractory actions of the women may have been shaped by gender-specific regimes which were more intolerably severe than those imposed on men. According to Mary Carpenter, who was active in the prison reform movement in the 1860s, there was a 'remarkable disparity in the punishments inflicted on the two sexes' in that the punish-ments of women were 'peculiarly severe' (86) and more frequent.

Dobash, Dobash and Guttridge do not make much of the evidence that there were 'seemingly greater infractions of the rules and more frequent punishments of women' beyond suggesting that:

> It is very likely that penal regimes for women were being enforced in a more rigorous manner than those established for men. . . . Minor infrac-tions by women would be less likely to be tolerated than those of males.
> (1986: 86–7)

Nor do they have much to say about penal technologies and punishments deployed in institutions for women beyond indicating that they were 'part of a wide-ranging, innovative attempt to manage the poor and the criminal'. As for penal arrangements for women in British prisons during the last four decades of the nineteenth century, this forty-year period is collapsed into a single paragraph on the ground that no significant changes took place at that time. Rather, the 'important developments involved consolidation of the position of the new penal professionals and promulgation of new theories about female criminality and imprisonment' (87–9). While they do not substantiate these claims, their chapter on the role of penal experts in women's prisons clearly establishes the part played by the medical profession in the 'creation and assessment of technologies of correction and punishment'. It also highlights the importance placed on examining women by the new medical bio-psychologists inasmuch as 'women in their role as mothers were seen as the biological and social source of degeneracy' (111). From this, it was a short step to the emergence between the late nineteenth century and the 1930s of 'a new orthodoxy' that the majority of women prisoners were emotionally disturbed or in need of treatment to a far greater degree than male prisoners. Once again, no detailed analysis of this development is thought to be required: we are simply informed that while psychiatrists and psychologists entered the women's prisons system from the 1930s, no new prisons or regimes were created strictly for women in the first half of the twentieth century. The establishment of unique penal institutions for women offenders based on bio-psychological and therapeutic perspectives did not occur until the 1970s with the building of the New Holloway prison in London and Cornton Vale in Scotland (122–3).

This point goes to the heart of the book's main concern: not merely to 'provide a background for understanding the development of the imprison-ment of women today' but, more particularly, to explore the relationship between historical patterns and contemporary forms of imprisonment. According to the authors, the most direct links between the past and the present are to be found in the impact of the ideologies of the medical profession in the late nineteenth and early twentieth centuries on Home Office policy on the imprisonment of women. The key aim of their research on the contemporary period is therefore to demonstrate how policy-makers have been 'heavily influenced by psychiatric conceptions of the criminality of women which underpinned the establishment of the therapeutic regimes' within the women's prison system. More specifically, the aims are to demonstrate how the therapeutic ideals have been translated into the organ-isation of prison regimes for women; to analyse how contemporary women's prisons 'are still basically geared to disciplining and punishing women, regardless of the rhetoric of rehabilitation', and to see how medical professionals have colluded with 'traditional penal demands to tighten regulation and surveillance within prison and to ensure that women are closely confined and heavily scrutinised' (11–12).

Broadly speaking, the book achieves these aims. It provides a con-vincing account that therapy was the 'dominant theme' and the 'central purpose' of both Holloway and Cornton Vale. On the basis of a prevailing assumption of the supposed psychiatric needs of women prisoners, 'all aspects' of these two regimes were co-opted 'under the rubric of treat-ment'. The penal implications are clear: 'anything done to women in prison may be defined as "therapy"' (126–30). After all, women have been put there 'for their own good.' Underlying the treatment rhetoric, however, is the hard reality that women are punished for disciplinary offences twice as often as men. Indeed, 'punishment' levels have risen in both women's prisons since 'treatment'-orientated regimes were introduced (147–8). Most problematic of all, the evidence suggests strongly that the therapeutic approach has expanded the disciplinary net 'by extending surveillance and control to even the most intimate and mundane aspects of daily life'. Dobash, Dobash and Guttridge conclude that assumptions about gender have been critical to the development and implementation of this especially oppressive therapeutic-orientated regime within the women's prison system. For while the therapeutic model has played only 'a minor role' in most men's prisons and the scrutiny of their behaviour under confinement is less exacting, the therapeutic regime has a special purchase in the women's prison – namely, to transform the deviating woman into a 'proper woman'. If the therapy fails, the women 'become subjected to the equally extensive system of discipline and punishment' (157–8).

Although not fully spelled out, the research implications of *The Imprisonment of Women* are clear: Foucauldian analysts interested in tracing the genealogy of disciplinary regimes would do well to focus their research on women's prisons. Similarly, Marxists and others committed to economistic accounts of the prison as a form of punishment connected to the emergence of capitalist social relations need to reflect on the fact that 'women do not figure' in critical accounts of penality 'either as prisoners or as ordinary members of society' (159). In particular, very little research has been done on work in women's prisons, even by recent critical scholars. For example, Pat Carlen did deal with work, education and training in her study of Cornton Vale, but she is taken to task for not seeing them as important elements in the prison's control system (160–2). Carlen's work aside, Dobash, Dobash and Guttridge complain that prison regimes for women have not been the focus of analysis, at least in the United Kingdom. Furthermore, because British researchers have been preoccupied with the individual characteristics of women prisoners rather than the social organ-isations of prisons, it has not been possible to make comparisons with studies indicating that mock family structures strengthen bonds of solidarity between women inmates in North American prisons. Their analysis of Cornton Vale, however, suggests that no such prison culture exists there and, more broadly, that

> it would take extraordinary strength to resist the degree of control, surveillance and manipulation directed at preventing the foundation of such bonds or at breaking them once formed.

(1986: 186)

Once again then, the themes of control, surveillance and manipulation come to the fore, and once again the impression is given that women prisoners are more closely controlled than men. Indeed, in this historical reconstruction, women have been 'more closely observed and controlled, more often punished, and punished for more trivial offences' than male prisoners from the time that separate women's prisons were established (207). The New Holloway and Cornton Vale may have been planned as mental hospitals, but

> in practice, they turned out to be just like prisons, orientated to surveillance, control and work but with an expanded vision of rehabilitation and reform meant to penetrate the emotions, psyche and personality through therapy. With this double form of control of both the body and the inner person, surveillance and control penetrated still deeper, and confinement for women became even closer.
>
> (1986: 208)

In short, the demands of discipline won out. The policy implications are clear:

> The whole question of the role of 'punishment' and the existence of punishment blocks in what were supposedly set up as therapeutic establishments, and their implications for women in prison . . . needs to be aired. No official policy was ever stated regarding discipline for Cornton Vale or Holloway.
>
> (1986: 210-11)

Another policy implication is that 'the virtual abolition of prison should seem an achievable goal' for this prison population (241). But this is to get ahead of the story. For now, all we need to note is the significance of *The Imprisonment of Women*. Most crucially, the research is placed within a theoretical context. The book not only provides a rare overview of the range of perspectives which have informed studies of women's imprisonment to date; it also makes an impressive attempt to construct a critical paradigm in which to comprehend penality in relation to women as well as men. In addition, it addresses key issues, notably the way 'gender assumptions' have saturated penal ideologies and given rise to policies based on myths of women offenders as medical cases requiring therapy. Moreover, the field work study of therapy as practised at Cornton Vale provides an added dimension to the historically-informed study of nineteenth-century British prisons for women. Considered together, these two studies establish a solid basis from which to make policy recommendations relating to penal regimes for women in the United Kingdom.

The Imprisonment of Women, then, has provided a firm foundation for the development of a critical consideration of penal practices within the women's prison system in Britain today.[7] More broadly, the analysis of the lasting legacy of nineteenth-century penal ideologies and regimes clearly demonstrates the significance of historical analysis for understanding contemporary Western prison systems. While there is a somewhat problematic hiatus in the analysis from the late nineteenth century to the 1970s – justified on the grounds that no new prison regimes were created for women in this period – the book does highlight important connections between the ideologies of the late nineteenth-century penal experts and the dominance of therapeutic regimes within women's prisons in the mid-1980s. And notwithstanding the fact that much of the historical analysis is based on secondary material, this still serves to underline a point made in an earlier Canadian study of women's imprisonment – namely, the political usefulness of an historical perspective for recognising stalemating tactics on the part of prison planners and administrators faced with prison reform movements bent on improving the situation of women prisoners (Berzins and Cooper 1982). Dobash, Dobash and Guttridge should also be commended for making the effort to write a Foucauldian 'history of the present' which includes penal regimes for women. Yet despite the attempt to situate the study within a Foucauldian framework, the master's influence does not extend beyond a recognition of the especially demanding nature of disciplinary regimes within the women's prison system. And while Dobash, Dobash and Guttridge criticise Foucault for overemphasising control at the expense of documenting instances of resistance, they themselves do not do much to rectify this imbalance between discipline and control, on the one hand, and resistance and struggle on the other. Consequently, the overwhelming impression left by the study is that of an oppressive surveillance which renders resistance impossible within the women's prison system in the United Kingdom. Furthermore, if the Foucauldian implications of their study are left undeveloped, feminist questions about research methodologies and the protocols to be adopted when analysing oppressed groups of women are not even raised.[8] *The Imprisonment of Women* may be feminist in the sense allowed by Pat Carlen – it is concerned with righting the wrongs done to women prisoners – but the analysis is untouched by recent feminist inquiries into questions about the politics of research on women and even more searching questions about the existence of 'women'. A feminist Foucauldian approach surely needs to take account of such methodological and postmodern problematics.

Women's imprisonment: respecifying 'the social' of social history

Much has been made of 'the social' in the revisionist histories of punishment and critical sociologies of penality over the last ten to fifteen years, but, as we saw in chapters 2 and 3, 'the social' of these studies leaves something to be desired. They almost always left out penal regimes imposed on women and, somewhat surprisingly given their commitment to providing more fully 'social' accounts, they had little to say about prisoners of either sex. We now know a great deal about the emergence of penal regimes in Western societies, but what about the people on the receiving end of all those repressive institutions which have attracted so much critical attention? Michelle Perrot was one of the first to notice the 'absence of the prisoners themselves' in accounts of nineteenth-century penal developments. We do not, she wrote, 'hear much from them' – they have 'disappeared from their own history, so that we must follow their traces in what is said about them' (Perrot 1978: 215). Perrot's observation about the silence imposed on prisoners in France could be extended to revisionist accounts of punishment systems in other Western countries, but as it happens, the most noted attempt to pursue this 'methodological concern' is O'Brien's history of prisons in nineteenth-century France. In *The Promise of Punishment* (1982), O'Brien argues that prisoners 'must be given their place in historical studies of inarticulate groups, along with women, children, workers and blacks' and she acknowledges the efforts of both Perrot and Ignatieff to 'put an end to the silence of the imprisoned, in particular through an examination of protests within prisons' (O'Brien 1982: 6–7). For his part, Ignatieff has returned the compliment, saying that O'Brien's text epitomised the new social history by shifting attention away from the administration of prisons to the prisoners themselves, 'to prisoners' tattoos, communication systems, contraband networks and covert sexual lives' – in short, to 'the living battles of the confined against their suffering' (Ignatieff 1983b: 168–9). In fact, it is far more accurate to say that O'Brien's efforts to flesh out the faceless, inarticulate mass of prison inmates in nineteenth-century France serve to highlight the poverty of the category of 'the social' in Ignatieff's and other self-professed 'social' histories of punishment.

Interestingly, O'Brien begins her revisionist history by singling out Foucault's work as having opened up an understanding of punishment as a complex social structure, even though she claims he was 'not a social historian at all'. She places *Discipline and Punish* at the centre of the debate over 'the role and meaning of the prison in modern society' (presumably, Western society). Evidently too, it was this text which alerted her to methodological issues. To understand the prison as a social institution we need first to examine 'how the prison operated and how it was organised'. Second, we need to place it in a broad time frame, 'extending the field of historical vision beyond the moment' – the 1840s in Western Europe – when the institution 'received its full institutional articulation'.

Third and crucially, we need to write prison history 'from the inside out, in the same way that crowds have been studied from the bottom up'. In a most relevant way, O'Brien explains why:

> prison populations continue to be discussed as undifferentiated, faceless masses. Incidents involving men, women and children are often cited interchangeably to exemplify *general* characteristics about the prison system rather than to highlight differences in response of particular prison populations. There is a significance to being a man, woman or child in prison . . . (her emphasis)

> (O'Brien 1982: 9)

We therefore need to determine who the prisoners were and how they reacted to the specific penal regime imposed on them. Only by examining the prison 'from the inside out' will we understand 'the place of the prison in the social system'. The objective, however, is not simply to write another history of the inarticulate, but rather to 'provide a missing element in connecting institutional change with the establishment of a new social order and stability' (1982: 7–9).

Thus, in a most original way, *The Promise of Punishment* sets out to explore that missing social element in the social histories of punishment of the 1970s – the specificity of being a man, woman or child in prison. Interpreting the prison as a 'social space' and subcultural adaptions of the different prison populations as 'a form of active participation' in the punishment process (1982: 10), O'Brien remains faithful to Foucault's injunction to see the prison not as 'an inert institution' but rather as 'an active field' (Foucault 1977a: 235). Her study encompasses changing penal forms in nineteenth-century France, but without focusing exclusively on the reformers and changing penal practices, nor on prison administrators. While the details need not detain us, it is relevant to note that when she turns to the still-novel question of men and women in prison, she discovers that, while women prisoners were always a minority in France, their numbers fluctuated dramatically. By the close of the nineteenth century they represented only 12 per cent of the total prison population, compared to 16–18 per cent twenty-five years earlier, and their numbers had been reduced to a third of their mid-century total, a development she attributes to the more lenient sentencing of women and a new emphasis on deinstitutionalised punishments in the second half of the nineteenth century, which led to an overall decline in both female and male prison populations. A similar fall in the number of women prisoners has been noted in other Western jurisdictions at that time, but O'Brien is exceptional in pausing to reflect on the impact of this decline on women's prisons. She argues that it had an especially strong impact on these institutions. By 1885 the number of central prisons for women was reduced from eleven to five and the new institutions had an enhanced capacity to 'categorise and differentiate' prisoners. For women prisoners this meant a particularly close surveillance, focusing on their morality and sexuality, which had effects qualitatively different from those on men. They were more frequently diagnosed as mad or depressed, just as they have been in late twentieth- century prisons. Still, O'Brien insists that despite differences in women's and men's prisons, 'we can speak of a single, centralised and highly homogenous prison regime that took shape in France before mid-century' (1982: 54–74).

But what of O'Brien's commitment to writing social history from the bottom up, from the perspective of the prisoners themselves? What about her self-imposed task of providing a fully social historical analysis of the prison – one which addresses what Ignatieff later came to call the 'true subject' of the social history of institutions, that of examining 'the historical relation between the inside and outside' and of throwing light on 'the exercise of power in society as a whole'? Once again, it is noteworthy that Ignatieff acknowledged the importance of Foucault's work in daring to study the prison and asylums 'not in and for themselves, but as sites' for the analysis of power relations in the wider society. The 'essential question', in his view, is to ask what part the institution plays in the 'reproduction of social order in the world beyond its walls' (1983b: 169). Unfortunately, O'Brien does not make much headway here: her account throws little light on the part played by the prison in the reproduction of gendered power relations in the wider society. But then her analytical framework cannot bear the weight of such a complex task, premised as it is on a highly problematic interpretation of social relations between women prisoners as being based predominantly on 'homosexual relations'. The problem is not only that the picture O'Brien draws is 'impressionistic', based as it is on the dubious evidence of letters purportedly written by women prisoners. More troubling still, while O'Brien questions the authenticity of these documents, she nevertheless sees them as providing a 'textured description of life in the prison' just as sociologists have found women's prison correspondence to be a rich source for understanding 'the nature and function of lesbianism in the prisons of our own society' (1982: 99–107). Here the objectifying, heterosexist gaze of the self-proclaimed gender-sensitive scholar appropriates the sexuality of lesbian women inside and outside the prison, translating it into functionalist terms. Such a reduc-tionist and essentialising approach is scarcely capable of providing a nuanced account of women's active resistance to penal repression, let alone of affording insights into the gendered order outside the prison walls. Thus, notwithstanding its methodological sensitivity to the question of 'the social' of social histories of punishment, *The Promise of Punishment* is not capable of delivering a viable picture of the historical relations between the 'society of women' inside and outside the walls.

The most recent contribution to the project of writing a history of the prison which includes women prisoners is Lucia Zedner's *Women, Crime and Custody in Victorian England* (1991), an examination of 'how Victorians perceived and explained female crime, and how they responded to it – both in penal theory and prison practice'. In the course of exploring these issues in relation to the evidence pertaining to local as well as national prisons, Zedner engages critically with the revisionist historians, notably Rothman, Foucault and Ignatieff. In her view, they have all concentrated too narrowly on penal ideology and the national prison system, thereby losing sight of 'the reality of continuing administrative chaos and human error'. Ignatieff, for example, overstated the influence of the model prison at Pentonville because 'he failed to examine just how far down the prison system this influence extended'. Ignatieff did, however, come to recognise that the revisionists had 'over-schematised' the complexities of prison history in his 'counter-revisionist critique', a critique which Zedner develops further in relation to evidence indicating that, long after the 1850s, English penal policy remained 'a multi-faceted, often contradictory and always problematic' operation (Zedner 1991: 1–4; 94–7). Equally important, with the exception of O'Brien, the revisionists ignored gender. They failed to see

> how notions of appropriate male and female roles figured in the development of penal theory; how far penal policy was directed towards one sex; and how, in practice, the very presence of women in prison generated major anomalies. In fact, gender distinctions affected the whole of the penal system.
>
> (1991: 97)

Indeed, assumptions about gender lay at the heart of fundamental differentiations in nineteenth-century English penal policy.

As Zedner notes: 'Very little *history* has been written about women's prisons in England' (my emphasis). Most studies have had a sociological orientation and the historical section of Dobash, Dobash and Guttridge's study does, as she points out, serves mainly as a background to their analysis of women's imprisonment in the late twentieth century. Consequently, their historical account is sketchy, leaping across long spans of time and, just as crucially, failing to differentiate between the long periods of servitude served by serious offenders and the brief terms served in the local prisons to which 'the mass of women prisoners were committed'. In Zedner's view then, a history of custody in nineteenth-century England must take account of the fact that the vast majority of women offenders – 98 per cent – were incarcerated for brief terms in local prisons. Moreover, it is imperative to note that they constituted as much as a quarter of all offenders sent to local prisons, compared to only an eighth of those sent to convict prisons, up to the 1880s. It follows that women prisoners were hardly invisible to penal administrators in nineteenth-century England, as most historians seem to assume. On the contrary, the question of the treatment of women prisoners was a central concern of Victorian penal policy (1991: 98–100). Accordingly, Zedner proceeds to document the differential treatment which women received in the local as well as national prisons. But importantly, her history is an attempt 'to write the history of women in local prisons not only from above but, more ambitiously, from "within"' (1991: 132). She therefore provides an account of the prisoners themselves – their backgrounds, their relations with warders and other prisoners (including, of course, their sexual relationships) and their inmate subcultures. She also reflects on the evidence that some women preferred the local prison to destitution or 'the more punitive level of provision in some workhouses' and suggests that if they did regard the local prison as less than a powerful deterrent, we will need to modify 'our understanding of the prison as a penal institution' (1991: 115; 131–70).

Zedner's account then, is not only very suggestive about the direction which women's prison history should take; it serves as a role model for the kind of close empirical study which is required if we are to transform our understanding of what counts as a properly 'social' history of the prison. Not that she claims to be writing social history herself; on the contrary, she is critical of that project. She does however, demonstrate the importance of examining how penal policy has been 'differentiated by sex', establishing clearly that the prison was a place touched by 'issues of gender' (1991: 99–100). However, analysts have not yet begun the task of collating the information amassed in the disparate studies of women's imprisonment in Western countries in the nineteenth century, let alone of addressing their sometimes contradictory observations. For example, Zedner claims that English women prisoners were not punished as severely as the men (1991: 169), yet, as we have seen, Dobash, Dobash and Guttridge present evidence that women's penal regimes were more repressive. Clearly, we need more precise accounts of specific penal regimes and of changes over time. More broadly, feminist historians have begun to critically engage with the older masculinist social histories, but they have yet to begin the task of systematically addressing questions raised by histories of the punishment of women. Not until the still-disparate studies of women's imprisonment have been consolidated into a new theoretically-grounded paradigm will they be able to provide a fully 'social' history of punishment, one capable of challenging the restrictive theoretical boundaries of masculinist studies untouched by a consideration of gender relations.

BEYOND A PENOLOGY OF WOMEN?

Historical lessons

In chapter 5 we will consider postmodern feminist contributions to the analysis of penality, but first let us assess the potentiality of recent critical accounts of women in prison to transform the analysis of penality. As revealed by all the studies considered here, two key factors in the continuing neglect of women prisoners are the insignificance of their numbers and of the offences they commit relative to male prisoners in Western jurisdictions. It is precisely because they pose such a small threat to social order that women prisoners in North America, France and the United Kingdom have simply not been considered to be a 'social problem' warranting close attention. In the face of such indifference on the part of prison administrators and critical theorists alike, the revisionist histories of the 1980s which we have explored here have contributed enormously to the task of fleshing out some of the details of prison life for the shadowy figure of the incarcerated woman. They have also provided very useful directives for research on penal regimes for women in other Western countries. For example, historians would do well to draw on the findings of these studies when they come to write the still largely unwritten history of women's imprisonment in Australia. The records we have access to suggest that similar themes of neglect, substandard conditions and refusals on the part of statutory bodies to take women prisoners seriously, even when their numbers were high, as they were at the turn of the nineteenth century (Braithwate 1980), have shaped the development of penal regimes for women in Australia.

More crucially, the new revisionist histories raise new questions about the historical significance of women's prisons in Australia. For example, did any major penal developments originate in the women's prison system, like those which Rafter documented in the United States (Rafter 1983: 288–90)? Again, this has not been researched, but, thanks to the revisionist histories of the 1980s, this much is assured: when we come to write a history of women's imprisonment in Australia from a feminist perspective, it will be sure to include many neglected dimensions of penality. For example, the aim will not be restricted to shedding still more light on dimensions of penality which have been ignored by the plethora of masculinist studies of 'our' convicts (read: male convicts) in that premier penal colony, New South Wales. We need historical accounts of prison populations other than the always already universalising white one, in states like Victoria which did not originate as penal colonies. We also need to know more about imprisonment in Australia after the much-studied convict period. As Mark Finnane has argued, the time has come to acknowledge the diversity of institutions and regimes 'which come under the prisons umbrella' and to shift the focus away from the white male prisoner inhabiting the single-cell maximum security prison designed in the nineteenth century (Finnane 1991: 108–9). Certainly, it will not suffice merely to correct those studies which purport to be general histories of punishment in Australia, studies in which it could be claimed, and indeed has been claimed, that 'one person in seven' transported to the penal colonies were women and that, on the question of whether these women were mainly 'whores', 'doubtless some were' (Hughes 1987: 71).[9] Rather, as the new revisionist histories have made clear, what is required is an excavation of the distinctive configurations of penality as they applied to women prisoners and a consideration of the ways in which an attention to women may change the overall image of penality.

Here Paula J. Byrne provides some insightful suggestions in her study of the criminal law and the colonial subject in early nineteenth-century New South Wales. In a most significant way, Byrne has demonstrated that white women were punished differently from white men in that penal colony, at least in the twenty-year period between 1810 and 1830, because of the lower value placed on their labour. Convict men were employed predominantly as labourers on public works while convict women were assigned to domestic service. Noting that convict men were corporally punished and minimally incarcerated, while recalcitrant domestic servants were sent back to the Female Factory at Parramatta, Byrne argues that the labour of convict women related more closely to incarceration than to waged labour (Byrne 1993: 38–50). Her point is that it is all very well to describe the Female Factory as a brothel and marriage market: first and foremost, it was a place of imprisonment for women. Her broader point is that the emphasis placed on punishing women with imprisonment positioned them closely to the development of the prison. Indeed, convict women were more 'closely linked to the prison as an institution' than male convicts: they were 'the first to experience nineteenth-century prison relations in the colony' (1993: 278).

Interestingly, related points have been made in other studies about women prisoners having a distinctive relationship with the emergence of penal regimes. As we have seen, Rusche and Kirchheimer saw differential modes of punishment for men and women as evidence that the rise of imprisonment under Western capitalism was bound up in part with the need to provide special treatment for women (1968: 65–6). A related but slightly different point was made by Dobash, Dobash and Guttridge. They noted that the British Penal Servitude Acts led to changes in the 1850s in the treatment of women prisoners who were not permitted to go out to labour, were not automatically released on licence and were sometimes sent to another institution such as a refuge after the expiration of their sentence.

They were 'subjected to a tighter regime' than male inmates. Tellingly, their observation, already noted above, that British women prisoners were 'more closely confined in this new regime created specifically for them' (1986: 60–1) is remarkably similar to Byrne's point about Australian women convicts. However, the implications of these rare insights into the close relationship between the punishment of women and the emergence of imprisonment as the dominant penal form in the West in the nineteenth century have yet to be developed by feminist analysts in ways which might challenge masculinist narratives of the 'master patterns' of social control. Thus it could be said that in the 1980s studies of women's prison history have established an empirical foundation for theory about the punishment of women which Rafter predicted, but to date the theorisation has not proceeded very far. It has not moved beyond control theory, as in the case of Rafter and Carlen, or beyond a Foucauldian interpretation of disciplinary regimes within the women's prison system, undertaken almost exclusively from the top down, as in the case of Dobash, Dobash and Guttridge. So while it can no longer be said that feminist discussions have 'hardly touched on women in prison' (Heidensohn 1985: 82) or that 'the female prison community has been overlooked', the new revisionist historical studies have not actually done much to 'add to the growing body of *theory* on group behaviour' which Giallombardo called for over twenty-five years ago (1966; my emphasis).

Toward a feminist theorisation of penality?

Several factors have inhibited a feminist theorisation of penality. First, very few critical or revisionist analysts in the field appear to be deeply committed to a feminist politics or methodology. Dobash, Dobash and Guttridge cite feminist work without actually claiming that perspective themselves; Rafter claims a socialist feminist perspective but subverts this identification by discussing disagreements about the position of women in class analysis in a footnote, without committing herself to a position on this crucially important question (1990: 251), and Carlen is satisfied to label as feminist any researcher concerned about injustices done to women in the criminal justice or penal systems. Second, while feminist historians have taken masculinist social historians to task for ignoring the question of gender, they have been less prepared to engage critically with historical accounts of women's imprisonment.[10] Third, there has been a failure to engage with the central debates within feminist theory, including and especially feminist debates with postmodernism. Certainly, revisionist studies of sentencing practices such as Mary Eaton's are informed by feminist perspectives, but studies of women's imprisonment – which predominate in the slowly-growing field of the punishment of women – remain locked into the now somewhat outmoded question of 'gender'. Analysis continues to be framed in terms of the problem of missing 'gender dimensions' or the lack of 'equality' between men's and women's prisons (e.g. Rafter 1990: 185–207).

To formulate the 'feminist' penal question in this way is to betray a certain naivety about the potentiality of a gender-sensitive study of the punishment of women to transform the analytical field of penality. First, as Dawn Currie amongst others has observed, 'the introduction of gender does not represent an advance in theorising' – at least, not necessarily. One problem is that theorists, including critical theorists, have failed to distinguish between the value of gender or sex as a descriptive variable and 'its limitations as an explanatory variable' (Currie 1986: 235–6). To take an example from the studies of punishment outlined above, the conceptual framework in Pat Carlen's *Women, Crime and Poverty* is informed by control theory which asks the question: 'why do people conform?' (1988: 11). But translating this question as: 'why do women conform?' does not necessarily lead to a satisfactory account of the relationship between gender and social control. As Deborah Baskin and Ira Sommers point out, Carlen does not explain how women's criminal careers are 'circumscribed specifically by *gender*' (1990: 152; their emphasis). Moreover, they argue that Carlen's repetition of the 'timeworn and functionalist rhetoric that only women experience dual exploitation' in the public and private spheres adds little to the analysis. On the one hand, she fails to see that working-class men also have to make 'class and gender deals' which include being regulated within the family; on the other hand, she does not distinguish the 'gender-specific ways' in which women are exploited and controlled by familialism and consumerism. In short, Carlen's analysis, gendered though it purports to be, does not address the precise ways in which social reactions are gender-specific and thus affect women's lives differently from men's (Baskin and Sommers 1990: 153–4). Second and connected, critical, gender-sensitive penal analysts do not seem to have realised that a consideration of gender cannot be reduced to a study of women. At least, no study has yet taken up Michelle Perrot's intriguing suggestions that the 'castrating prison was the ultimate, intensified image' of sexual repression in mid-nineteenth-century France or that contemporary writing on the penitentiary 'fairly overflows with phallic anxiety' about sexual promiscuity, nocturnal masturbation and homosexuality, or that the designers of penitentiary systems were 'haunted by sexual obsessions' (Perrot 1978: 225–35). At a more mundane level, Nicole Rafter is one of the few revisionist historians to have observed that 'the discipline of male convicts was shaped by notions of masculinity' as well as by organisational ideas about control and labour (1985b: 234). But we still await the emergence of feminist studies of the role of ideas about masculinity in the development of men's prisons.

In sum, feminist analysts of the punishment of women still have a considerable way to go. They may have come to recognise that women's prisons are, as Rafter put it, of 'theoretical interest' because they have been and continue to be 'a point of juncture between widely disparate types of social control', ranging from the formal to the informal, the overt and the inconspicuous, the brutal and the gentle, inflicted 'by government and by those trusted and familiar' (Rafter 1990: xi–xii). But they have not taken what might be called the project of theorisation very far. In particular, they have barely begun to tackle the dilemma confronting the very idea of a feminist penology – a dilemma which corresponds closely with the one outlined by Victoria Greenwood and Angela McRobbie and other British sociologists over a decade ago in relation to the then emergent project of a feminist criminology. The problem, as Greenwood put it, is that while the attempt to raise gender issues in the broad area of crime and punishment is laudable, feminist work which 'locates its critique at the level of sexism' is problematic. Such work seems to rely on the assumption that, if criminological theories could be somehow 'emptied of sexism', they might 'in themselves be valid' – an assumption which was decisively challenged by a wide range of critical expositions of criminology undertaken in the West in the 1970s. Furthermore, an obsession with 'sexism' might obscure 'more elemental issues' such as the role of the state 'in creating deviant populations' (Greenwood 1981: 75–7).[11] Elaborating on Greenwood's argument, Angela McRobbie expressed concern that feminist researchers might get trapped into asking the sorts of questions that have been discarded by contemporary critical work in the field. This could lead, and indeed has led, to 'the resurrection of old issues like the female criminal personality type being debated from an ostensibly "feminist" position'. Worse, it led to 'the reduction of the whole question of women, crime and social disorder to the lonely figure of the female offender' (McRobbie 1982: 218).

Notwithstanding the pertinence of these observations to those contributing to the field of feminist penality, it is salutary to note that the prediction that an ultimately uncritical approach will become hegemonic in the 'women and crime' trajectory is not borne out by the research on women's imprisonment surveyed in this chapter. This work is not marred by that 'veneer of "contemporaneity"' which McRobbie feared would produce 'regressive work' on the position of women within discursive and non- discursive practices in the 'crime' field (McRobbie 1982: 219). As we have seen, critical analysts have been concerned to highlight the harshness and injustice of past and present penal regimes for women in order to support progressive penal policies.[12] Moreover, some critical analysts have provided a platform for women prisoners themselves to speak out about criminalisation processes and penal practices (e.g. Carlen 1985). Nevertheless, McRobbie's reminder that 'a simple concern with gender is by no account necessarily progressive' is still pertinent today and the conclusion she drew in 1982 – that feminist work on women and crime still had a lot to learn from the more historical and theoretical writings of the 'recent radical tradition' of the 'new' or critical criminologists – could be extended to cover much of the work on women and punishment which has emerged over the last ten years (1982: 218–19). For this work has, for the most part, failed to engage with the theoretical issues raised by the new 'social' analysis of penality. For example, Rusche and Kirchheimer's text, 'seminal' though it may have been to its masculinist admirers, is mentioned only in passing, if at all, in critical accounts of women's imprisonment. The revisionist studies of Rothman and Ignatieff have also been tangential to the concerns of most researchers studying the punishment of women. And if Foucault's *Discipline and Punish* is the sine qua non of non-feminist critical approaches to penality like Stan Cohen's, it figures only peripherally in most recent research on women in prison.

One explanation for this disengagement on the part of analysts of the punishment of women with the critical masculinist theorisations of penality of the 1980s is that they have been so preoccupied with plotting the empirical and historical realities of women's imprisonment – with writing women into the historical and sociological picture – that they have not had time to gaze across disciplinary boundaries to assess the range of contributions being made in the field. Certainly, the new research, especially the British research, on 'the female criminal' – now designated as female lawbreakers, or, better still, offending women (Worrall 1990) – has provided her with an identity, agency, political and even theoretical respectability, thereby ensuring her a place in any seriously progressive penological text. They have also provided a firm knowledge base about the development of punishment regimes specific to women. However, it needs to be said that the theoretical but ahistorical sociological studies of women's imprisonment which emerged in the 1980s have yet to mesh with the empirical, atheoretical histories of the women's prison system which appeared over the same decade. This disjunction has helped preclude the development of a coherent, feminist analytical framework within which researchers can engage with the theoretical challenges put up by critical yet non-feminist analysts of punishment.

One final problem besets the development of a theoretically-informed feminist analysis of punishment. As we have seen, critical scholars, from Rusche and Kirchheimer through to the new 'social' analysts of penality, have insisted on the need to disconnect the study of punishment from the study of crime: penality, in their view, must be regarded as an object of analysis in its own right. Yet studies of women's imprisonment continue to connect changing patterns within the women's prison system to changing patterns of women's lawbreaking. This conundrum is apparent in Carlen's work. In *Women, Crime and Poverty* (1988) she analyses women's law-breaking *and* official responses to it, while in her earlier study of Cornton Vale she includes an account of women's offending patterns in Scotland. Yet just a few years earlier Carlen herself was calling for a methodological commitment to Rusche's and Foucault's directive to break the 'imaginary bond between crime and punishment' (Carlen 1980: 14–15). So somewhere between discussing critical approaches to penality and doing research on women's imprisonment Carlen either lost sight of her own theoretical perspective or changed her mind about the need to cut the cord between crime and punishment, at least in relation to women. Similarly, Freedman, Rafter, Zedner and Dobash, Dobash and Guttridge dutifully note shifts over time in patterns of women's criminality. The latter typify this crime-and-punishment orientation when they declare that the history of the imprisonment of women in Britain '*must* be considered . . . relative to the criminality of women' (1986: 11; my emphasis). Clearly, Foucault's in-junction to release the question of punishment from the question of crime has been ignored in *The Imprisonment of Women*, which ironically remains one of the few books on Western penal regimes for women to have been influenced by *Discipline and Punish*.[13]

Thus, it could be argued that the failure of feminist researchers on women's prisons to fully engage with theoretical issues raised by critical, non-feminist theorists of penality has had the unfortunate effect of reconnecting punishment to crime within analytical frameworks deployed to address questions about the punishment of women. However, it is possible to take another tack here, one which reads the research on women's imprisonment as raising questions about the universal validity of masculinist theories about penality, theories which, after all, are based on studies of punishment regimes imposed on men. It may be that the great disconnection between crime and punishment effected by Rusche and Kirchheimer's *Punishment and Social Structure* and Foucault's *Discipline and Punish*, and hailed by their followers as an astounding epistemological achievement, does not have a purchase when it comes to studying the punishment of women. Indeed, it may well be that the task of unearthing the specificities of women's imprisonment actually requires a crime-and-punishment approach.

First, it is possible that fluctuations in women's imprisonment rates are more intrinsically related to offending patterns than men's imprisonment rates which, as political economies of punishment have suggested, are tied to changes in labour market conditions. Given that women's labour continues to be devalued in capitalist economies, women's unemployment levels may not give rise to the same control concerns as men's, leaving women's offences as the key determinant of sentencing practices. Conversely, women's imprisonment rates may well provide a more significant measure of changing lawbreaking patterns than men's rates in so far as changing penal responses to women offenders may be more directly tied to changing perceptions of 'female crime'. In any event, it is surely significant that historians of women's imprisonment have insisted that, 'in examining the treatment of women in prisons, it is essential to consider how women were regarded as criminals' (O'Brien 1982: 64) and that critical observers argue that penal practices today are 'intelligible only by reference to a set of ideas' related to the nature of women's criminality – ideas which 'result in women and women's crime being defined and responded to in qualitatively different ways to men and male offending'. As these feminist researchers point out, an 'epistemology of female crime' which is over-determined by value-laden psychologically-based assumptions about 'female deviance' is very directly implicated in the organisation of prison regimes for women (Genders and Player 1986: 368–70). It remains to develop the implications of these observations for a fully 'social' theoretical understanding of penality.

Second and related, Western states have rarely had to resort to penal sanctions to keep women in place. Given that the role played by the prison in the larger story of the disciplining of men's lives has already been questioned (Donnelly 1986: 24), we certainly need to determine whether it is indeed the prison that should play the central role in our accounts of the disciplining of women. We might well choose another institution as the exemplary instance of the discipline of women – perhaps psychiatric hospitals or heterosexuality.[14] But returning to the question of those women who are incarcerated in penal institutions: it is precisely because women are so rarely placed in prison that studies of their imprisonment may have to be related to their offending patterns for, arguably, these patterns provide a more revealing measure of the failure of socially-based disciplinary regimes imposed on women than do men's offences about social control mechanisms directed at men. Furthermore, an analysis of the offences women commit may indicate that women have a qualitatively different relationship to punishment than men. For example, does the fact that the majority of women in Western prisons today have been incarcerated for drug-related offences have any theoretical significance for the analysis of penality?[15] Could women's drug-related offending be seen as a form of punishment itself? Does this offending give rise to the notion of a punishment continuum, rather than a crime-and-punishment equation, especially when women's drug-taking practices continue unabated inside and outside the prison walls? Are women's crimes and punishments bonded in such a way that they simply cannot be pulled apart to satisfy the theoretical requirements of critical masculinist analysts?

Speculation aside, it is clear that women prisoners constitute a major empirical and analytical hurdle for the great theorists of penality who devised their analytical schemas in relation to men. Alternatively, it is clear that a properly 'social' analysis of punishment – one which explores the social foundations of penality in relation to women's as well as men's lives – must start outside the narrow confines of the prison *and* of crime statistics if it is going to have any chance of decentring that intriguing preoccupation with criminality which continues to characterise critical studies of the punishment of women.

CONCLUDING NOTE

The questions which are raised by a consideration of what a feminist theorisation of penality may look like return us full circle to the view expressed by Barry Smart and Carol Smart over a decade ago, that the social control of women takes many forms. It may be 'internal or external, implicit or explicit, private or public, ideological or repressive'. Indeed, the 'primary sources' of such control are 'outside or even beyond, judicial influence' – they are located within seemingly innocuous social processes (Smart and Smart 1978: 1–2). From this perspective, a 'model for the study of the structural coercion of women' must be built outside conventional approaches to the question of women, crime and punishment. As I have suggested, such a model may also need to be constructed outside the analytical boundaries of recent non-feminist approaches to penality. The point of departure must be 'women's material conditions' and the first issue is to 'find a language in which women's experiences can be communicated and understood'. Once we have a language, we can develop an analysis which shifts the focus from an etiological concern with female offenders or a political concern with the conditions of women's imprisonment, to an understanding of 'the coercion of privacy' – a coercion which restrains women to the point where we can speak of them 'living their lives in a private prison' (Dahl and Snare 1978). The concept of the 'private prison' is an important one for understanding the restraints placed on women's lives all along the 'freedom'–'imprisonment' continuum. It suggests that an historical analysis of the social control of women should shift away from the formal custodial institutions to informal sites of social control. Yet although, as the song says, 'Joann is you, Joann is me / Our prison is the whole society' (Freedman 1981: 1), we must avoid the absurdity of infinite relativism: we must not forget that incarcerated women are more coerced than those outside the prison walls and that some women, notably black and other minority women, suffer from the coercion and oppression of institutionalised racism within Western criminal justice systems. The challenge ahead, then, for feminist analysts is to address the difficult questions – such as whether or not to effect a disengagement of crime and punishment, or whether a consideration of the specificities of the punishment of women demands a fundamentally different kind of theoretical approach – but to do all this without losing sight of women prisoners, and also without limiting the focus to the penal sphere. Yet another challenge is that presented by postmodern attacks on the analytical category of 'woman'. How can a feminist who is informed by a postmodern sensibility that women no longer exist, speak for women prisoners? Must she risk losing sight of women prisoners, just when they are beginning to become visible?

These questions take us beyond the scope of this chapter, which has been concerned to survey new developments in the study of the punishment of women. We have not yet dealt with the implications for a progressive analysis of penality of critical studies of girls and young women at risk of state intervention – studies which have gone a long way towards recognising and following up Victoria Greenwood's insight that the 'particular condition of women requires a specific form of analysis which cannot be similar to that used for men' (Greenwood 1981: 78). But because they intersect at several points with feminist postmodern inquiries into the disciplining of women, we will consider these critical accounts of the control of young women in the next chapter.

5 Postmodern feminism and the question of penality

By now we have accumulated a number of problems whose resolution depends on a consideration of methodological and epistemological issues. As we have seen, there have been several major contributions to the study of women prisoners over the last decade. However, they have not, for the most part, paid much attention to recent theoretical developments. On the one hand, analysts of women's prisons have ignored the theoretical issues which have concerned revisionist masculinist discussions of penality. They have not, for example, engaged with debates within political economies of punishment, let alone developed their own political economies in the field; nor have they paid attention to critical issues raised by the purveyors of a 'social' analysis of penality. Furthermore, whereas masculinist scholars have enquired about the possibility of a Marxist penology or moved beyond penology altogether, analysts of penal regimes for women have not directly addressed the question of a feminist penology: the dynamics of correctional penology, state power and penal relations remain untheorised in their accounts. On the other hand, feminist analyses of punishment lack that self-conscious attention to methodology, and thus to theory, which has come to characterise feminist analysis in other knowledge fields in the late twentieth century. There, a confrontation with postmodernism has helped transform the direction and nature of feminist scholarship. For example, in criminology, which has been seen as the closest field to penality, the theorisation of the implications of anti-essentialist critiques of positivistic constructions of 'the criminal woman' has proceeded apace (e.g. Brown 1986 and 1990; Worrall 1990). Moreover, arguments for and, more crucially, against the development of a feminist criminology have been widely can-vassed by analysts informed by a postmodern sensibility (e.g. Smart 1990). Certainly, it can be said that, in recent years, studies of women's imprison-ment, especially in the United Kingdom, have adopted 'a more robust theoretical perspective' than can be found in the traditional, pathologising, positivistic and liberal approaches which continue to collude with 'regulatory

discourses' (Cain and Smart 1990). Yet the deeper questions of punishment
or even of a more broadly conceived penality as objects of analysis have
not attracted critical feminist attention, save for an occasional recognition
of the implications of Foucault's analysis of disciplinary regime for a study
of women's imprisonment (e.g. Dobash, Dobash and Guttridge 1986). As
we saw in chapter 4, critical approaches to the punishment of women are
still organising themselves into a coherent framework, and they remain
marginal to the so-called 'social' analysis of penality. Consequently, both
punishment and penality languish behind the locked doors of masculinist
(albeit revisionist masculinist) frameworks.

In this chapter I am concerned to move beyond a critique of the masculinist nature of recent critical work in the field of penality in order to open
up the question of what a postmodern feminist engagement with penality
might look like. Beginning with a consideration of some of the implications
of postmodernism for a feminist penal politics, I move on to explore some
pertinent questions arising from critiques of the feminist criminology project. I will then consider recent feminist studies of young women at risk of
state incarceration – studies which decentre the state and, in the process,
open up the possibility of fundamentally reconceptualising critical
approaches to penality. Finally, and connectedly, we need to consider
feminist Foucauldian analyses of the 'disciplining' of women which are
forging new understandings of the policing and punishment of bodies and,
in the process, transforming the meaning of penality.

POSTMODERN PENAL POLITICS?

It could well be said that the coming of the postmodern has raised interesting questions for feminist and other progressive politics. On the one hand,
the deconstruction of modernist ideas such as 'truth' and 'reason' has led
to a questioning of the very idea of a politics founded on notions of justice
or equality. On the other, the announcement of the death of the subject has
led to an insistence that we move beyond the now antiquated, time-warped
subject-based feminism of the 1970s. But the problem with such a construction of the reception of new ideas is that it privileges the impact of an
intellectual movement which was largely white and, at least initially,
masculinist. A more critical historiography would point out that if the
feminist dilemma of the 1990s is that the notion of a taken-for-granted
universal subordination of women is now under siege, the initial challenges
came from self-defined women of colour, amongst other minority women,
in the 1970s (e.g. Combahee River Collective 1983). While the power of
these early critiques of universalising feminist assumptions passed most
white Western feminists by, it seems that the emergence of a more

intellectually acceptable, fashionable movement has made the anti-universalising thrust of the earlier critiques accessible to them. At any rate, the cumulative challenge, first of women of colour and later of Third World women and other post-colonial critics, to the analytical categories of white Western feminism is finally having effects – better late than never. At long last, the very category of 'woman', resting as it does on the assumption of an already constituted and coherent group, is now being rejected by Western feminists who have taken the 'postmodern turn'. Thus 'Woman' and even 'women', having become unstable categories, will no longer do as self-evidentiary bases for feminist claims. For as Teresa de Lauretis amongst others has pointed out, it has been the fate of the second-wave feminist movement – surely, one of the most ironic twists of fate in the history of social movements – to have discovered, in the process of pressing claims on behalf of women, 'the nonbeing of *woman*' (her emphasis). She describes this 'nonbeing' as:

> the paradox of a being that is at once *captive* and absent in discourse, constantly spoken of but of itself inaudible or inexpressible, displayed as spectacle and still unrepresented or unrepresentable, invisible yet constituted as the object and the guarantee of vision; a being whose existence and specificity are simultaneously asserted and denied, negated and controlled.
>
> (de Lauretis 1990: 115; my emphasis)

For de Lauretis it is this 'paradox of woman' which is the necessary starting point of feminist theory inasmuch as the constitution of the social subject depends on the nexus of language, subjectivity and consciousness. It follows from this that feminism's field of knowledge and 'modes of knowing' are 'caught in this paradox of woman'; that is, they are both: 'excluded from the established discourse of theory and yet *imprisoned* within it or else assigned a corner of their own but denied a specificity' (1990: 115; my emphasis).

'Captive' beings, 'imprisoned' in dominant discourses? Penality per se may not yet have become a focus of concern for postmodern feminist theorists, but it is surely significant that 'captive' women as well as modes of knowledge perceived as being 'imprisoned' within dominant discourses have been marked for interrogation. It is, then, very relevant to the project of developing a feminist analysis of penality to note that de Lauretis characterises the current preoccupation of the postmodern feminist as the releasing of 'woman' from her discursive imprisonment, and the postmodern political agenda as the reconceptualising of 'woman' as a shifting subject, 'multiply organised across variable axes of difference' (1990: 116). What all this means for the feminist political future has yet to be determined or, in postmodern parlance, fully 'mapped'. At this historical 'moment', analysis has not proceeded very far beyond the recognition that it has become *de rigueur* to kiss foundationalism goodbye and engage with postmodernity's tropes and other rhetorical ruptures. But such playful courting of uncertainty is not to every feminist's taste. Indeed, it is hardly surprising, given the unfinished nature of modernist feminist political projects, that postmodernism's seemingly wilful disregard of feminism's founding conceptual category – gender – has given rise to anxiety that second-wave feminist projects are to be abandoned. Nor is it surprising that this anxiety has led to a serious misreading of the postmodern political agenda.

This is not the place to engage with the seemingly endless debates for and against postmodernism which have preoccupied feminist theorists in a number of disciplines – sociology, philosophy, literary theory, linguistics, legal theory – over the past decade (e.g. Diamond and Quinby 1988; Nicholson 1990; Butler and Scott 1992). Our concern is with the implications of these debates for feminist theoretical and political intervention in the field of penality. Here we have a carte blanche, a virginal space untouched by feminist postmodern hands, on to which I want to project an imaginary conversation between postmodernists and their opponents on the question of the potentiality of postmodernism to transform feminist approaches to penality. Indeed, it is precisely because this question has not been addressed that such a scenario becomes possible.

Imagining conversations

Adopting, then, the conversational mode – one of the favoured formats of the postmodernists – let us engage in an imagined conversation between postmodern feminism and its sceptical detractors.[1] It is not difficult to imagine the opening salvoes of those sceptical of, or even scathing about, the potentiality of postmodernism to transform our understanding of penality. Their conversation would begin something like this: postmodernists may luxuriate in discursive armchair splendour, mapping out the postfoundational future, but what, in the meantime, are we to do about the pressing social needs and political demands of modernity's underprivileged groups? How, for example, would the committed postmodernist (a contradiction in terms?) have the would-be progressive feminist analyst of women's imprisonment sort out a postmodern penal strategy, if there can be no resorting to, or at least no unquestioning resorting to, that discredited founding category: 'women'? More crucially, when the dust has settled, what implications will postmodernism have for women in prison?

First, let us consider women prisoners themselves. At face value, the sceptic's question is a valid one: just what would women prisoners make of the postmodern conundrums (assuming, for the sake of argument, that they had access to them)? One could hazard a guess – not much. What else could they be but bemused by the question: 'Am I that name?' (Riley 1988) – assuming again that they had the luxury of asking it? For women prisoners are always already constituted as women. They are 'women prisoners' – 'female offenders' no less – whether they like it (or more likely despite it) or not. Surely theirs is a designation which no postmodern sensibility can evacuate. What might the postmodern feminist reply to this? One line of reply might be to note that while an over-totalising categorisation of women prisoners as 'female' appears to be the fate of women incarcerated in Western prisons, alternative subjectivities are possible. Importantly, Barbara Harlow has drawn attention to women's prison writings from the Third World which she believes are 'potentially constructive' of a new discursive category. She claims that these writings describe a collective experience emerging from a position within a set of social relations that gives rise to a 'secular ideology' not based on bonds of race, ethnicity or, crucially, gender.

> Based exclusively on neither issues of gender or race nor, strictly speaking, based on questions of class, they outline the possibilities of new secular forms of social organisation.
>
> (Harlow 1986: 502–7)

Harlow is referring to the prison writings of Nawal El Saadawi, Ruth First and other political prisoners who have sought to develop 'new bases of affiliation' with fellow inmates and other political detainees (1986: 508–20). By contrast, with a few important exceptions – notably, black American and Irish political prisoners – there is not much evidence of such bids for ties of affiliation being made by women in Western prisons. French women's prison writings, for example, have been described as neither 'transcendental' nor rebellious. Elissa Gelfland found little evidence in them of a political voice: 'there is at best a sense of weakness inverted into irony or solitude glorified as martyrdom' (Gelfland 1983: 20). Similar comments have been made contrasting the silence of women prisoners with the vocal and active male prison reform tradition in other European countries, notably Norway (Dahl and Snare 1978). In Australia too, a strong political tradition has yet to emerge within the women's prison system. Occasionally, muffled voice are heard, as they are today especially in the states of Victoria and New South Wales, but they are still no match for the 'authentic' (because louder and documented) male prison tradition.[2] We rely on outside lobby groups such as the state coalitions against women's imprisonment for information about conditions 'inside' for women. Official sources, especially in Victoria, Queensland and Western Australia, provide little information about women's prisons: without the lobby groups we would not know, for example, about the death of Aboriginal women in custody (Howe 1988).[3] Yet in all this, one thing is clear: the woman imprisoned in a Western penal institution is not a stable subject. She is constituted as part of a highly diversified population of long- and short-term prisoners, ethnically and racially mixed, heterosexual and lesbian women.

Returning to our sceptic's question: what would women prisoners make of the postmodern condition, which appears to be productive of an 'anxiety about claiming theoretically what we know experientially' and an 'anxiety about accounts of post-gendered subjectivities' (Miller 1986: 115)? It is difficult to say, and anyway, who are *we* to say anything, we who have learnt from Foucault 'the indignity of speaking for others'? Following Foucault, all we can do, apparently, is to help create the conditions which permit prisoners to speak for themselves and 'appreciate the fact that only those directly concerned can speak in a practical way on their own behalf' (Foucault 1977c: 206–9). To be clear: my concern here is not to create a futuristic scenario in which (with apologies to Carol Smart), Atavistic Woman Prisoner meets Postmodern Feminist (Smart 1990). Rather, it is to reflect on our imagined sceptic's suggestion that while postmodernists sort out the ramifications of the epistemological crisis of modernism, women prisoners languish in sub-standard and over-crowded conditions which provide no opportunity for contemplating the death of the subject, the demise of truth or the errors of universalism. Certainly, one could reply, these conditions are not conducive to an engagement with the dilemmas of postmodernism.[4] But it is salutory to recall that it often used to be said by those opposed to earlier feminist theoretical projects that singularly oppressed women such as prisoners had no time for the luxuries of feminism, let alone of feminist theories. But, the sceptic persists, what relevance could a theoretical anxiety about gender identity being 'a regulative ideal' (Butler 1990) have for women prisoners when their every moment is always already regulated? What interest could they possibly have in post-gendered subjectivities when they haven't come close to winning a rights-based modern subject position? The feminist penal analyst who has suffered no such deprivations and who is mindful of current intellectual debates is surely obliged to take these questions seriously.

So much then for the imagined claims of postmodernism's sceptics on behalf of women prisoners against the ravages perceived to have been wrought by the postmodern onslaught on feminism's foundational categories. It is time now to stop hiding behind 'imagined others' and to confront the political implications of the postmodern problematic. Let us turn, then, to the case of the would-be feminist penal analyst who, having suffered none of the deprivations of imprisonment, is confronted with the task of theorising penality in ways which are both strategically useful for women prisoners and sensitive to postmodernism's conundrums. The case-study I want to consider is my own.

'Social injury'

Over the past few years I have been concerned to develop a 'social injury' strategy for women at risk of further injury, notably women prisoners and young women at risk of state intervention. The strategy is premised on what I have described as a distinctive aspect of women's experience – namely, 'our' injuries. I meant the hidden injuries of all gender-ordered societies, the injuries associated with lower gender status, the once privatised injuries which we have begun to name over the last twenty years, such as domestic violence (now criminal assault in the home), incest (now father–daughter rape) and sexual harassment which is now, at least in the workplace, sex discrimination. I have argued that while these injuries have become public issues they are still trivialised in the wider culture because we missed a crucial step in our argument. Insisting that our private injuries become public issues has not been enough: to ensure that our distinctive mode of alienation as women is not lost in its translation into a legal claim, we need to demonstrate that the injuries we feel at a private, intimate level are socially-created, indeed, social injuries, before we demand that they become public issues (Howe 1987, 1990a and 1990b).

I have suggested two specific areas of application for this social injury strategy. First, I suggested that it might be useful for empowering young women at risk of state intervention in the child welfare and juvenile justice arenas because it provides them with a language for naming their more injurious life experiences, such as sexual abuse, exploitation and dis-criminatory treatment in their homes, in schools, in the workplace and in the 'welfare' system itself. It seemed to me that if they could name these injuries, young women could begin to develop a sense of injury and a sense of entitlement to redress. The social injury strategy provides them with a sense of entitlement because it addresses the problem of the privatised nature of their pain by creating a language in which to communicate that pain and make it public knowledge. This appeared to be especially import-ant at a time when the concept of 'harm' – 'significant harm' – was entering the discourse of child welfare and status offender statutes in Australia (Howe 1990b). Second, I have begun to develop a feminist reductionist–abolitionist strategy for women prisoners which is also dependent on the concept of 'social injury'. While the question of political strategy and its relationship to theory is more appropriately raised in the concluding chapter, it is relevant to discuss it briefly here. Building on the concept of 'aggregate social harm' cultivated in the abolitionist programme of the

Prisoners Action Group in New South Wales in the early 1980s, I have suggested that this injury-based approach has a potentiality which could be more fully developed in relation to women prisoners. Its purpose would be to measure the injuriousness of imprisonment against the social injuries of women's daily lives by drawing attention to the specific, concrete circumstances of women's criminalised actions and of their imprisonment. It must address the particular localised regulatory issues which impact on these women – such as access to community-based orders or the abolition of pre-release and the replacement of remission with 'merit time' – in the context of their socially-injurious life experiences (Howe 1990c).

By now, postmodern aficionados must be in a state of apoplexy. A distinctive aspect of *women's experience*? *Our* injuries? *Our* private injuries? *All* gender-ordered societies? And '*our distinctive mode of alienation as women*'? Havn't such foundational universalising myths withered before the postmodern onslaught? Mercifully, I did not smuggle the most forbidden vocabulary – 'identity' and 'unity' – into the social injury strategy, but I came close: 'women can share injury and recognise difference' (Howe 1990a). This will not do, it will not do at all, as a response to the problem of dealing with women's class-differentiated and race-differentiated socially-injurious experiences. Furthermore, some women may not recognise, or may not wish to recognise, their life experiences as injured ones, however socially based these may be represented to be. More critically, the social injury strategy ignored the problems raised by the postmodern pressure on the capacity of the category of 'woman' to act as the foundation of a feminist politics. At a time when the capitalised 'Woman' is 'in blatant disgrace' and even 'woman' is 'troublesome' (Riley 1988: 1–2), thereby creating uncertainties about the relationship of 'women' to feminism, the starting point for my social injury strategy was an unabashed 'women's pain' (Howe 1990a: 148).[5] Subject-based politics, gender identity and shared experiences may be falling by the postmodern wayside, but I will have to live with a strategy premised on 'gendered harms' for 'women' who are, or appear to be, characterised in my analysis as 'a singular group on the basis of a shared oppression' – their social injuries – and 'somehow socially constituted as a homogenous group identifiable prior to the process of analysis' (Mohanty 1988: 65).

Can anything be salvaged from this kind of strategy, fraught as it appears to be with modernist errors? Or must we scrap it, return to the drawing board and start again? Two possibilities currently present themselves. On the one hand, we could take the path of those feminists who question whether a postmodern politics is seriously conceivable and insist that theorising needs some closures or 'stopping points', and that gender is one of them (Bordo 1990). We could agree, for example, that 'gender is basic in ways that we have yet to fully understand' (Di Stefano 1990: 78). And we could go along with the charge that postmodernists want to ignore women, and then point out that to ignore women prisoners just when they are beginning to become visible is to risk losing sight of them again. That is, we could join the Hartsock chorus and ask:

> Why is it that just at the moment when so many of us who have been silenced begin to demand the right to name ourselves, to act as subjects rather than objects of history, that just then the concept of subjecthood becomes problematic?
>
> (Hartsock 1990: 163)

It would seem to be relatively simple to take this line on behalf of women prisoners and their feminist penal researchers, and to claim that it is crucial that we extend visibility and legitimacy to women prisoners as political subjects, thereby refusing the postmodern problematisations of the subject and of the politics of representation. At least, it would be quite simple to take such a stand if it were not for the fact that this is a caricature of postmodern feminist interrogations of the foundational categories of feminist politics, interrogations which do not lead to a refusal of representational politics on behalf of oppressed groups of women.

At this stage in the dialogue, it might be useful to introduce Judith Butler's careful articulation of the political effects of the claims of poststructuralist feminism. Preferring the term 'poststructuralism' to 'postmodernism', Butler argues that those whom I have called here 'the sceptics' are engaged in a 'self-congratulatory ruse of power' which seeks to lump together a diverse range of critical perspectives under 'the sign of the postmodern', thereby missing the point of poststructuralism which is precisely to question what it is that authorises such an 'act of self-mastery'. The point of poststructuralism, she explains:

> is that power pervades the very conceptual apparatus that seeks to negotiate its terms, including the subject position of the critic; and further, that this implication of the terms of criticism in the field of power is *not* the advent of a nihilistic relativism incapable of furnishing norms, but, rather, the very precondition of a politically engaged critique.
>
> (1992a: 5–7; her emphasis)

The aim then, is not to abolish foundational categories but rather 'to interrogate what the theoretical move that establishes foundations *authorises*, and what precisely it excludes or forecloses'. For example, a political or representational strategy which resorts to a universal 'we' must be 'exposed for its highly ethnocentric biases'. The poststructuralist understands that the position articulated by the subject is 'always in some way constituted by what must be displaced for that position to take hold' (1992a: 7–8; her emphasis). Subjects are 'constituted through exclusion, that is, through the creation of a domain of deauthorised subjects, presubjects, figures of abjection, populations erased from view' (1992a: 13). Within a feminist context, the point of post-structuralism, as Butler would have it, is to interrogate whom it is that the foundational category 'woman' authorises and whom it excludes and de-authorises. In her view, the insistence on 'a stable subject of feminism, understood as a seamless category of women' – 'a generally shared conception of "women"' – encapsulates this exclusionary process. But she is adamant that the interrogatory project of poststructuralism does not mean that we should 'refuse representational politics – as if we could' (Butler 1990: 5). Indeed, she is emphatic on this point:

> Within feminism, it seems as if there is some political necessity to speak as and for *women*, and I would not contest that necessity. Surely, that is the way in which representational politics operates . . . lobbying efforts are virtually impossible without recourse to identity politics. So we agree that demonstrations and legislative efforts and radical movements need to make claims in the name of women.
>
> (Butler 1992a: 15)

At the same time however, we must be constantly on our guard against those ruses of power and universalising self-authorising moves which seek to ground a right to speak for all women. Not that the category 'women' is dead: rather, it would be vastly preferable to see it as 'a site of permanent openness and resignifiability' – a site, that is, of continuous yet open and productive con-testation between different groups of feminist women (1992a: 16).

Women prisoners then, would not be bereft of representational efforts or radical movements on their behalf, at least not from Butler's post-structuralist perspective. A feminist penal politics informed by post-structuralist theories we could insist, following Butler's lead, would still be able to demonstrate and make claims on behalf of women prisoners. Moreover, such a politics would be in a strong position to specify race and ethnic differences between women prisoners in a bid to ensure that minority women do not get erased from view in the act of speaking on behalf of 'women' prisoners. Indeed, the most effective strategies on behalf of women prisoners will be those which persistently contest the categories 'woman' and 'prisoner' as well as the subject-position of the feminist prison activist outside the walls. At this point however, our postmodern feminist might despair of defending the intricacies of poststructuralist feminism and simply call a halt to the sceptic's parodies and misreadings, refusing to engage further with the 'chant of antipostmodernism', with its reductionist refrains condemning postmodernists for failing to understand 'the material violence that women suffer' (Butler 1992a: 17). Shaking her head in despair at the sceptic's blindness to the political purchase of poststructuralist feminism's self-reflexive searching, she could take sanctuary in what might be called the pragmatism of those postmodern feminists who admit that, despite all their efforts to move beyond the politics of creating counter-identities and 'the torments which spring from speaking for a collectivity', they grind to a halt when they confront the problem of feminist political strategy today (Riley 1988: 110–11). Denise Riley's response to this dilemma is expressly to stake out a 'territory of pragmatism', suggesting that we can know 'amongst ourselves' that 'women' don't exist, while 'maintaining a politics of "as if they existed" – since the world behaves as if they unambiguously did'. The problem of the category of 'woman' is thus side-stepped by means of a 'a strategic willing-ness to clap one's feminist hand over one's theoretical mouth and just get on with "women" where necessary' (Riley 1988: 112–13). Or we could follow Judith Butler's suggestion that we at least imagine what it might look like to work free of the constraints of representational politics. Such a move to liberate feminism from 'a singular notion of identity' and 'a premature insistence on a stable subject' could, Butler argues, facilitate a politics which might contest 'the very reifications of gender and identity' which are stifling feminist strategising today (Butler 1990: 5–6).

Yet none of the feminist positions elaborated above fully satisfies. The postmodern pragmatists may at least be trying to show that there are 'alternatives to paralysis' in the face of uncertainty about the relationship of 'women' to 'feminism' (Tyler 1990). But in the process, they undermine the power of their own deconstructive critiques. For if Butler is right that the task of a radical postmodern politics is to interrogate the theoretical moves of established foundations, including those of feminism, and to determine what these moves authorise as well as what they exclude and foreclose – if the aim is to contest all foundational moves (Butler 1992a) – then it won't do simply to reinsert 'women' for strategic purposes as Riley suggests. Nor does it suffice to declare 'a new sort of feminist politics' to be desirable, one which has purposes other than the articulation of identity (Butler 1990: 5), without working through the practical problems of speak-ing for women here and now. On the other hand, the defensive moves of the modernist sceptics also fail to satisfy. Holding on fast to identity politics and the right to speak for a unified category of 'women' cannot save feminism's foundationalist assumptions from the devastation wrought by the opposition of women, whom feminism claims to represent, to the assertion of a common gender identity, a universal 'Woman'. This devastation has been fully explored elsewhere and need not detain us.[6] My concern here is with the fate of the social injury strategy. Can it survive the kind of interrogation of foundational categories which Butler calls for?

Briefly, the defence I would mount of the social injury strategy is that, contrary to appearances, it can meet several of the criteria set by the postmodernists for an adequate political strategy. First, it need not rest on a universal, essentialising notion of 'women'. The whole point of the strategy is that it be utilised by groups who recognise a socially-based injury to themselves – that is, an injury to them as members of a particular social group. Women prisoners and young women at risk of incarceration are two such groups. But inasmuch as a specificity of application is built into the strategy, it is therefore open to any group who perceive a socially-based injury to themselves. Second, and related, the strategy is not dependent on gender identity: any member of a marginalised group who recognises a harm or discrimination as an injury to themselves as members of that group could deploy the strategy. In terms of custodial populations, an obvious group which springs to mind here is Aboriginal men in police custody in Australia. After all, the social injury strategy built on the concept of 'aggregate social harm' developed by the New South Wales Prisoners Action Group – a male prisoners' action group – in the early 1980s. 'Aggregate social harms' – all those injuries and material losses which are a consequence of deliberate policy or intentional behaviour (Prisoners Action Group 1980: 46–65) – are surely, on the evidence of the inquiry into Aboriginal deaths in custody, exactly what Aboriginal men continue to experience in custody.

Returning to women prisoners, the social injury strategy, as I elaborated it, was not intended as a strategy for all women prisoners. It had a very specific application: namely, women prisoners in one Australian state – Victoria. One of the important particularities of this specific group of prisoners today is that they are at last winning attention in policy statements. According to Office of Corrections policy pronouncements, women prisoners are, evidently, now part of a new corporatist strategy in Victoria. It is policy developments such as these which provoke those opposed to postmodernism feminism to call for action now. This, in turn, returns us to our imaginary conversation with postmodern feminism's sceptical detractor. The sceptic's agenda is clear: it is imperative that progressive penal analysts intervene to represent women prisoners in any new developments designed to reorganise the penal order. Anxiety about the dubious nature of a 'single authenticating truth of female experience' cannot get in the way of ensuring that new policy developments, even those proclaiming to prioritise women, do in fact best serve the interests of women prisoners. Nor is it hard to imagine the sceptic's final retort to the feminist postmodernist: sisters, forget Foucault and forget about formulating a critique of 'the categories of identity that contemporary juridical structures engender, naturalise and immobilise' (Butler 1990: 5). Forget all that: we need to get on with the job of advocating the interests of women prisoners now. But the job specifications could be broad – they could read: 'equal opportunity employer, even postmodernists may apply'.

ON THE NON-EXISTENCE OF THE CRIMINAL WOMAN

It is not that I intend to give the sceptic the final word: in chapter 6 we shall return to the question of forging a postmodern-sensitive penal politics. Indeed, all questions pertaining to the supposed havoc wrought by postmodernism on the foundational categories of representational politics are best deferred to the final chapter. There we will reconsider the purported dangers of postmodernism – for example, the allegation that, in the process of destabilising the subject and questioning a subject-based politics, we will lose sight of a politics of the 'everyday world', in our case the everyday world of the prison, especially of the women's prison, just when it is 'returning to sight' (Brown 1989). Leaving aside the vexed question of 'the everyday' (which figures in positivistic and essentialising constructions of 'the real' as some kind of gold standard against which to measure the supposed shortcomings of postmodern theorisations),[7] we will need to return to some key issues. For example, we need to ask: who are the 'we' behind this interrogation – the disembodied, abstract voice of the commentator; the politically-embedded voice of the prison reform activist, or even the experientially-privileged voice of the prisoner herself? All these quandaries are taken up in chapter 6 when we come to consider the vexed question of the relationship between research, politics and policy – a relationship thrown into disarray by the postmodern challenge to those too casually assumed relations between 'the real' and the researched.

For now, I want to underline the broader point of the above exercise in conversational fantasy: it was to predict some of the contestations which will occur when postmodern feminists finally turn their attention to the question of penality. The shake-up which will then ensue is likely to resonate with some of the postmodern refrains which have been heard in the related field of criminology for over a decade. For while studies of women's imprisonment, including revisionist ones, remained largely untouched by the postmodern quandaries of the 1980s, there has been a concerted effort to deconstruct the category of 'the criminal woman'. As adverted to earlier, postmodernism has already impacted on criminological studies to the point where Pat Carlen, for one, has been able to deny categorically 'the existence of the criminal *woman*'. More exactly, she has declared that the 'essential criminal woman does not exist' (Carlen 1985: 10; her emphasis). While the details of this postmodern interrogation of the feminist criminology project fall outside the scope of this book, there is one question we should ask here. To put this question bluntly: what's in it for penality? That is, how will the problematisation of 'the criminal woman' contribute to a theoretically-enriched study of penality, one which will not only include women prisoners as subjects but which will also transgress the boundaries of the hermetically-sealed masculinist analytical frameworks? Two points are salient. First, it is relevant to note the striking contrast between developments in feminist criminological studies (where postmodernists have questioned the validity of the feminist 'successor science' project)[8] and feminist studies of punishment, which remain un-marked by such debates, save for the occasional recognition of the impli-cations of Foucault's analysis of disciplinary regimes for any analysis of women's imprisonment (e.g. Dobash, Dobash and Guttridge 1986). Accord-ingly, a demarcation between postmodern-sensitive feminist criminologies and unreconstructed feminist prison studies must surely be refused if we are to advance the analysis of penality. Second, we should take note that the attack on the notion of an essential criminal woman commenced over a decade ago. The starting-point is usually taken to be Mark Cousins's pronouncement in 1980 that analysts in the crime field should follow the example of the more advanced (that is, postmodern-sensitive) theorists in other fields who had already abandoned stable referents for the categories of 'male' and 'female' and 'masculine' and 'feminine' on the grounds that such categories are 'produced as definite forms of difference by the parti-cular discourses and practices in which they appear' (Cousins 1980: 117).

Taking up what we may call the Cousins gauntlet, Carlen declared war on the idea of a feminist criminology project in the mid-1980s, announcing that:

> *any* explanations of a taken-for-granted 'female criminality' – whether those explanations be styled feminist, radical, marxist or whatever – *must*, by the nature of the project, be as reductionist and essentialising as the much-maligned biological ones.
>
> (Carlen 1985: 9; her emphasis)

This 'anti-essentialist' attack on the foundational assumptions of the feminist criminology project has become theoretically very dense. Indeed, it has injec-ted – (or as Carlen would no doubt have it, 'inseminated'[9]) – a theoretical density, or perhaps opacity, into the 'woman-and-crime' field. A case in point is Beverley Brown's indictment of feminist criminologists' 'mistargeted cri-tiques' of the criminological enterprise. In her view, an 'overfocusing on biologism' – which she claims feminists see as the cardinal sin of crimino-logical positivism – has derailed the feminist analytical project. For example:

the critique of biologism has led to an extraordinary effacement of the specificity of the ways that women have actually been dealt with in conventional criminological and legal discourses on women's crime.

(Brown 1990: 42)

The problem, as Brown presents it, is not only that the attack on the purportedly biologistic foundations of criminology leaves unexamined essentialist assumptions about the existence of a universal 'female' essence which may be presupposed in non-biological terms. More pertinently, the feminist critique of the biologism of criminological discourses has helped perpetuate the belief that women's prisons are organised on a psychiatric or therapeutic basis. A closer reading of Lombroso's work indicates that his was not a 'medicalising strategy': the pressure to medicalise crime came from his opponents (Brown 1990: 53–4).

Brown's complex critique of feminism's faulty 'syllogistic' reading of criminology typifies the approach taken by those on the postmodernist anti-essentialist crusade against the feminist criminological project (Brown 1986 and 1990). Admittedly, Brown's work does not appear to have impacted very much on that project: it occupies a marginal, arguably 'extreme' position along a range of perspectives on the 'feminist criminology' project. Thus, Brown's denunciation of this project could be placed at one end of the spectrum, close to Carol Smart's defiant statement that as the 'core enterprise of criminology is problematic', feminist attempts to transform criminology 'have only succeeded in revitalising a problematic enterprise' (Smart 1990: 70). Maureen Cain's is more equivocal. On the one hand, she insists that a feminist criminology is 'impossible' (Cain 1989: 3); on the other, she claims that a 'transgressive' feminist criminology – one which aims to 'transgress criminology, to break out if it' – *is* possible if we start the analysis outside the discursive boundaries of criminology' (Cain 1990a: 10; my emphasis). Moving further along the spectrum of opinions on the feminist criminology project we find Loraine Gelsthorpe and Allison Morris claiming that the development of 'feminist perspectives in criminology' is still a 'project under construction' (1990: 4). And at the far end of the spectrum, light years away from Beverley Brown's intense theoretical interrogation of essentialising manoeuvres, empiricist studies are still being undertaken in the name of 'feminist criminology' (e.g. Heidensohn 1987).

It is not our brief to enter this debate, nor to concern ourselves with the theoretical and political ramifications of the anti-essentialist critique for analyses of offending women and men.[10] What is of interest, however, is whether feminist problematisations of 'the criminal woman' have implications for the study of penality. Surely they do. First, critical analysis has reached a point where genealogies of 'the female criminal' have become a possibility. The way has been opened for the emergence of a genealogical excavation of the discursive manoeuvres which have constituted women offenders in Western jurisdictions, holding them in place in a powerfully stereotyping, homogenising and demeaning fashion low down on the social hierarchy. Such a development could challenge the masculinist Foucauldian framework's stranglehold on the theorisation of penality in that the very different trajectories implicated in the criminalisation of women will increasingly demand their theoretical place in the 'master patterns' of punishment. At the same time, however, we need to keep in mind the problem adverted to in chapter 4; namely, that a focus on criminalisation, or the production of the 'female delinquent', could have the paradoxical effect of reconnecting punishment to criminality. But as we shall see below, recent feminist investigations in the social control field have found ways around this problem. Second, the application of feminist poststructuralist theories to feminist criminological studies presents an important challenge to self-consciously 'social' analysts of penality. Clearly, empirical studies undertaken in the name of 'women' offenders have become problematic. A simplistic, untheorised appeal to 'women' or 'women's experience' will no longer do in the face of challenges by feminist poststructuralists as well as post-colonial and older, long-standing challenges by black and other women of colour to the category of 'women'. Marcia Rice, for one, makes this point clear in her insistence that feminist criminologists notice that black women are over-represented in women's prison population in many Western jurisdictions.[11] As she says:

> Almost without exception the bulk of research carried out on women in custody has referred to 'women' as a homogenous category and has ignored the interaction of gender, race and class.
>
> (Rice 1990: 60)

But what about black female offenders who are caught between 'black criminology' which has focused on black men and feminist criminology, which is 'largely concerned with white women' (1990: 58)? Almost without exception, studies of women and the criminal justice system, including feminist studies, have been studies of white women and the criminal justice system.[12] The lesson is clear: if criminology must, as Rice argues, 'avoid the use of universal, unspecified categories of "women" and "blacks" in theoretical discussions and in research' on black women offenders (1990: 68), so must studies of penality. Rice insists that homogeneity cannot be assumed for women offenders and, as we have seen, white poststructuralist feminists like Judith Butler agree – any universaling project must have its ethnocentric biases exposed.[13]

Clearly, the main point to be drawn from this brief discussion of poststructuralist and other critical encounters with criminology is that we do not need a feminist penology which repeats the problems of a feminist criminology. It would surely be much more productive to develop what Tove Stang Dahl and Annika Snare have called 'a model for the study of the structural coercion of women', one which starts with an analysis of the coercion of privacy. In a neglected yet pivotally important paper written in the late 1970s, they argued convincingly that in order to move beyond the narrow, pathologising discourses of criminology, we need to shift the analytical focus from 'an etiological concern with women offenders' to 'legal *nonintervention* in the private sector' – that is, to judicial ideologies and legal rules which protect the privacy of the family from legal intervention (Dahl and Snare 1978: 8–13; their emphasis). Included here for consideration are the economic and physical coercions experienced by women who cohabit with men, as well as women's use of tranquillisers, 'a more privatised strategy of control' than the criminal sanctions imposed on the predominantly 'male pattern' of alcohol abuse. But while Dahl and Snare read these forms of coercion as evidence that many Western women live their lives 'in a private prison', claiming that the nuclear family 'represents a prison comparable to the public institution carrying this label', they do not lose sight of the 'public' of women's prison. Noting that the privatised nuclear family and the public women's prison have many institutional features in common, notably the silence enshrouding their prisoners, they argue that the links between these two 'institutions of confinement' merit attention (1978: 14–23). While we still await studies making these links in a rigorously theoretical manner, other analysts, notably Frances Heidensohn, have at least taken up the refrain that 'the best way to understand women and crime' is not through feminist criminology but by studying the social control of women in the wider society (1985: 197).

Certainly, British feminist social control studies which analyse 'how the social control of women leads to state control, thus consolidating the process by which women are criminalised' have proved to be a promising line of research for feminist analyses of criminalisation processes (Chadwick and Little 1987: 255). Specific studies have included the policing of women 'at the margins' – welfare claimants, prostitutes and political activists, such as the peace women at Greenham Common. But the focus has also broadened to include all the ways in which women are regulated; by state power and also within 'the broader contexts in which women and women's behaviour' are socially defined and controlled. While feminist researchers have yet to sort out the theoretical implications of the fact that the policing of women is less formal and less frequent than that of men, their empirical findings indicate a clear pattern. As Kathryn Chadwick and Catherine Little state:

Recent feminist research shows overwhelmingly that gender divisions
and women's regulation begin with the process of primary socialisation
in the family and, secondly, socialisation in the peer groups, school and
the media.

(1987: 257)

Furthermore, as Gelsthorpe and Morris point out, feminist studies which
prioritise 'alternative modes of social control and their interconnections
with criminal justice controls' have revealed 'correspondences between the
policing of everyday life and policing through more formal mechanisms
(1990: 3). On this crucial issue, it is studies of the policing of young women
which are setting the standard in the field and providing new exciting
directions for a feminist analysis of penality.

THE POLICING OF YOUNG WOMEN – NEW DIRECTIONS FOR PENALITY

Breaking out

Studies of young women at risk of state intervention in Western jurisdictions have come a long way since the days when criminologists got on
with the business of pathologising and thus accounting for 'the female
delinquent'. The female juvenile offender, always rendered a pathetic,
marginal figure within positivistic criminology, has made way for what
Annie Hudson has called the 'elusive subjects' of feminist ethnographic
research – 'young women in trouble' (Hudson 1990: 115). Over the last
two decades, feminists researching the social control of girls have dis-
pensed with the usual focus on delinquency and punishment, as traditionally conceived, or even on 'penality' as reconceptualised by masculinist
'social' analysts, in order to discover how girls are policed in their everyday lives. Concentrating on the policing of the sexuality of girls and the
sanctioning of their infractions of sexual codes, they have produced evo-
cative and now comparative ethnographies of girls' cultures, most of them
working-class, as well as studies of penal practices in juvenile justice
systems. By moving away from a limiting concern with the sex discrimination of juvenile justice statutes to the policing and punishment of
young women's transgressions of the gender orders in which they live, they
have demonstrated an enormous but as yet untapped potential to release
penality from the crime–punishment trajectory and, most crucially, to
transform our understanding of the 'social' analysis of penality.

Collectively, this feminist research could be described as a bid to 'break out
of' or 'transgress' the narrow confines of conventional criminological analyses

of so-called 'female delinquents' in order to explore the continuities in the ways in which girls are 'socially controlled across a range of institutions and settings' in Western societies (Cain 1990a: 6). Because of this transgressive effort, we now know a great deal about how girls in Western Europe are policed in everyday life (Cain 1989). The evidence analysed by feminist analysts suggests strongly that girls are sanctioned in their families more than boys; that they are discursively policed by boys and other girls inside and outside their families by a language which focuses on their sexuality. We know too that they are policed into marriage, not least by their precarious employment prospects. Moreover, feminist studies revealing the connections between the policing of the everyday life of girls with policing by and within official agencies has apprised us of intersections between 'the penal structure and the sex/gender structure' (Cain 1986).

Studies of girls have, then, made considerable advances since the 1970s. In particular, European ethnographic studies of the past decade have built on the firm foundations laid by Angela McRobbie's innovative analyses of working-class girls, their subcultures, 'the culture of femininity' and especially her insight that over and above the material limitations placed on girls which are experienced through 'the ideological apparatuses they inhabit', particularly the family, education and the media, 'there is an invisible level of oppression which stems directly from their explicit experience of sexual relationships' (McRobbie 1978: 107). A decisive and productive shift has taken place from a preoccupation with 'youth as deviant, youth as spectacular, youth as a peculiarly and unproblematically male genus' to questions about gender and about 'the ordinary', and to explorations of the ways in which 'commonplace relations, experiences and representations of youth are quite crucially related to questions of the masculine and the feminine' (McRobbie and Nava 1984: ix). This objective is being achieved with the publication of research on the distinctive ways in which girls are regulated, once again especially in the United Kingdom.[14] What has not been previously recognised, however, is that one of the most significant aspects of this 'new' research on the policing of girls is its reworking of concepts of sanctions and penalties – that is, its contribution to a deeper understanding of penality. Thus, for example, we learn that if girls 'are not in need of the same kind of regulation as boys' and if girls are 'less insurrectionary than boys' this is at least in part because:

> On the whole parental policing over behaviour, time, labour and sexuality of girls has not only been more efficient than over boys, it has been different. For girls, unlike for boys, the *principal* site and source for the operation and control has been the family.
>
> (Nava 1984: 10–11; her emphasis)

Furthermore, the processes of regulating girls do not only operate within the family; they also take place in schools, youth clubs, on the streets and in other public places where:

> the regulation of girls is enforced largely by *boys* through reference to a notion of femininity which incorporates particular modes of sexual behaviour, deference and compliance. In this culture outside the home, . . . boys are observers and *guardians* of girls' passivity. . . . It is therefore not only through the family, but also through the interaction of girls with boys outside it, that the femininity and thus the policing of girls is assured.
>
> (Nava 1984: 12; her emphasis)

Thus gender, conceived as a *'relational* concept', one involving 'power relations *between* boys and girls', is central to an understanding of 'the differential regulation of boys and girls both inside and outside the family' (Nava 1984: 13; her emphasis). However, as penality per se is not a focal concern in these ethnographic studies of girls' cultures, the implications for an understanding of penality have not been developed. Mica Nava's objective, after all, was to highlight the failure of the British youth service to provide amenities for girls, not to theorise penality. To take another example, Barbara Hudson's 1984 study, 'Femininity and adolescence', was not primarily concerned with the question of penality but rather with the effects on girls of institutional definitions of femininity and adolescence. However, her insights about the differential effects of these discourses on the constitution of the status 'girl' have a considerable potential to alter our conceptualisations of penality. Deconstructing the discourse of social workers in an East Anglian town, Hudson discovered that whether the illegalities of girls were perceived in terms of adolescence or femininity 'made a considerable difference to the seriousness with which they were regarded'. Her explanation warrants a close reading because of the clarity it brings to a gendered understanding of penality:

> If something can be seen as a 'phase', as normal albeit undesirable youthful behaviour, then the expectation is that increasing maturity will bring about its end; but if a form of behaviour is regarded as gender-inappropriate then there are fears that a girl is seriously disturbed, that she is not following the pattern of normal social and emotional development, and the behaviour comes to be judged not by its own seriousness in terms of consequences, social harm done, degree of delinquent motivation, or any other common-sense notion of seriousness, but it comes to be overblown as predictor of future, more serious trouble. Adolescence is, after all, the status a teenager is moving out of, so that adolescent failings can be tolerated; but femininity is what a girl is supposed to be acquiring, so that any signs that she is

rejecting rather than embracing the culturally-defined femininity are treated (by those whose professional vocabulary enables them to read the signs and offer such interpretations) as necessitating intervention and urgent resocialisation.

(Hudson 1984: 43–4)

The penal practices which flow on from this preoccupation with girls' gender-inappropriate behaviours are well known: girls have been found to be disproportionately institutionalised on grounds of 'moral danger'. The political consequences for girls of the tyranny of culturally-defined femininity are just as clear: they feel 'that whatever they do, it is always wrong' (Hudson 1984: 53).

Taking account of these experiences surely entails a radical reconceptualisation of penality. Hudson herself has contributed further to this project in her comparison of developments in the English and French juvenile justice systems. Here she considers the question: 'justice or welfare for girls?' – that is, are their prospects likely to be enhanced by reforms such as those in France in the late 1980s in the direction of a more welfare-orientated system or by the 'return to justice' policy in England? The answer, she says, is complicated by the fact that girls in Western jurisdictions have been 'disproportionately committed to institutional care for reasons other than offending' (Hudson 1989: 107). Hudson's study can be usefully read as illustrating the ways in which the policy dilemma over the question of punishing girls challenges masculinist theorisations of penality. She formulates the dilemma in this way. On the one hand, she claims that there have been so many blatant inequities in the institutionalisation of girls under welfare proceedings that the justice model would seem to be the way to go for girls. On the other hand – and this goes to the heart of the matter – we must face the problem which is inherent in the 'justice' strategy:

if we rescue girls from the rigidities of notions of orthodox femininity embodied in our judgements of girls as 'beyond control', or in 'moral danger', we do not eliminate girls being judged by the double standard we apply to girls' and boys' behaviour; rather we transfer judgement from a set of stereotypes connected with girls' behaviour within the family to another set connected with female delinquency.

(1984: 108)

For the illegalities of girls are constituted very differently from the norm of boys' delinquency. Most notably, youthfulness appears to be irrelevant to the discursive construction of female offenders: the female young offender is a 'female criminal' as much as the adult woman. The problem is not seen to be her youth so much as her failure to behave in an appropriate 'feminine' way. Consequently, her delinquent acts, Hudson argues, are regarded as more serious 'because they are taken as indications of worsening future trouble'. Why this is so bears repetition:

> Femininity, after all, is something that girls are supposed to grow into, not out of, so signs of thwarted feminine development or maladjustment to femininity will be treated very seriously indeed. Intervention, both drastic and prompt, is thought necessary before things get even worse.

As far as policy is concerned, it follows that

> the justice model approach, with its emphasis on the offence rather than the individual characteristics of the offender, erodes the distinction between juveniles and adults, so will tend to encourage even further this judgement of girls' delinquency against standards of adult femininity rather than juvenile immaturity.
>
> (1984: 110)

As far as the theorisation of penality is concerned, it is imperative that Hudson's insights into the differential penalising of girls must, like the girls themselves, be taken into account.

Barbara Hudson is not the only commentator on the policing of girls to draw out the implications of recent feminist research on young women for a study of penality. Reflecting on research on working-class girls' disclosures about their lives and expectations, Maureen Cain has also made clear the relevance of these studies to theorisations of penality when she says:

> There are real rewards for conventional living, and real penalties for eschewing it. It is therefore necessary for researchers to recognise these realities and the discourse of sexually appropriate behaviour which expresses and constitutes them . . . it is clear that discourses can be used to authorise and justify painful and even penal practices, and that sometimes the use of language can constitute a pain itself.
>
> (Cain 1990a: 7)

Here Cain begins the task not only of transgressing the boundaries which have held penality in place but of broadening its analytical scope to encompass a much wider field of application. In view of the fact that her insights have been informed by Sue Lees's work, it might be useful to take it as an example of recent Western European feminist analysis in the field of social control. To be sure, this has the unfortunate effect of seeming to privilege yet another British study of English girls over studies of marginalised young women in other parts of Western Europe. Much is to be learnt from studies of Spanish girls (Maquieira 1989; Andrieu-Sanz and Vasquez-Anton 1989), or girls' street gangs in Paris (Lagree and Lew Fai 1989), or Dutch girls in a subculture of 'heroin-prostitution' (Blom and van den Berg 1989) or of gypsy girls in an Italian juvenile court. This last study, for example, reminds us that girls are punished by penal interventions as much as by non-penal supervisory measures, and informs us that gypsy girls are more likely than Italians to be arrested and detained than summonsed, and then sent to formal trial, at least in Rome (Cipollini, Faccioli and Pitch 1989: 126–7). As Cain remarks, we have a long way to go with theorising the intersection of gender and race in this field, and the theorisation we need 'depends on a great deal more careful empirical mapping' of the kind found in this Italian study (Cain 1989: 10).

Equally, the study of a failed attempt in the early 1980s to integrate girls with boys in a juvenile prison in southern Italy has important implications for the study of the penal administration of girls. What is powerful about this study is its insistence that the gendering of boys 'is at least one half of gendering' (Cain 1989: 11), and also its elucidation of the process by which integration involved 'the taken-for-granted subordination' of women in everyday life. Gabriella Ferrari-Bravo and Caterina Arcidiacono argue convincingly that 'platitudes of the feminine' which place the feminine 'in a logic of subordination' overdetermine the position of women staff and inmates in this Italian prison (1989: 149–55). Surely no other study of imprisoned women pinpoints the specificity of that penal experience quite so eloquently as in the following passage.

> The presence of women in a male total institution allowed the spectre of the feminine to haunt the prison. We call it a spectre, since we are not referring to a relationship between real men and women, but to the image that the men have of the feminine and that the women themselves have of themselves, which tends to be amplified in a closed institution.

And:

> The institution was preparing at an organisational level to welcome the girls, but on the level of fantasy and imagination it was Woman that was being awaited. The actual girls themselves thus stayed hidden and obscured behind the imaginary Woman. . . . Moreover, if the prison institution relocates girls in a context of institutional subordination, what this induces and elicits is the behaviour characteristics of subordinate groups. The logic of seduction and of sexual challenge is characteristic of someone who is in a position in which there is no other possibility of being seen.
>
> (Ferrari-Bravo and Arcidiacono 1989: 155–6)

In the face of clear evidence within this institution of the pervasiveness of 'perceptions of the "normality" of the feminine dimension that totalises' the young women inmates, Ferrari-Bravo and Arcidiacono conclude that a progressive penal policy for girls must aim for a 'liberation from the oppression of the platitude' and also be informed by a 'specific historical knowledge about both women and Woman' (1989: 156–7). Clearly, their research has done a great deal to open up new sites for excavating the specificities of the impact of punishment regimes on those once 'elusive subjects' – young women in trouble – who are at last becoming, thanks to all these European ethnographies, subjects indeed. Moreover, Ferrari-Bravo and Arcidiacono, while refusing to credential their analysis with poststructural or, indeed, any theoretical reference points,[15] offer a pathbreaking and distinctly 'postmodern' perspective on the punishment of girls – one which sets an example for other feminist interventions in the field of penality. In the light of all this, my justification for focusing on Lees's work may seem feeble: it is simply that her Foucauldian framework forges critical links with other feminist Foucauldian interventions which are currently revolutionising the study of penality.

Going the Foucauldian way – Sue Lees: *Losing Out*

Losing Out: Sexuality and Adolescent Girls (1986) is Lees's account of research based on interviews with fifteen- and sixteen-year-old girls in three London schools in the early 1980s. The aim of the research was to discover the meanings which the girls attached to school, friendship, boys, sexuality and their expectations for the future. More specifically, the aim was to probe the ways in which girls constructed their experience, especially their sexual experience which, as Lees says, is crucial to a girl's identity. In brief, her research findings were that 'girls live in a very different social world to boys – one where being a girl determines everything they do'; that sexually girls are labelled passive objects and that, more specifically to English girls, the 'slag' label is 'largely unquestioned but perpetrates the control of female behaviour by males' (1986: 15 and 26). What is of most relevance here, however, are the possibilities for a new understanding of penality which are hinted at in the conclusions which Lees draws from her research. First, she suggests that, in order to understand the power exercised over girls by the language of sexuality, we need to examine the way terms like 'slag' are actively used as moral censures. Second and related, she suggests that 'the effectiveness of "slag" as a term of moral censure rests on its uncontested nature as a category and on its elusiveness and its denigrative force'. Third, she claims that language has to be seen as a material practice with its own determinate effects, and that one of the most important of these effects is 'the lack of a language in terms of which girls can talk about their own sexuality and experience in a way which does not already define them as the objects of male gaze' (1986: 28). Fourth, Lees deploys a Foucauldian methodology. The Foucauldian influence is apparent in her early declaration that: 'How sexuality is talked about, thought about, displayed and structured is a crucial aspect of social life' (1986: 13). But later the debt to Foucault, this time to his concept of power as 'self-carried', becomes explicit when Lees deploys Foucault's understanding of power as productive of subjectivities to explore the 'power of male dominance which is not "exercised" by boys over girls, but which girls carry with them and which penetrates their lives and their recreations' (1986: 82). Lees's method of discourse analysis – understood as 'a particular way of analysing how ideas, or ideology, function as a system of power and domination' – is also derived from Foucault. What is most significant and novel about Lees's Foucauldian methodology is the way she applies it to those material practices, 'the discourses of sexist power', which constrain girls' lives. As she demonstrates, the policing of women through sexual reputation takes place in language.

> The actions and evaluations and labelling of one another by girls and of girls by boys is the operation of a particular *discourse* about sexuality and moral worth. The language of slag is not exercised by boys over girls, rather both sexes inhabit a world structured by the language quite irrespective of who speaks to or about whom. The double standard of morality is so embedded in language and in the conceptions of masculinity and femininity that girls rarely contest them.
>
> (1986: 160)

If the relevance of this to a study of penality is obscure, Lees spells it out. Drawing on an idea developed in Colin Sumner's sociology of censures, she suggests that the term 'slag' is most usefully understood as a category of 'moral censure' – that is, as part of a discourse about behaviour which departs from, as she puts it,

> male conceptions of female sexuality which run deep in the culture, so deep that the majority of men and women cannot formulate them except by reference to these terms of censure that signal a threatened violation.
>
> (1986: 161)

Lees's agenda is different from ours here – her interest is in developing a language 'through which the legitimacy of slag as a way of censoring girls can be contested' (1986: 162) and with changing social relations and sex education practices in schools (Lees 1989). Nevertheless, her work provides some new and exciting directions for a feminist study of penality.

First, she suggests that the language of sexual reputation, and in particular gender-specific slurs like 'slag', control girls (or at least her English girls) by steering them into marriage as 'the only legitimate expression of sexuality' (1989: 31). At the very least, it is imperative to prove that you are not a slag. Thus it could be said that moral censures like 'slag' cross the boundary established in masculinist frameworks between policing and punishment, inasmuch as the use of this language – as Cain says – constitutes a pain itself. The discursive policing of girls becomes their punishment. Certainly, there are 'real penalties' for breaches of the language of sexual reputation. Second, it is important to emphasise that it is girls, and not boys, who are policed and punished through this discourse. There is no equivalent discourse controlling boys, as 'virtually all of the terms of abuse available are ones which denigrated women' (1986: 167). It follows that a thoroughly 'social' analysis of penality will have to be apprised of the differential effects of sexed discourses which can be used, to repeat Cain's point, 'to authorise and justify painful and even penal practices'. If moral censures like 'slag' are penal in their effects on girls – and Lees shows that they are – then their role in constituting the gendered subjectivities of girls must become as central to theories of penality as conventional, male-focused penal practices.

Thus, while her sociological agenda is different from ours, Sue Lees nevertheless opens up the question of penality to new forms of analysis. Indeed, in its deployment of a Foucauldian framework, Lees's study can be seen as following a lead from the master himself to move away from 'penality in the strict sense'. For what Foucault had in mind in *Discipline and Punish* was an analysis of penality where 'the carceral circles widen and the form of the prison slowly diminishes and finally disappears altogether'. After all, the 'great carceral network reaches all the disciplinary mechanisms that function throughout society' (Foucault 1977a: 298) – including, presumably, moral censures of girls' sexuality. Indeed, it is the development of a Foucauldian approach to gendered censures which has been the most productive in terms of moving beyond the 'women and social control' paradigm (e.g. Hutter and Williams 1981) and responding to Heidensohn's injunction to study 'the production of conformity' (1985: 108). For example, in *Welfare, Power and Juvenile Justice* (1987), Harris and Webb adopt a Foucauldian framework in order to consider 'the social purpose' of the supervision of juveniles. Part of their agenda is to understand how within an 'ensemble of legal welfarism' and assumptions about gender, offending girls 'find themselves subject to a particular regulatory censure . . . they are subject to the attribution of multiple waywardness' (Harris and Webb 1987: 134). Foremost amongst these attributions is that of so-called 'gender deviance'. Drawing also on Jacques Donzelot's work on the policing of families (1979), they suggest that girls' 'gender deviance' is subject to 'a stronger form of that tutelary process which is also directed at working-class boys' (but not, apparently, at middle-class boys). That is, some girls are subjected to 'additional forms of censures' – to 'gender-related prescriptions'. While Harris and Webb are at pains to argue that there are no sharp differences between the treatment of girls and boys within the juvenile justice system, they do concede that there are differences when it comes to the regulation of sexuality. Here again *Discipline and Punish* is found to be helpful. Following Foucault's suggestion that a failure to control, including a failure to control sexuality, justifies more control, Harris and Webb argue that the state's failure to control the sexual behaviour of girls 'creates its own rationale for yet more control and for even finer calibrations of that control which already exists'. Even here, however, they insist that it is possible – although this is unsubstantiated – that similar controls are placed on homosexual boys and that the sexual behaviour of institutionalised boys is liable to censure (1987: 135–40).

What Harris and Webb want most to say is that the juvenile justice system does not systematically discriminate against girls.[16] They manage to concede that 'some girls' are 'more quickly sucked into the tutelary system than boys' and that girls 'seem more likely to be sentenced to tutelage' – that is, more likely to be institutionalised or placed on supervision or on probation orders than boys (1987: 141–2). But still they insist that the tutelary process is not strongly gendered in that there are more boys than girls in care, at least in the United Kingdom. Furthermore, their research indicated that this imbalance could be found across all categories of care orders, with one significant exception: the moral danger category. By making an exception of this the most notoriously gendered criterion for placing girls in care, Harris and Webb are able to press on with their main claims, namely that,

> the evidence for a committed, feminist argument that there is systematic and *generalised* discrimination against girls seems weak, though there are clear indications that *particular* forms of discrimination have occurred historically and probably still do in still to be defined circumstances.
>
> (1987: 143; their emphasis)

At this point we will take leave of this masculinist Foucauldian analysis, marred as it is by an obsession with debunking notions of discrimination against girls, by its reluctant concessions to clear evidence pertaining to the 'penological consequences of being a delinquent, female, child' and by its begrudging admission that, notwithstanding the authors' best efforts to conclude otherwise, the effect of juvenile justice tutelary processes '*is* a disproportionate exercise of power over girls' (1987: 152–4; my emphasis). Let us turn instead to studies which are filling the gaps in our understanding of those still to be defined circumstances in which girls are censured in gender-specific ways.

Sumner's master-censures

Perhaps the most self-conscious attempt to combine a feminist with a Foucauldian approach to penality is that displayed in Colin Sumner's move to establish a sociology of social censure and regulation.[17] This project, which commenced within the sociology of deviance, began as a reworking of that field by means of the centring of the concept of censures. Censures, he argued, 'mark off the deviant, the pathological, the dangerous and the criminal from the moral and the good'. As such they are 'clearly moral and political in character' and therefore of sociological interest (Sumner 1983: 195–6). More recently, Sumner has sought to elaborate his sociology of censures by filling the space left by Foucault's androcentric framework: the new aim is to provide an account of the 'gendered character of disciplinary procedures'. Developing Foucault's ideas about normalisation processes, Sumner argues that normalisation involved the imposition of 'master-censures', including a master-censure of deviance, and that

> most hegemonic censures of deviance are, at a minimum, coloured at a deep-structural level by the master-censure of femininity, in connection with other master-censures.
>
> (Sumner 1990: 26–7)

Sumner takes as his starting-point one which, as we saw in chapter 3, has proved to be fruitful for social analysts of penality: Foucault's argument that the carceral archipelago which was established in Europe in the nineteenth century transported the 'penitentiary technique . . . from the penal institutions to the entire social body' (Foucault 1977a: 298). To reiterate, Foucault's point was that the extension of the carceral and its 'mechanisms of surveillance and punishment' beyond legal imprisonment has important effects. Not only does the spread of the carceral network help link 'the punitive and the abnormal', as well as organise 'disciplinary careers', it also 'succeeds in making the power to punish natural and legitimate, in lowering at least the threshold of tolerance to penality'. Recall that it is 'the extra-legal register of discipline', played off by the carceral system against the legal register of justice, which is crucial to this legitimation of the power to punish. And recall too that disciplinary power is linked with 'the normalising power' – 'the universaling reign of the normative' (1977a: 299–304).

Elaborating Foucault's argument, Sumner describes discipline as 'a strategy of cost-efficient domination that homogenises, simplifies, regiments and scientises an otherwise messy practical world of hungry, passionate and creative human beings'. While discipline is imposed by the state it is not confined to state apparatuses, operating rather 'across the whole social field, infiltrating, linking and extending other modalities and mechanisms of power' (1990: 27–8). Moreover, it is through these processes of normalisation that 'social censures', which encapsulate Sumner's understanding of discipline's response to deviations from normality, emerge. At this point however, he parts company with Foucault. The problem is that in his analysis of normalisation, Foucault not only fails to consider 'the censure of women and femininity'; he never seems to realise that disciplinary power is 'based on a military masculinity' – 'an awful masculinity'. Normalisation, in *Discipline and Punish*, produces 'an apparently gender-neutral, political and economic subjection', but how can this be when the modern subject is formed in 'profoundly gendered' ways and modern social censures and forms of social regulation are 'fundamentally gendered'? More particularly, the censure of gender which, Sumner adds, includes the censure of 'subversive' or 'alternative' masculinities (whatever that may mean) is crucial to the formation of gender division and hegemonic masculinity (1990: 30–5). Foucault writes that men were confined during 'the great confinement' of the classical age, but, Sumner adds, so were women, and much more so in the period which established the capitalist state and, simultaneously, 'the state of hegemonic masculinity'. Foucault saw that capitalism and disciplinary power were interdependent, but is oblivious to what Sumner sees as central: that 'the normalisation process concomitant with capitalist development contains within it the censure of femininity and of deviant masculinities'. Thus it is men's as well as women's bodies and speech that are censured: we are all 'confined by the tyrannical censure of femininity' (1990: 37).

Sumner's appropriation of Foucault's analysis of normalisation usefully opens up a space for a consideration of the gendered nature of disciplinary power and, by extension, of penality. But paradoxically, in opening up one space he prematurely closes off another. Sandra Bartky's suggestion that Foucault was blind to gender-specific disciplines which produce 'a modality of embodiment that is peculiarly feminine' and that he overlooked the forms of subjection which 'engender the feminine body' is given short shrift in Sumner's account. So too is her emphasis on women's distinctive bodily experiences of disciplinary power (Bartky 1988: 63–4). Sumner exhorts us to understand that hegemonic masculinity 'censures *both* the feminine and alternative masculinities' (1990: 38; my emphasis). Yet, while it is well to be reminded that men have a gender too, we must not allow feminist analyses of the effects of disciplinary power on women's bodies to be glossed over so quickly. For these analyses have a potentiality to transform our understanding of penality in ways which seem to have passed our theorist of 'master-censures' by. It is then to these studies that we will now turn.

DISCIPLINING BODIES – TOWARDS A FEMINIST ANALYSIS OF PENALITY

Feminist appropriations of Foucault have occupied a privileged place on feminist reading lists for several years now. His analyses of power, sexuality and bodies have been applied within feminist frameworks across several discursive fields and found to be very productive indeed. In centres for criminological studies, in sociology, politics, legal studies, history, linguistics and philosophy departments and even in law schools, no post-modern feminist academic worth her salt scorns the grand master of disciplinary societies. He may have his faults; indeed he can be found to be contradictory (e.g. Butler 1990: 96–7), and his androcentrism has long been notorious. But he is too alluring to be bypassed altogether. Conversely, those feminists sceptical of the postmodern push are hard pressed to resist taking a passing shot at feminist analysis which succumbs to the seductions of the maestro of micro-power, the doyen of discipline (e.g. Hartsock 1990). Yet, for all this assiduous attention, Foucault's more than passing preoccupation with punishment and his reworking of the moribund field of penology as 'penality' appears to have escaped feminist notice.

This feminist neglect of penality is all the more surprising in that Foucault begins to speak of bodies and penality almost simultaneously in *Discipline and Punish*. Bodies are the surface of emergence for penality. Indeed, the whole point of the opening chapter, 'The body of the condemned', could be said to be the centring of the body within a political economy of punishment. This body–punishment nexus is nowhere more clear than in the following passage on the 'decline of the spectacle'.

The disappearance of public executions marks therefore the decline of the spectacle; but it also marks a slackening of the hold on the body . . . punitive practices had become more reticent. One no longer touched the body, or at least as little as possible, and then only to reach something other than the body itself. It might be objected that imprisonment, confinement, forced labour, penal servitude, prohibition from entering certain areas, deportation – which have occupied so important a place in modern penal systems – are 'physical' penalties: unlike fines, for example, they directly affect the body. But the *punishment–body relation* is not the same as it was in the torture during public executions. The body now serves as an instrument or intermediary: if one intervenes upon it to imprison it, or to make it work, it is in order to deprive the individual of a liberty that is regarded both as a right and a property. *The body, according to this penality*, is caught up in a system of constraints and privations, obligations and prohibitions. Physical pain, the pain of the body itself, is no longer the constituent element of the penalty.

(Foucault 1977a: 10–11; my emphasis)

I have cited this passage in full because its concern with punishment, or more precisely the 'punishment–body relation', has been overlooked in feminist appropriations of Foucault. These have been preoccupied with disciplined rather than punished bodies. Accordingly, the chapters on 'Docile bodies' and 'Panopticism' are the ones which have commanded feminist attention in *Discipline and Punish*. These have been taken to lead logically to the passages on bodies, power and sexuality in *History of Sexuality*, rather than back to Foucault's initial question – that of penality. What has not yet been attempted is a feminist appropriation of Foucault's ideas about penality as opposed to discipline.

Bartky – gendering docile bodies

But we are already way ahead of the story. If we had started at the beginning, we might by now have noted that while feminist scholars have not pursued Foucault's ideas about punishment, several could be described as dutiful disciples in so far as they have moved away from 'penality in the strict sense' in order to trace the ways in which the carceral network imposes disciplinary grids on women's as well as men's lives. Alternatively, we might want to contend that a feminist interest in tracing non-penal forms of control emerged simultaneously with, but independently of, Foucault's. Dahl and Snare's analysis of the coercion of privacy, noted above, is a case in point (1978). But however one chooses to read recent feminist work on the control of women, it is pertinent to observe that, on the question of the 'punishment–body relation', the docile female body has in fact become the core concern of several recent feminist studies which acknowledge a debt to Foucault. One is Sandra Bartky's piece, 'Foucault, femininity and the modernisation of patriarchal power' (1988). Bartky takes as her starting-point Foucault's theory about the emergence in the modern era of a new disciplinary power directed against the body. Gravitating to his chapter on the production of 'docile bodies', she picks up his thesis about the ways in which the disciplined bodies of modernity are subjected to the 'micro-physics of power' which 'fragments and partitions the body's time, its space and its movements' (1988: 62). She also adapts his Panopticon imagery to consider the ways in which women are constituted as self-policing subjects by disciplinary techniques:

> the disciplinary power that is increasingly charged with the production of a properly embodied femininity is dispersed and anonymous. . . . The disciplinary techniques through which the 'docile bodies' of women are constructed aim at a regulation that is perpetual and exhaustive – a regulation of the body's size and contours, its appetite, posture, gestures and general comportment in space and the appearance of each of its visible parts.
>
> (Bartky 1988: 80)

What Bartky fails to note however – and this is a significant omission in terms of developing an analysis of penality – is that Foucault's 'micro-physics' is a micro-physics of 'the *punitive* power' (1977a: 28; my emphasis). Indeed, this oblivion to punishment – to Foucault's captivation, as it were, with prisons – is also apparent in Bartky's rendition of panopticism.

> Jeremy Bentham's design for the Panopticon, a model prison, captures for Foucault the essence of the disciplinary society. . . . In the perpetual self-surveillance of the inmate lies the genesis of the celebrated 'individualism' and heightened self-consciousness that are hallmarks of modern times. For Foucault, the structure and effects of the Panopticon resonates throughout society.
>
> (1988: 63)

Yet Bartky misses the significance of the fact that the Panopticon was, in the first instance, a model prison. Foucault's aim in *Discipline and Punish* was, as he said, to write a history, if not of the prison as an institution, then certainly a history 'of the practice of imprisonment' (Foucault: 1981: 5). So he would not want to say only that Panopticism captures 'the essence of the disciplinary society'. His fascination with theoretical schemas such as Bentham's Panopticon was not that they could stand as a metaphors for modern society, but rather that they had effects – that they were themselves 'fragments of reality' which had effects on penal regimes (1981: 10–11). Bartky's interest, however, is with discipline, not punishment. Her agenda is to chastise Foucault for treating the disciplined, docile body 'as if it were one, as if the bodily experiences of men and women did not differ'. She asks: 'Where is the account of the disciplinary practices that engender the "docile bodies" of women, bodies more docile than the bodies of men?' And she answers:

> he is blind to those disciplines that produce a modality that is peculiarly

feminine. To overlook the forms of subjection that engender the feminine body is to perpetuate the silence and power of those upon whom these disciplines have been imposed.

(1988: 63–4)

Bartky then proceeds to provided a gendered account of docile bodies – an account of 'those disciplinary practices that produce a body which in gesture and appearance is recognisably feminine', focusing on those which govern the size, gestures, postures, movements and decoration of the female body. Her concerns are the nature of these disciplines, how they are imposed and their effects on female identity and subjectivity. She scans dietary regimes, exercise and make-up regimens, photographs, medical discourses, fashion magazines, and concludes that these disciplinary technologies produce 'the feminine body-subject', one on which 'an inferior status has been inscribed'. For Bartky the logical question becomes: 'who then are the disciplinarians?' – who is inscribing the feminine body-subject as inferior (1988: 71–4)? This may well be her most un-Foucauldian moment – *he* was not interested in investigating the agents of control – but Bartky nevertheless makes headway with her analysis of discipline. While her list of disciplinarians – the law, parents, teachers, the media, beauty experts, movie stars – hardly breaks new ground, Bartky makes the interesting suggestion that while Foucault tended to conflate the imposition of discipline on the body with the operation of institutions such as the prison, the school, the factory, discipline can be 'institutionally *unbound* as well as institutionally bound' (her emphasis). Furthermore, the 'anonymity of disciplinary power and its wide dispersion have consequences that are crucial to a proper understanding of the subordination of women'. To be specific:

insofar as the disciplinary practices of femininity produce a 'subjected and practiced', an inferiorised body, they must be understood as aspects of a far larger discipline, an oppressive and inegalitarian system of sexual subordination.

(1988: 75)

In case this picture seem too totalising, Bartky suggests possible sites of resistance such as the transgressive bodily images created by women body builders. Our interest, however, is in the implications of her analysis for the development of a feminist theorisation of penality. While penality is not her concern, relevant themes occasionally emerge. For example, in Bartky's conceptualisation, women who do not submit to the appropriate body discipline face heavy sanctions – they are refused 'male patronage' which may sink employment prospects and deprive heterosexual women of intimate relationships with men. She also notes how women punish themselves if they fail to measure up (or more usually down) to standards of bodily acceptability. Consider too the notion of 'a generalised male witness' structuring 'woman's consciousness of herself as a bodily being'. Importantly, this is not the personalised gaze of a particular male: it represents the anonymous surveillance of panopticism under which a woman takes on the job of self-policing. In this Foucauldian scenario, disciplinary power is orientated towards the production of isolated and self-policing social subjects (1988: 75–7). Such self-surveillance is for Bartky the stuff of women's subordination, but our interest is in the penal or rather non-penal repercussions for women. By now these may be obvious: given all this bodily discipline, self-policing and regulation – a regulation, recall, which is perpetual and exhaustive – is it any wonder that so few of the docile bodies of women end up in prison? In Bartky's narrative, they are always already imprisoned within an internalising, self-disciplining gaze.[18]

Yet if this is so, if women's subordination within an inferiorised body is so total as to be self-imposed, how is resistance possible? How is it that some women break out of the inegalitarian system of sexual subordination, thereby signalling that their not so docile bodies require sanctions such as incarceration? Bartky's discussion of resistance is less than compelling, but her account of the disciplinary technologies which produce specifically feminine forms of embodiment makes this much clear: the idea of the gaze, whether it be designated a 'male gaze' (Kaplan 1983) or a disciplinary gaze (Fraser 1989: 22–3), is Panopticism's gift to feminist analysis of the control of women. For example, in her discussion of authority, Kathleen Jones privileges the concept of the gaze in a way which opens up some interesting possibilities for reconceptualising penality. In order to critique authority 'as a specific form of male privilege', or more particularly to understand why women are 'not entitled to speak', Jones suggests that authority is currently conceptualised in such a way that 'female voices are excluded from it'. Once again a debt to Foucault is acknowledged, this time to his genealogical method. Following this method, we can see how 'the dominant discourse on authority silences those forms of expression linked metaphorically and symbolically to "female" speech'. Significantly, this discourse is 'constructed on the basis of a conceptual myopia that normalises authority as a disciplinary, commanding gaze'. Female speech, then, is patrolled by a gaze – authority's gaze. Genealogy enables us to deconstruct the ways in which 'the subject of authority is constituted so that "female" bodies, gestures, and behaviours are hidden by authority's gaze' (Jones 1988: 120–2). Such an exclusion of the 'female' from 'the practice of authority', as elucidated in Jones' account, is reminiscent of Dahl and Snare's notion of the coercion of privacy. Linking them together is a shared but yet-to-be-articulated conceptualisation of women's lives and of the subject position, 'female', being constrained by such powerful non-penal measures that penal sanctions are rendered redundant in most cases.

Once again, a feminist appropriation of Foucault, this one a study of the control exercised over women by the 'ordered discourse of authority', opens up new dimensions of surveillance. But once again too, the study is not concerned with penality, nor even with discipline for that matter. Nevertheless, it remains germane inasmuch as Foucauldian analyses, like Foucault's work itself, must be judged – as Jana Sawicki argues – 'on the basis of the effects that it produces' (1988: 176). The effect of the analyses of Bartky and Jones is to create a space for further theorisations of penality. Another case in point is Irene Diamond and Lee Quinby's statement that Foucault failed to examine the impact of 'a society of normalisation' on women's lives. They suggest that 'the routinisation of battery, sexual exploitation, harassment and sexual abuse in contemporary society' are perhaps the most oppressive by-products of Foucault's 'technologies of sex' (Diamond and Quinby 1988: 197). But while feminist analysts have yet to consider the implications of such suggestions for a feminist theorisation of penality, the effect of all these studies is clear. Collectively, they constitute yet another one of those breaches of self-evidence which Foucault called for, a breach of 'those self-evidences on which our knowledges, acquiescences and practices rest' (Foucault 1981: 6). Only this time, the self-evidence breached is that of masculinist theoretical frameworks, including that of the master himself. Foucault enjoins us to examine how power and discipline produces docile bodies 'at the extreme point' of their exercise, and to explore punishment and the power to punish at the local level, especially how they are embodied in 'local, regional, material institutions' (Foucault 1980d: 96-7). But in Foucault's texts, these 'extremities' are still discovered within a hermetically-sealed masculinist framework in which the male remains the norm, encased in a de-gendered docile body. This framework must give way to new questions, new fields of inquiry. For example, if, as Bartky suggests, we understand that discipline can be institutionally unbound as well as institutionally bound, we may want to discover noteworthy instances of the disciplining of women not only in psychiatric hospitals, nor even in the institutions of heterosexuality or the family, but rather within the whole range of discursive and non-discursive constraints placed on the female body.

Bordo – disciplining the female body

Here Susan Bordo's work on gender-specific 'disorders' such as hysteria, anorexia and agoraphobia is exemplary. Once again, it is Foucault's work which generates the stimulus for this feminist analysis, but this time *The History of Sexuality*, volume one, provides most of the reference points. His unstable, denatured body is the starting-point, although it undergoes an important transformation here as Bordo shifts attention to the corseted or caged female body. And it is Foucault's concept of 'nonsubjective' power relations which operate without the benefit of a presiding 'headquarters' (Foucault 1979: 94–5), which Bordo draws upon in her study of anorexics, 90 per cent of whom, she notes, are women. What is of immediate interest is Bordo's discovery that the anorexic body is experienced in part 'as *confinement* and *limitation*', as 'prison' or a 'cage', while 'the soul or will is described as being trapped or confined in an alien "jail"' (Bordo 1988: 92; her emphasis). Further, the anorexic 'experiences her life as well as her hungers as being out of control'. Indeed, the feeling that her life is 'fundamentally out of control' in conjunction with 'the feeling of accomplishment derived from total mastery of the body' lies at the heart of this disorder. Themes of confinement, control and even the jail are thus all raised by Bordo's image of the self-policed, tortured figure of the anorexic who, in a bizarre, paradoxical exercise of agency, not only destroys her health but also '*imprisons* her imagination' (1988: 96–8, 109; my emphasis).

Crucially too, Bordo applies Foucault's notion of the body as a 'direct locus of social control' to the female body, a body whose 'forces and energies are habituated to external and internal regulation, subjection, transformation, "improvement"'. Indeed:

> the discipline and normalisation of the female body – perhaps the only gender oppression that exercises itself, although to different degrees and in different forms, across age, race, class and sexual orientation – has to be acknowledged as an amazingly durable and flexible strategy of social control.
>
> (Bordo 1989: 14)

Furthermore, Bordo maintains that the political, that is feminist, discourse about the female body, which is required today to combat the contemporary tyranny of a gender-imbalanced obsession with appearance and circumscribing aesthetic ideals currently prescribed for women, must be a discourse adequate to the task – the task, no less, of analysing 'the insidious, and often paradoxical, pathways of modern social control' (1989: 14–15). Here again, Bordo draws on Foucault, calling for a 'feminist appropriation' of some of his 'later' concepts of power. These concepts, pertaining to the constitutive dimensions of power, are familiar enough. What is new is Bordo's insistence on the applicability of Foucault's injunction to study power 'from below' (1979: 94) to the 'realm of femininity, where so much depends on the seemingly willing acceptance of various norms and practices'. Her particular interest is to account for the 'subversion of potential rebellion' and to confront 'the mechanisms by which the subject becomes enmeshed, at times, into collusion with forces that sustain her own oppression'. To test the utility of Foucault's account of power, she considers three test cases to demonstrate how 'potential resistance is not merely undercut but *utilised* in the maintenance and reproduction of existing power relations'. Her cases are chosen from a 'group of gender-related and historically localised disorders' – hysteria, agoraphobia and anorexia nervosa (Bordo 1989: 15; her emphasis).

The details of Bordo's account of what she calls the 'pathologies of female protest', which function 'as if in collusion with the cultural conditions that produce them', fall outside the scope of this study. What is relevant is Bordo's conceptualisation of the female body as 'a locus of practical cultural control', a control which she insists must be situated in the 'practical lives of bodies' – the 'practical' world of dieting and fasting (1989: 22–7). The repercussions for extending the social analysis of penality to embrace coercions placed on women's lives may become clearer if we substitute policing for 'practical cultural control' and punishment for women's gender-specific forms of pathologised protest. If Bordo's concern with the female body as a site of practical cultural control were read as saying something about policing *and* punishment – as well they might given the close proximity of all these themes in Foucault's work – we might get a different, and certainly gendered, handle on the question of penality. Her case-studies of gender-related disorders can be read as offering the beginnings of a radically different approach to this question – one which starts with the practical lives of gendered women's bodies, rather than with the degendered (read: male) docile bodies which abstract their way through Foucault's androcentric world. Punishment understood as a generative or productive force takes on a new meaning when placed in the context of the realm of femininity elucidated by Bordo and others. In this realm, as they have demonstrated, so much depends on the seemingly willing acceptance of various norms and practices. Penality in this sphere encompasses mechanisms, which enmesh the subject in her own oppression in ways which Foucault could not foresee – mechanisms, nevertheless, which are properly described as coercive and punitive.

More broadly, if Bordo's and other feminist studies of the disciplined female body have been more concerned with the ways in which women's lives are circumscribed rather than penalised, disciplined and policed rather than punished, then it follows that penality must be reworked to incorporate a wider range of controls and sanctions as its subject-matter. Further, if feminist control studies focus more on policing than punishment, it may be that it is time to reconceptualise them both, or, better still, refuse the discursive boundaries which separate policing from punishment. Reading their effects in this way, it is possible to see that feminist Foucauldian studies of the disciplining of women and girls are not only the sophisticated current end point of analyses of the social control of femininity; in the process of deepening our understanding of the ways in which women's bodies are disciplined and controlled they are also transforming penality as an object of inquiry.

Young – hystericised female bodies

Let us take as our final example of a feminist postmodern inquiry into the disciplining of women's bodies one which provides several opportunities for linking discipline back to penality. In *Femininity in Dissent* (1990), Alison Young explores how the Greenham Common women's anti-nuclear protest involved 'unusual deployments of the body'. In order to discuss the ways in which the Greenham women 'presented their bodies as both objects and subjects for the deployment of political power', Young draws on Foucault. After all, she is particularly interested in Foucault's idea of the body 'as the object of the operation of technologies of power and control, while simultaneously remaining the site for potential strategies of resistance' (Young 1990: 14). Furthermore:

> The deployments of the body at Greenham Common are located on the edge between the effects of that 'political technology' of the body described by Foucault, in which the body experiences the effects of control strategies such as 'dressage', discipline, surveillance, analysis; and the potential afforded for resistance to such oppressive conditions.
>
> (1990: 15)

Discipline and now dressage as control strategies deployed against women: this is definitely moving away from penality in the strict sense – just as the master ordered. In true Foucauldian fashion, Young is intent on reworking the boundaries, analytically speaking, of the carceral circle. But there is more. Young is concerned with 'bodies, with the efforts and constraints made around the individual, physical, fleshy body'. Indeed, she insists it is important to begin with that,

> especially as the body has often been the focus of surveillance and control, subjected to the desire to normalise and homogenise through strategies that spill over into the wider social realm over the last 150 years.
>
> (1990: 61)

But the body – 'the individual, physical, fleshy body' – is not the only target of control strategies: 'the individual is also the site for the impregnation of *moral* principles'. It is then not only the physical bodies of the Greenham women which are attacked in the press but also 'their *moral* selves' (Young 1990: 62; her emphasis). At this point in the analysis, Young turns to 'the social', or rather, the notion of 'the social body'. Interestingly, in the shift in the press discourse from reports on individual incidents at the camp to generalised moralising about dirty and unhealthy women, she detects the operation of a social body which, 'like the physical one, is vulnerable to disease and pollution'. In a most relevant way to the study of penality, Young interprets the media discourse as producing the image of a social body which has unhygienic parts which are marked for control 'by the police, by moral reformers, by hygienists'. Indeed:

> The Greenham women have been so policed: in the general, literal sense through the increasing deployment of personnel at the base, and in a less usual sense through the repeated accounts in the press of their dirtiness, their insanitary habits, their morally defective values.

> (1990: 62)

Herein lies the seeds of a new mode of analysing penality. For transgressing 'lines of gender, territoriality, sexuality, familiarity' – for violating 'the symbolic content of the dominant discourse'- the Greenham women must be patrolled *and* punished simultaneously. They are 'subjected to defilement through the language and images of revulsion and disgust which equate them with excrement, dirt, blood and disease'. At the same time, the press also renders this filth an object for consumption by its readership.

> This consumption is the very force of *repression*, which also incorporates an internal displacement or representation. Thus the 'low' life at Greenham is digested by the reader, then thrown out with the rubbish as yesterday's news, a bio-degradable symbol that lives on in the comforted and complacent mind of the reader long after the moment of censure is over.

> (Young 1990: 63–4; her emphasis)

Censure, our understanding of censure – even of the 'master censure of gender' – is transformed here. It becomes a process which is at once punishment and patrol, physical and symbolic; it traverses the discursive and non-discursive. And lest the point is lost, Young returns to Foucault in a section on 'the pains of the female body'. To elucidate the attribution of hysteria to the Greenham women in the press, she draws on Foucault's notion of the 'hysterisation of women's bodies' which he specifies as one of the 'mechanisms of knowledge and power centring on sex' originating in the eighteenth century. Clearly, the 'hysterisation of women's bodies' begs for a feminist appropriation. What might feminists make of that multi-layered process, whereby the feminine body was analysed – qualified and disqualified – as being thoroughly saturated with sexuality; whereby it was integrated into the sphere of medical practices, by reason of a pathology intrinsic to it; whereby, finally, it was placed in organic communication with the social body . . . the family space . . . and the life of children . . .: the Mother, with her negative image of 'nervous woman', constituted the most visible form of this hysterisation.

(Foucault 1979: 104)

While all three of these processes identified by Foucault have obvious uses for feminist analysis, it is medicalisation, or rather therapy, which Young selects to inform her response to the hystericisation of the Greenham women's bodies. Importantly however, she extends the analysis beyond social control theories and also beyond Foucault's 'strategy of hysterisation' which she dismisses, without elaboration, as 'ahistorical'. However, she is not interested in 'conscious interventions' to cure or control the hysteric. Her interest is rather in processes operating at 'a deeper level than that of deliberate labelling'. In conjuring up the image of the hysteric to dismiss the Greenham women's protest, the press drew on a cultural code associating 'feminine psychic crisis' with hysteria. Young therefore shifts the focus away from 'conscious strategy' to the 'culturally unconscious level of a *wish* to condemn, a recourse to gendered notions of reason/unreason, men/women, legitimate protest/hysteria' (Young 1990: 83–5; her emphasis).

Young next turns to consider the question of the hysteric's potential subversiveness, but our interest is in her elaboration of the notion of censure – the censure of the Greenham women 'took root at the very fact of their womanhood' (1990: 7). The censure of the Greenham women had a historical specificity as did the censure of the suffragettes (Young 1988), yet the conclusion to be drawn from both case-studies of 'wild' women protesters is that our understanding of censures must be transformed. Young hints at how:

The conception of censure to which I would adhere recognises that the very fact of existence within the category defined as femininity *implies* the potential for the generation of particular series of condemnatory discursive moves.

(Young 1990: 151–2; her emphasis)

For Alison Young, the 'deviance' which is seen as inherent in femininity has important implications for the study of the 'criminality' of women. But by extension, and more crucially here, her analysis of the censure of femininity has implications for a gender-sensitive, theoretically-grounded social analysis of penality. Young herself hints at these implications when she claims that what is camouflaged by the media discourses attributing hysteria to the Greenham protesters is 'the *control* which is coupled to the cure: alongside the therapy is the means to re(s)train' (1990: 85; her emphasis). Control, censure, therapeutic restraints, and now the capacity of the category of the feminine to produce specific sets of condemnatory discursive moves designed to hold women in place and to punish those who transgress, must surely be included in any future theorisations of penality claiming the mantle of 'the social'. Interestingly, Young's conceptualisation of the category of femininity as implying censure or potential condemnation takes us back to de Lauretis's notion of the 'nonbeing of woman', a being which is at once captive and absent in discourse, a being whose existence and specificity are simultaneously asserted and denied, negated and controlled – a being which, as Young has it, exists discursively within the always already censured category of the feminine. The analytical implications of all these feminist Foucauldian studies of docile female bodies are clear: no theorist of penality claiming a critical, let alone 'social', perspective can afford to ignore them. The political implications are also clear: a progressive penal politics in the 1990s cannot preoccupy itself solely with representing the interests of women imprisoned in public prisons; it must also strive to confront and interrogate those censorial discursive constraints which lock women within the category of the feminine. At the same time, having strayed way outside the walls of the prison, we must not be oblivious to the dilemmas associated with the invisibility of women prisoners, especially now when they are becoming politically visible in many Western jurisdictions. It is, then, to the question of generating a postmodern-sensitive progressive penal politics that we turn in the final chapter.

Concluding note

As long ago as 1979, Steven Spitzer had occasion to observe that:

> Regulations which are generally considered to lie outside the punitive realm may actually be far more important in establishing a structure of domination than the most visible and documented forms of legal coercion.
>
> (Spitzer 1979: 225)

Over the last fifteen years, feminist studies of the non-legal, non-penal coercion of girls and women in Western societies have burgeoned. We now know a great deal about the discursive and non-discursive ways in which Western women are regulated. However, a disjunction remains between feminist analyses of the social control of women and masculinist analyses of penality which for the most part continue to privilege the punitive realm as it has been traditionally conceived. Penality thus finds itself locked into a paradoxical situation. On the one hand, critical analysts of penality have been driven by a desire to make punishment an object of knowledge, but their studies remain imprisoned within the confines of a narrowly-construed, legally-defined penal arena where they continue to focus almost exclusively on men's prison systems. On the other hand, feminist research on questions ranging from the coercion of privacy to the disciplining of the female body, as well as condemnatory discursive moves which hold the category of 'woman' in place, have contributed immensely to the project of developing a feminist, and thus more nuanced, social analysis of penality. Yet none of the feminist studies which we have considered here were primarily concerned with the question of punishment or even penality. We still await a sustained critical engagement between masculinist analysts of the penal realm with feminist analysts of the disciplining of women which will transform our understanding of punishment. However, a useful start in this direction has been made by David Brown and Russell Hogg in their Foucauldian reading of contemporary Australian prison struggles as struggles conducted around and through the body – struggles against bashings, self-mutilations and deaths of women as well as men in custody (Brown and Hogg 1985a: 63). Also, in a more recent development, Hogg has opened up the concept of penality to include punitive policing practices. Hogg has called for a recognition that police stations frequently operate as 'a penal agency', particularly when they are preoccupied with petty public order offences such as those committed by Aboriginal people in Australia. Noting that 'levels of Aboriginal over-representation in police custody signficantly outstrip those in the Australian prison system', he suggests that such discriminatory police practices should be conceptualised as instances of disciplinary power and as a form of penality which he defines as 'a domain of summary penality'. Hogg comments that it has taken the issue of Aboriginal deaths in custody 'to open up this realm of penality to some scrutiny'. Crucially, his scrutiny includes noting that Aboriginal women as well as Aboriginal men are massively over-represented in Australian police cells (Hogg 1991: 3–5, 15).

It has been the purpose of this chapter to demonstrate that feminist studies of the disciplined female body have an as yet untapped potential to transform our understanding of punishment in the Western world fundamentally. In my view, the task ahead is to pursue Sandra Bartky's suggestion that discipline and punishment can be institutionally unbound as well as bound. At the same time, we need to extend the parameters of Hogg's conceptualisation of what constitutes the 'domain of penality'. The challenge, then, is to continue the project of exposing and enlarging our vision of what constitutes discriminatory penal practices, while remaining cognisant of the theoretical and political significance of critical feminist analyses of the private prisons of docile yet rebellious bodies, drugged and tranquillised bodies, famished self-policing bodies in which many women live their lives, 'free' from penal control.

6 Towards a postmodern penal politics?

> So many awkward theoretical, political and practical problems confront anyone who gets off the fence of 'pure' theory to intervene in the rather 'impure' politics which constitute the social response to law-breaking.
>
> (Carlen 1983b: 208)

Throughout this book I have been concerned to highlight a series of theoretical disjunctions or disengagements which may be discerned within the range of critical approaches to Western penal regimes which have emerged over the last twenty-five years. Thus for example, I have pinpointed disjunctions between political economies of punishment which focus almost exclusively on men and feminist analyses of the criminalisation of women; between 'social' histories of prison regimes imposed on men and feminist histories of the imprisonment of women; between masculinist 'social' analyses of penality and feminist empirical research on the punishment of women and feminist theorisations of the disciplining of women's bodies; between research on oppressed groups of women, including women prisoners, and postmodern (or poststructural) feminist problematisations of the very category, 'woman'. Now I want to reflect, briefly, on another disjunction – that between theory and practice. More specifically, I want to conclude by considering two relationships: that between the theorisation of penality and the lived experience of punishment regimes, and that between critique and the construction of a progressive penal politics. Both relationships are fraught, and I cannot hope to resolve here the theoretical and political problems which they raise, let alone canvass all the emergent penal issues of the 1980s and 1990s. But we can at least 'get off the fence of "pure" theory', as Pat Carlen put it, and confront some of the hard political questions.

Of course, it hardly breaks new ground to raise the theory/praxis conundrum in the field of penality. The analysts whose work has been considered in this book have all been concerned to critique penal regimes in Western societies in order to challenge them. Indeed, this has been a continuing theme since Rusche's call for a 'social policy' which would improve criminogenic socioeconomic conditions (Rusche 1980: 44). For example, the theoretical movement to transform the study of punishment into the social analysis of penality claimed to be 'characterised by a healthy appreciation of the need to discuss policy' and to 'intervene in the practical'. Its message was clear: any theory calling itself 'social' had to be 'irrevocably tied to practice' (Garland and Young 1983: 5). Foucault too, as we have seen, saw his role as providing 'instruments of analysis' for 'those who do the fighting' (1980b: 62). The intellectual's role was to set up possible strategies. As Foucault's framework was masculinist, the strategies he had in mind privileged the men's prison struggle, but on the question of linking theory to the penalisation of women, Pat Carlen's work is exemplary. Foucault and Carlen then, can be our case studies of analysts who have shown a great commitment to making theory practical in the penal arena.

FOUCAULT REVISITED: THEORY IS PRACTICE

We left Foucault waxing eloquent about the 'counter-discourse' of prisoners and introducing the concept of 'problematisation' in relation to penality. *Discipline and Punish*, he finally decided, was a study of historical changes in 'the problematisation' of relations between crime and punishment (1988c: 257). Elaborating this theme in yet another final interview, he described the GIP, the Prison Information Group he established in France, as

> an enterprise of 'problematisation', an effort to make problematic and to throw into question the practices, the rules, the institutions, the habits and the self-evidences that have piled up for decades and decades. And that in relation to the prison itself, but also, across it, in relation to penal justice, the law, and, still more generally, punishment.
>
> (Foucault in Gandal 1986: 127)

Moreover, his work on 'the historical relativity of the "prison" form was an incitement to try to think of other forms of punishment', not an attempt to discover 'some substitutes'.

> What is to be radically rethought is what it is to punish, what one punishes, why punish and, finally, how to punish . . . the problem cannot be resolved by some theoretical propositions . . . . We don't have a solution.
>
> (in Gandal 1986: 132)

Thus, when it comes to the prison, one does not lay down theoretical guidelines, let alone solutions. One writes books to problematise self-evidences, to throw them into question or, more graphically, one writes books which can be used as 'Molotov cocktails' (Foucault in Megill 1985: 243). Foucault's histories of the present were to be used in just this way – to expose 'lines of fragility in the present' in order to show 'why and how that-which-is might no longer be that-which-is'. As he saw it, this was the task of the intellectual – 'to describe that-which-is by making it appear as something that might not be, or that might not be as it is'. Moreover, showing 'how that-which-is has not always been' (Raulet 1983: 206) in the field of penality is not merely academic: it is immensely practical work, an incitation, no less, to rethink punishment and penal politics.

On the question then, of the relationship between theory and practice, Foucault is clear: the distinction between theory and practice must be collapsed. That is, 'theory does not express, translate or serve to apply practice: it *is* practice' (Foucault 1977c: 208; my emphasis). Applied to penality, this means that a theorisation of penality is itself a critical penal intervention. But what of the prisoners, the subjects of emancipatory penal discourses? In 'The intellectuals and power', Foucault gives them a privileged voice in relation to the prison. They have a 'counter-discourse', even 'an individual theory of prisons' which, in Foucault's view, is what ultimately matters, and not any 'theory *about* prisoners' (1977c: 209; his emphasis). But if, by a sleight of hand, Foucault can get away with collapsing theory into practice, thereby clearing the critical analyst of any allegation of fence-sitting, his valorisation of the subject position of the prisoner cannot go unchallenged. Foucault's remarks about the privileged speaking position of the prisoner may have provoked Gilles Deleuze to pay homage to the master for teaching us 'something absolutely fundamental' – 'the indignity of speaking for others'. Yet while Deleuze was content to learn from Foucault 'the theoretical fact that only those directly concerned can speak in a practical way on their own behalf' (1977c: 209), others, notably Gayatri Spivak, have been less convinced. For Spivak, the question: 'can the subaltern (read: prisoner) speak?' requires a close analysis.

Spivak's deconstructive Marxist articulation of an anti-imperialist 'subaltern' political movement lies beyond the scope of this book.[1] So does her analysis of intellectual practices which consolidate the international division of labour. But without wishing to do 'epistemic violence' to these her focal concerns, what is of vital relevance here is her critique of Foucault's valorisation of the oppressed as subject in 'Intellectuals and power'. In Spivak's calculation, Foucault's tactic of 'brandishing the concrete experience' of the oppressed group does not stand up to critical interrogation. First, it forecloses the difficult task of 'counterhegemonic ideological production' – ideology being for Spivak a much more analytically and politically potent concept than discourse in class-divided societies. Second, 'the concrete experience that is the guarantor of the political appeal' of oppressed groups like prisoners helps to justify 'advanced capitalist neo-colonialism' inasmuch as it is under the sign of 'concrete experience' that exploitative economic and social relations become 'reality' or 'what actually happens'. Third, and more crucially for our purposes here, when referring to 'lists of self-knowing, politically canny subalterns', Foucault and other left intellectuals 'represent themselves as transparent', that is, as merely reporting on those who speak for themselves (Spivak 1988: 274–5). At the same time they reintroduce a constitutive subject – the self-representing prisoner – thereby subverting their own critique of the sovereign subject. Thus, while the privileging of a sovereign subject is obviously problematic from a poststructuralist perspective, Spivak extends her critique to 'individualistic refusals' on the part of the intellectual 'of the institutional privileges of power bestowed on the subject'. The critic (in our case, the penal analyst) has an 'institutional responsibility' to interrogate his or her own relationship to the oppressed or 'subaltern' group (in our case, prisoners): an abstention from representation, such as allowing the subaltern to know and speak herself, is not a solution (1988: 279–80). Without such an interrogation, without challenging the way in which the intellectual privileges himself or herself by 'selectively defining an Other', we are left with 'the first-world intellectual masquerading as the absent nonpresenter who lets the oppressed speak for themselves' (1988: 292). And through all this, the Third World subaltern woman remains 'as mute as ever' (1988: 295).

Spivak's prognosis for a speaking-for-ourselves prison politics is bleak. It is not merely that, theoretically, she can find 'no space from which the sexed subaltern can speak' in the Third World; also, 'the oppressed under socialised capital have no necessary unmediated access to "correct" resistance' (1988: 307). Still, her enquiry does have political implications for 'radical practice' (1988: 279) in that such a practice must attend to its own ruses of power if it is to avoid underwriting a delusionary politics of self-representing subalterns speaking for themselves. Spivak's point is clear: in his rush to commit himself to the prison struggle, Foucault has left his own theory behind. Anyone who subscribes to the view, as he did, that the critic must represent and analyse 'the texts of the oppressed', while disclosing 'one's own positionality in the process', should have perceived that theorising his attempt to represent the oppressed as 'letting' them speak for themselves is doomed to theoretical and, ultimately, political failure. More specifically, Foucault fell for 'the privileging of "concrete experience"', which is something that is also used by the other side, capitalism' (Spivak 1990a: 56). What then would Spivak say to those, like Foucault, who are in a position to be 'able to speak in the interests of the privileging of practice against the privileging of theory' (Spivak 1990b: 9)? She would say, or at least she has said, this:

> It is not a solution, the idea of the disenfranchised speaking for themselves, or the radical critics speaking for them; this question of representation, self-representation, representing others, is a problem. On the other hand, we cannot put it under the carpet with demands for authentic voices; we have to remind ourselves that, as we do this, we might be compounding the problem even as we are trying to solve it. And there has to be a persistent critique of what one is up to . . . . I think as long as one remains aware that it is a very problematic field, there is some hope.
>
> (Spivak 1990c: 63)

Certainly, the development of a radical penal politics is one such problematic field. In the light of Spivak's comments, the declaration of the GIP that it did not 'propose to speak in the name of the prisoners in various prisons' seems theoretically feeble. So too is its claim (or was it Foucault's)[2] that the GIP aimed to provide prisoners

> with the possibility of speaking for themselves and telling what goes on in prisons . . . we hope that prisoners may be able to say what it is that is intolerable for them in the system of penal repression.
>
> (in Eribon 1991: 227)

That Foucault came to think that the GIP 'had accomplished nothing' (Deleuze in Eribon 1991: 234) is beside the point. We still need to grapple with the highly pertinent issues raised by Spivak's critique of a speaking-for-themselves politics which disavows any representational voice on the part of the critical 'outsider'. Yet, at the same time, we need to ask how 'those of us who have not experienced the pains of imprisonment claim to understand them' (Ward 1991: 225). Is a persistent critique of what one is up to the only available option? Should the would-be progressive penal analyst admit the collapse of critique before the experience of penal confinement? Should the outsider concede to the prisoners, the privileged voices in this field, the impossibility of even imagining their experience, let alone of representing their interests? Should the politically-committed theorist retreat deferentially behind the immediacy and authenticity of the prisoners' narratives and declare a political (if not theoretical) allegiance to the standpoint of inmates and ex-inmates? For example, according to Blanche Hampton, an ex-prisoner and editor of a recent Australian collection of experientially-based stories by women ex-inmates, women are 'usually loath to discuss their experiences' of prison and she is pessimistic that 'much can come out of doing so'. But she asks: 'who other than inmates have such an intimate understanding of Corrective Services and its policies, or lack thereof, with respect to women?' (Hampton 1993: viii). Who else indeed? But what a dilemma for the postmodern feminist who understands that experience, including that of imprisonment, 'is at once always already an interpretation *and* in need of interpretation' – that what counts as experience 'is neither self-evident nor straightforward; it is always contested, always therefore political' (Scott 1992; her emphasis). The question of the relationship between theoretical critique and the experientially-based but untheorised account of the prisoner thus remains an analytical and political problem today, long after Foucault sought to resolve it by allowing the prisoners to 'speak for themselves'.

CARLEN – THEORY AND PRACTICE

As we have seen, Pat Carlen came at the question of developing a progressive penal politics from a different starting point – her research on women's imprisonment in England and Scotland. Indeed, one of her focal concerns has been to formulate a policy which will improve the situation of women prisoners. Carlen's position could be characterised as a 'theory-and-practice position', inasmuch as her considered view is that feminist analysts can combine a poststructuralist theoretical stance with a pragmatic, hands-on policy orientation:

> feminists might both engage in the deconstructionist struggle *and* suggest principled ways in which the criminal justice and penal systems might become more *woman-wise*.
>
> (Carlen 1990a: 107; her emphasis)

And

> Principled commitment to an open-ended deconstructionist theoretical programme, *plus* political commitment to sets of collectivist (feminist and/or socialist) ideals is required . . .
>
> (1990a: 118; my emphasis)

Interestingly, Carlen singles out Carol Smart as her archetypical 'deconstructionist libertarian', a theoretical position which Carlen sees as implying 'a non-interventionist stance on women's lawbreaking and criminalisation'. In her reading, Smart's critique of law as a feminist strategy generates a 'reluctance to engage with the empirical reality of women's lawbreaking and criminalisation', let alone with penal policy. While Carlen wants to make the point that an avoidance of law is not an option open to women awaiting punishment, what is actually at stake here is a fundamental disagreement about the relationship between research and policy. In her view, which she distinguishes from what is presented as an anti-policy position, knowledge gained from theoretically-informed research can be used to inform policy. Carlen concedes that an interventionist politics cannot be read off from theory, but nevertheless maintains that 'neither can one read off from any theory a politics of *nonintervention*'. Academics must not let 'theoretical rectitude' deter them from 'committing themselves *as academics* and *as feminists*' to campaigns on behalf of women lawbreakers (1990a: 111–12: her emphasis).

This position is reminiscent of Denise Riley's pragmatic and strategic directive 'to clap one's feminist hand over one's theoretical mouth, and just get on with "women" where necessary' (1988: 113), in this case with women lawbreakers. Clearly, Carlen is not deterred by poststructuralist scruples about either the politics of representation or the politics of letting women prisoners speak for themselves (e.g. Carlen 1985). Clearly too, she reads Smart's poststructuralist feminism as a disavowal of policy. Yet if Carlen is right that Smart's elaboration of a poststructuralist feminist approach to law reform in *Feminism and The Power of Law* (1989a) gives rise to ambiguities as to her stance on political intervention, Smart's later clarifications indicate that Carlen has misread her position. For Smart is emphatically not a non-interventionist. Rather, she puts poststructuralist theory to work in order to raise questions about the relationship between theory and practice. Her agenda is to question the idea that policy can be read off from either theory or empirical investigation. Interrogating the 'modernist assumption' that once we have the right theory we will know what to do, she argues that modernism's positivistic paradigm, resting as it does on a belief in the capacity of the intellectual to divine the answers through 'bigger and better theories', simply cannot withstand poststructuralism's challenge to its epistemologically naive truth claims (Smart 1990: 72–6). It follows that feminist analysts need to scrutinise their practice and their law reform strategies, particularly those which aim 'to impose a different unitary reality' such as an alternative truth about women's experience (1990: 82).

Returning to women offenders, Smart has no trouble recognising the value of research exposing the harsh material realities of poverty, inadequate welfare, police racism and drug addiction which overdetermine women's lawbreaking. Carlen's research demonstrates that such material realities are 'outlawing factors'. What worries Smart is that Carlen's policy recommendations, promoted on the basis that they may produce more conforming behaviour, entail a compromising preoccupation with vulnerable women who are already marginalised and criminalised. Such policy-driven feminist research simply repeats criminology's will to truth or, rather, its will to power, carried out on the backs of marginalised people.

The danger here is that such research may be used to increase controls over the lives of women at risk of criminalisation. However, Smart's critique of the committed researcher who feels compelled 'to intervene with sweeping policy proposals' in order to 'justify the enterprise of singling out already criminalised women for further interrogation' does not imply a disavowal of either policy or politics (1989b: 521–4). The problem is rather that the feminist 'desire to be political has been confused with the desire to be practical'. The point is not to abandon law or policy as sites of a radical practice but rather to recognise 'the power of law as a technology of gender', without being 'silenced by this realisation' (Smart 1992: 40). Clearly too, Smart agrees that the feminist researcher and policy-maker must interrogate her own theoretical ruses of power, for that, as we saw in chapter 5, is the whole point of poststructuralism (Butler 1992a).

TOWARDS A POSTMODERN PENAL POLITICS

This book has canvassed a wide range of socialist, postmodern and feminist transgressions in the field of penality. Some analysts, as we have seen, believe that it is now time to move beyond this transgressive impulse. They suggest that those committed to the critical project developed over the last two decades have gone too far along a control-orientated, even power-obsessed path in their bid to claim theoretical space from the empiricist studies and punishment philosophies which once constituted criminology's 'sister' discipline, penology. The implication is that social analysis, having transformed punishment into an object of analysis called 'penality' with its own critical history, has not only come a long way – it has gone far enough. In my view, however, the critical analysis of penality has not gone nearly far enough. The evidence for this view is devastating. In the twenty-five years since the re-publication of Rusche and Kirchheimer's *Punishment and Social Structure*, labour market contractions have been matched by a documented increase in incarcerated populations which have stretched prison capacities to breaking point in Western countries, especially in the United States, which in the 1980s experienced record levels of incarceration. In the two decades which have elapsed since the English translation of Foucault's *Surveiller et punir*, Western states have introduced new panoptical modes of surveillance, such as home detention. In the ten years since Pat Carlen put 'the moment' of women's imprisonment firmly and decisively on the critical penal agenda, women's prison conditions have deteriorated and women's prison rates have continued to rise in many Western countries. Clearly, these are all pressing issues: the question is how to address them – how to bridge the gap between critique and progressive penal intervention.

This is not the place to review all those continuing efforts on the part of critical analysts to expose harsh penal regimes and to suggest alternative penal practices. Nor is there space here to trace shifts in progressive strategies from, for example, the heady abolitionist platforms of the late 1960s and 1970s to the more sober reductionist and reformist penal politics of the 1980s and 1990s.[3] Certainly some diehards are still calling for the abolition of prisons. Yet while attempts have been made to devise a strategy for abolishing women's imprisonment (Carlen 1989 and 1990b; Howe 1990c), abolitionists have barely begun the task of addressing the question of the appropriate punishment for violent men, especially men who have been convicted of killing or assaulting women and children.[4] However, rather than addressing this question here, or even the broader question of devising a progressive political response to the emergent penal issues of the 1990s, I want to conclude by reflecting very briefly on the conditions of emergence of an emancipatory postmodern feminist strategy in the field of penality.

Poststructuralist feminists maintain that an interrogation of one's own theoretical position and a refusal of subject-based or identity politics are the preconditions of radical practice. In yet another clarification of this position, Judith Butler argues that 'the political efficacy of feminism' does not rest on the capacity to speak on behalf of a unitary category of 'women'. Feminism's force comes rather from a confrontation with 'its own constitutive crisis of representation'. She sets out two different 'discursive tasks for feminist practice' which have an immediate relevance here. One is that of wielding 'the abstraction of "women" in the service' of policy; the other is that of subjecting our generalisations and arguments to 'internal scrutiny'. So even as we intervene on behalf of women prisoners, we must persistently subvert the 'we' which would objectify and erase these women who are the objects of our representations. Significantly, none of this entails denying that women exist. Indeed, Butler claims that 'women exist socially at sites where power converges in both typical and unpredictable ways' (Butler 1992b: 163–4). One such power site where women undoubtedly exist is that of the prison. Another is the so-called private prison in which many women live their lives. Analyses of the social control of women reveal that discipline and punishment as well as power relations cross over institutional boundaries, impacting on the female body within and without the prison walls. A postmodern feminist penal politics must therefore not only look for examples of contemporary prison struggles conducted through and on bodies; it must extend its ambit to cover all those corporeal experiences of discipline and non-penal punishment.

But what about the matter of punishing lawbreakers? How can postmodern feminism inform a radical practice in relation to the state's power to punish? It can, and must, in the same way that it informs all feminist politics – by engaging in a persistent critique of what one is up to when one calls on the state to punish women or men; by speaking for prisoners while simultaneously engaging in an interrogation of one's universaling self-authorising moves; by constantly scrutinising what our representational politics authorises and who it erases; by always working to breach the self-evidence of 'women' *and* of coercive and disciplinary practices, whatever form they take, and by seeking to overcome the disjunction between postmodern critique and feminist practice. And even as we refuse essentialist notions of already given groups, we will have to tackle the difficult penal questions, such as how to rethink punishment for violent offenders. This may seem like a lot of work. It might also seem dangerous, this self-scrutinising refusal to ground a radical politics in a universal oppression or a common identity, this constant flagellation in the name of postmodern theorisations of the political. But these are the preconditions of a radical practice which does not fall into the universalising and essentialising traps which have constrained feminist, socialist and other progressive representational efforts on behalf of oppressed groups in the past. Besides, 'everything is dangerous' and if everything is dangerous 'we always have something to do' (Foucault 1983b: 231–2). Our work is set out for us. One day it may be reported in another book.

Notes

1 POLITICAL ECONOMIES OF PUNISHMENT

1   Durkheim's supporters include Baxi (1974); Cotterrell (1977); Blumstein *et al.* (1976); the critics include Schwartz and Miller (1964) and Greenberg (1977).
2   See for example, Garland and Young (1983: 7); Zdenkowski and Brown (1982: 6); Lowman *et al.* (1987: 5); Garton (1988: 311).
3   David Garland provides a thorough critical assessment of Rusche and Kirchheimer's work in *Punishment and Society* (1990a), which was published during the writing of this book.
4   Melossi surmises that Rusche's theory does not extend to this later period because his original programme was limited to the period from the breakdown of feudalism to laissez-faire capitalism.
5   The 'stability-of-punishment' argument nevertheless continues to find favour (e.g. Tremblay 1986).
6   But see Chiricos and Bales (1991) and Lessan (1991) for recent salvoes in this interpretative battle.
7   See for example, Cain and Hunt (1979); Ratner (1986) and Jessop (1980).
8   In a similar vein, O'Malley, noting accelerating processes 'blurring the perimeters of state intervention' evident, for example, in the development of 'civil offences' – civil law sanctions which operate punitively – has argued that 'this ideological sublimation of state penal intervention' has to be considered in any theory of punishment (1983: 163–6).
9   See the brief references to women in Rusche and Kirchheimer (1968: 43–5) and Melossi and Pavarini (1981: 35).
10 Presumably, women are more likely to be found in his 'social junk' grouping of passive, relatively harmless elderly, disabled, 'mentally ill and mentally retarded' folk (Spitzer 1975b: 645).
11 The feminist literature is vast, but see for example, Barrett (1980), Sargent (1981) and Acker (1988).

2 'NEW' HISTORIES OF PUNISHMENT REGIMES

1   Larry Ray labels arguments as 'more or less exclusively Euro-centric or really West Euro-centric' when they 'address problems encountered by the Western

left, and make no reference to developments or forms of struggle elsewhere in the world'. The effect of such arguments is to perpetuate 'the patronising and neo-colonialist illusion' that 'historical developments of any significance take place in the West' (Ray 1988: 74).

2 See for example Cohen's list of revisionist texts (1985: 283–4).

3 From Robert White's perspective, one critical of the Eurocentric and colonialist bent of Western historiography, the Algerian War of Independence is of more paradigm-shifting significance than 1968 (White 1990: 1).

4 I have here borrowed unashamedly from Beverley Brown's intriguing critique of the term 'society' in feminist sociologies of crime written in the 1980s (Brown 1986: 363).

5 For an interesting assessment of 'the uses and abuses' of the concept of social control in histories of incarceration see Rothman (1983).

6 The debate over Douglas Hay's now classic social history of eighteenth-century English criminal procedure is a case in point. See for example Langbein's critique (1983) and Linebaugh's response (1985).

7 See especially Spitzer (1983) and also Snyder and Hay's comparative study of social relations involving labour, law and crime in Europe and the Third World (1987).

8 There is now a considerable literature critiquing masculinist constructions of female convicts in Australia. See for example Oxley (1991) and Garton (1991). For a critique of the omission of gender issues in social history and the importance of analysing the construction of female populations by new penal regimes see Garton (1988: 324–5).

9 Daniels notes another dilemma – 'in Australia social history did not ever grow as an indigenous product'. It had to be imported from Britain, North America and Europe (1985: 34–5). For an adaption of this historiographical tradition to New Zealand penal conditions see Pratt (1991).

10 See for example McMullan (1987); DeLacy (1981) and (1986); Beier (1985) and Spierenburg (1984).

11 In an interesting recent development, a mainstream criminologist, Marvin Wolfgang, has joined the Ruschean-instigated debate about the origins of the prison, claiming that the evidence of the records of a Florentine prison constructed in 1301 'pushes back the use of imprisonment as a form of punishment to the early fourteenth century' (Wolfgang 1990: 576).

12 However, they will be raised again in the next chapter, as a large part of this critique of social history's periodisation has been directed at Foucault.

13 Indeed, several critics have questioned whether it counts as history at all. Ignatieff has been amongst the most scathing. In his view *The Prison and the Factory* is not simply bad history; it is not even worthy of the name 'history'. It is so dependent on secondary sources and an 'almost touching positivism' that penal facts can be read off from Marx's theory of primitive accumulation that it fails to produce new evidence or break any new ground (1981).

14 See for example the reviews by Wilkinson (1983), Ditton (1983) and Carlen (1982).

15 For this argument see Melossi and Pavarini (1981: 28–9, 145, 162–3, 188).

16 See also the revisionist-influenced Marxist histories of nineteenth-century penal developments in the United States (Petchesky 1981; Adamson 1983 and 1984).

17 It should be noted here that not all political economies of punishment are couched in a Marxist framework. For example, John Conley's work on the

economic role of the nineteenth-century North American penitentiaries (1980) has been read as Marxist (Garland 1990a: 106). However, while Conley agreed in general terms with the Rusche–Kirchheimer thesis about economic determinants of punishment, he explicitly rejected 'the rigid economic determinism of Marxism and the Rusche/Kirchheimer model' (Conley 1982: 33).

3 THE FOUCAULT EFFECT: FROM PENOLOGY TO PENALITY

1 Barret-Kriegel spoke these words at an international conference in Paris in 1988, three and a half years after Foucault's death in 1984.

2 Acknowledgments are due to Graham Burchell, Colin Gordon and Peter Miller who named their task (and their book) as the documenting of the 'Foucault effect' on studies in 'governmentality' (1991).

3 Foucault's angry denial of his relationship, let alone indebtedness, to structuralism is notorious, but it is not the subject of this book. See for example, his Foreword to the English edition of *the Order of Things*, where he rants against 'certain half-witted "commentators"' in France who have labelled him a structuralist (Foucault 1973: xiv). See also Raulet 1983: 198.

4 Of course, none of this parody of Foucault's problematisation of 'author' is original, either. 'What is an author?' has been subjected to many readings. One of the best is Daniel O'Hara's superb ironising of this piece as 'intellectual self-parody' – 'a recognisably self-contradictory conceit of defensive hyperbole that arises from the exuberance of critical productivity, as if the parodist were almost beside himself with self-opposing forms' (1988: 83).

5 See especially the accounts in Lemert and Gillan (1982); Cousins and Hussain (1984), Dreyfus and Rabinow (1983), Garland (1986 and 1990a) and Bernauer (1990).

6 Unless otherwise indicated, page references in this section are all to Foucault (1977a).

7 In Garland's view too, Foucault uses this concept 'to avoid using a more theoretical term of art that might seem to commit him to a particular psychology of one kind or another' (1986: 852).

8 In another interview Foucault dismissed critics who claimed that truth did not matter to him: 'All those who say that, for me, the truth doesn't exist are being simplistic' (1988c: 257).

9 While I have borrowed the idea of analysing the 'reception of Foucault' from Allan Megill, I can hardly be accused of having followed his example of using this reception as 'a surrogate for the work itself' (Megill 1987: 117).

10 For an extension of these arguments against Foucault in relation to the use of solitary confinement in the Netherlands see Herman Franke (1992). Jeff Minson provides an extensive critique of Foucault's account of the jurisprudence of torture and, more generally, his assumptions about the juridico-discursive underpinnings of penal transformations (1985: 83–91).

11 Bill Forsythe criticises Foucault's thesis and Garland's historical adaption of it in his study of British and German prison discipline in the 1930s (1989).

12 For example, Patricia O'Brien describes *Discipline and Punish* as 'the most important study yet to be done on prisons in the modern period' and then proceeds to catalogue its faults (1978: 512–18).

13 Compare Steinert's Marxist critique of Foucault's periodisation. He points out that Foucault failed to notice that the generalisation of discipline commenced under monarchic absolutism – an observation which raises questions about the claims made in *Discipline and Punish* that the origins of generalised discipline were vague and decentralised (Steinert 1983: 86–7).

14 A notable exception is Merquior's rabid tirade calling for the rejection of all Foucault's work, including the 'shoddy' *Discipline and Punish* (1985). In turn, Bové dismisses Merquior's critique as 'an example of uncritical arrogance that embarrasses everyone involved' (Bové 1988: xxxvi).

15 Steven Wilf's fascinating history of New York's anatomy act is a case in point. He reads the introduction of punitive dissection in late eighteenth-century New York against Foucault's claim that there was a shift to non-corporal modes of punishment (Wilf 1989).

16 I am grateful to Sarah Ferber for her translation of Foucault's 'La poussière et le nuage' (1980f).

17 Barry Smart provides a list of those in each camp. For example, he placed Bob Fine (1979) in the rejectionist camp and Poster, Patton and himself in the 'beyond Marxism' group (Smart 1986: 157–8 and 172).

18 In a review of several Foucauldian texts, Mike Gane names several works, including those of Allan Sheridan (1980), Dreyfus and Rabinow (1983) and Lemert and Gillan (1982) as adherents of the view that 'Foucault conquers all' (Gane 1986: 114). I would add Colin Gordon to Gane's list of sycophants (1980).

19 Michael Donnelly provides a more critical analysis of Foucault's account of the emergence of the prison and its role in the larger story of discipline. See his careful exposition of the shifts in the level and form of the argument in *Discipline and Punish* (Donnelly 1986).

20 While we will consider feminist receptions of Foucault later, the effect of this uncritical reception of the master's androcentric framework should be registered here. Perhaps nowhere is it more apparent than in the reaction to his collection of documents pertaining to the case of Pierre Rivière, the French peasant who killed his mother, sister and brother in 1835. For Foucault the killer's memoir is a text of such 'beauty' that it defies comment. 'Its beauty alone is sufficient justification for it today' (Foucault 1982: 199). His followers question neither this judgement nor his 'identification' with the killer (Bernauer 1990: 182). After all, Rivière's action could be explained by his determination 'to save his beloved father from the tyranny of a cruel, domineering wife' (Sheridan 1980: 132). One might expect this kind of statement from Allan Sheridan, Foucault's most slavishly loyal follower. But it comes as a surprise to find feminist poststructuralists like Chris Weedon going along with the interpretation of Pierre Rivière as 'a questioner of the system without the right to speak', a peasant hero no less, whose murder of his mother and siblings should be read as 'a bid to speak' in order to challenge the exclusion of the peasantry from social power (Weedon 1987: 116). Such a suspension of critical judgement characterises the Foucault effect on his followers who, clearly, have taken their adulation too far. Compare Julie Marcus's excellent deconstruction of the gender bias which litters the Rivière documents and commentaries (Marcus 1989).

21 See also Bottoms's critique of the 'dispersal of discipline thesis' (1983).

22 Garland and Young's collection of studies of penality and the formation of the disciplinary society frequently resorts to the 'penetration' mode. According to

Barry Smart, for example: 'The penal process, from investigation to judgement and to the exercise of penality, has been penetrated by the disciplines and its "tools"' (1983a: 72).

23 Mike Gane points out that the concept of 'beyond' is a favourite Nietzschean conceit. He identifies moves by Foucauldians to show that the master offered a way out of quandaries faced by other social theories, a way which moves in effect 'beyond' the problems faced by those theories (1986: 113). However, I am not joining that particular Foucauldian bandwagon: my usage of 'beyond' is quite different.

24 Garland is prepared to acknowledge that his analysis of criminology as a 'power–knowledge regime' is also indebted to Foucault (1990a: 149). Others have sought to venture beyond Foucault. See for example David Nelken's bid to transcend the Foucauldian-inspired debate between Cohen and Bottoms over the alleged growth of the 'disciplinary society' (Nelken 1989).

25 Garland has clearly failed to consider seriously feminist research in the field of penality. He makes only a fleeting reference to the role of 'gender differences' in structuring penal practices; the feminist research in the field is relegated to a footnote and the women's movement is referred to as a 'cultural movement' (1990a: 202–3). Wife-beating is presented as an anachronistic form of male behaviour prevalent in the sixteenth century, and masculinist researchers are quoted to the effect that such practices would be 'shocking to modern sensibilities' (1990a: 230–1). And finally, crime, including sex killings, is described as having a widespread appeal (1990a: 239) – yet another 'cultural sensibility', no doubt. A close reading of the vast feminist literature which has emerged over the last twenty years on gendered power relations and men's violence in Western countries would have provided a very different form of analysis.

26 Garland takes a similar view of *Discipline and Punish* which he claims 'works less well as a history of punishment than as a structural analysis of power', or more exactly of 'the peculiarly modern form of exercising power which Foucault calls "discipline"'. So his investigation of the emergence of the prison is 'actually a means of exploring . . . how domination is achieved and individuals are socially constructed in the modern world' (1990a: 134).

27 In this respect, Foucault was more explicit than other social historians about the Western focus of his work, declaring that while he could call his subject 'the history of penal policy in France', he allowed 'the frontier to wander about, sometimes over the whole of the West'. But if he needed to talk about the 'whole of Europe' to get at the specificity of the penal situation in France, he was nevertheless consistently clear that it was Western penality which was his concern (1980g: 67–8).

28 Always already covering himself, Foucault came up with a way out on the 'woman question'. Asked about whether his references to the 'hysterisation and psychiatrisation' of the female body would 'advance the women's question', he responded that these ideas were 'hesitant ones' open to discussion, but that 'it is not up to me to lay down' how to use his work (Foucault 1980e: 192).

29 The appropriation of his work by the right is a case in point. See Peter Dews for an account of the exploitation of his work by anti-Marxist intellectuals in France, a development Dews attributes to Foucault's 'assumption of a spontaneous affinity betweeen "radicalism" and socialist politics' (Dews 1986: 103).

30 In 'Intellectuals and power' Foucault mentions that he spoke to a woman ex-prisoner who said: 'Imagine, that at the age of forty, I was punished one day with a meal of dry bread' (1977c: 210). To my knowledge this is the only place that Foucault mentions a contemporary woman prisoner (at least it is the only such reference in English translations of his work), although there are occasional references to the imprisonment of women in *Discipline and Punish* (e.g. 1977a: 33 or 243, where the women's workshop at Clairvaux is described as the 'perfect image of prison labour').

4 FEMINIST ANALYTICAL APPROACHES TO WOMEN'S IMPRISONMENT

1 See Anne Edwards (1989) for an overview of the recent British feminist research.
2 See for example Eaton (1986); Carlen and Worrall (1987) and Allen (1987).
3 See David Brown's critique of critical masculinist analyses which ignore women prisoners (Brown 1987 and 1989).
4 She does however, refer to Foucault's work in her chapter on 'disordered' prisoners (1983a).
5 Prison planners in Victoria, Australia, ignored Carlen's study when they established a unit management system in the state's newest prison for women at Barwon. Reports indicate that this system is having the same deleterious effects which Carlen criticised almost a decade ago.
6 Elaborating on the comparative components of *The Imprisonment of Women*, it is claimed that conditions were more favourable for women in Britain than in North American prisons in the nineteenth century. We are informed too that the reformatory ideal with an emphasis on agrarian self-sufficiency and cottage-style living patterns did not take hold in Britain and, more broadly, penal arrangements in Britain, unlike America, changed very little in the late nineteenth century. On the question of whether imprisoned men and women have received comparable treatment, the book claims that women in prison were always 'treated differently from men, considered more morally depraved and corrupt and in need of special, closer forms of control and confinement'. Further, stereotyped images of 'the criminal woman' and theories about the causes of her crime informed the development of unique penal regimes for women (1986: 1–4; 60–1).
7 See also the section of women in custody in Carlen and Worrall (1987).
8 See for example the methodological issues raised by Janet Finch (1984) and Maureen Cain (1986).
9 As Deborah Oxley and others have argued, it is time to revise the conventional 'gendered images' of women convicts in Australia by moving beyond debates centring on an either/or dichotomy – were they prostitutes or good mothers and productive workers? In a context of widespread poverty and social dislocation, women could clearly be both productive workers and casual prostitutes (Oxley 1991; Garton 1991).
10 Perhaps the most remarkable disengagement is that between analysts of women's imprisonment in the two Western countries where the most work has been done – the United States and Great Britain. Reviews are the only place where engagements (such as they are) with other research can be found. Here

researchers take issue with each other's style. Thus, Rafter berates Carlen for her pompous style and for producing an 'obscure' text which reads like the off-spring of a coupling between a social work report and Foucault's *Discipline and Punish*, overloaded as it is with 'Foucaultisms'. Furthermore, Rafter finds the analysis 'neither coherent nor critical, in the political sense', not least because Carlen 'often seems uncertain of the relationship of her subject to feminism' (Rafter 1984: 388–9). Rafter finds nothing substantive in Carlen's analysis, and this notwithstanding the fact that she shares Carlen's interest in social control issues. Indeed, it is astounding that Rafter, who defines her perspective as a 'social control' one, can find no meeting point in Carlen's explicitly-defined 'social control' study of a Scottish women's prison. For her part, Carlen has continued to ignore Rafter's research along with other important feminist contributions to the study of women's imprisonment.

But nowhere is the parlous state of scholarly relations in the emerging field of feminist penality more in evidence than in a recent, belated North American critique of Rafter's research. In this scathing indictment of Rafter's work, Dorothy McClellan not only challenges Rafter's methodology and rejects the originality of her work, she also questions Rafter's integrity as a scholar, intimating that she has exploited research assistants and claimed their work as her own (McClellan 1990: 144–7). Further, in a misreading of Rafter's summary of the evidence pertaining to racial discrimination in the sentencing of women in nineteenth-century North American courts, she accuses her of coming to 'racist conclusions' (McClennan: 144–7). Certainly, Rafter does leave herself open to the criticism that she labours her point about possible discrimination in favour of black women. And it is methodologically problematic, to say the least, to suggest that the disproportionate imprisonment of black people was a 'function of higher black rates of offending' (Rafter 1985a: 136). However, Rafter's main point is emphatically not that the penal system discriminated against white women and in favour of black women; rather it is that regional variation within the women's prison system resulted in a tendency for black women in the North and Midwest to 'escape the negative effects of reformatory benevolence' which was directed at working-class white women. In the South, black women received harsher sentences than white women and black women everywhere in North America continued to fill custodial prisons in disproportionate numbers throughout the period, 1865–1935. Moreover, while Rafter claims that black women outside the South were 'sometimes sentenced more lightly than their white counter-parts', her conclusion about the impact of racism on the punishment of women in North America bears repeating: 'Nearly all aspects of treatment, then, were shaped by attitudes that devalued blacks' (Rafter 1985a: 147–55).

11   For a more recent 'sceptical look at sexism' see Loraine Gelsthorpe's consideration of the complexities of the notion of 'sexism' when it is 'placed in an organisational context' such as the juvenile liaison office in a British police station (Gelsthorpe 1986).

12   In addition to the Dobash, Dobash and Guttridge study, see Rafter's comments about sex discrimination in the women's prison system in her revised edition of *Partial Justice* (1990: 195–207).

13   To take another example, one of the few places where Rafter addresses theoretical issues is where she adopts control theory to explain changing patterns of 'female crime' (1985a: 128–9).

14 See Jill Matthews's reflections on the controlling effects on Australian women of the disciplinary regimes of both heterosexuality and psychiatric institutions in her now classic study of women psychiatric patients between 1945 and 1970, *Good and Mad Women* (1984). See also Bronwyn Labrum's analysis of gendered committal practices in the Auckland Lunatic Asylum in the late nineteenth century (1992).

15 To take one example, twenty of Carlen's thirty-nine criminalised women were convicted of drug-related offences (1988: 23–4).

5 POSTMODERN FEMINISM AND THE QUESTION OF PENALITY

1 This imaginary sceptical detractor is not to be confused with adherents of Susan Bordo's 'feminist gender-scepticism', a term she uses to designate feminists who are sceptical about the use of gender as an analytical category (Bordo 1990).

2 See for example, Zdenkowski and Brown (1982).

3 There are other Australian studies which analyse the criminalisation of Aboriginal women for example Parker (1987). See also Carrington's study of the over-represenation of Aboriginal girls in the juvenile penal system (1990a).

4 I have specified these conditions, at least for the state of Victoria in Australia, elsewhere (Howe 1986, 1990c and 1991).

5 True, I never fell into the unforgivable essentialist trap of capitalising 'Women' – the 'Women's pain' which made an embarrassing appearance in one American publication of 'The problem of privatised injuries' was an editorial indiscretion, not mine (the capitalised version of 'women's pain' appeared in *Studies in Law, Politics and Society*, 10, 1990). Moreover, when this article was about to reappear, I did insist that if it had to be placed in a section called 'Recognising pleasures and pains', it was not to be yoked to the preceding article which argued for the concept of 'authenticity' in evaluations of women's lives (Fineman and Thomasden 1990: 110–1). 'Women' and 'our pain' rule OK, but please, no authentic experiences. But while I avoided 'Woman' in all my elaborations of the social injury strategy and consciously distanced myself from 'authenticity', I am responsible for relentlessly pursuing a subject-based political strategy for women, one which a recent feminist legal text has catalogued, appropriately, under the heading: 'Gendered Harms' (Graycar and Morgan 1990: 272–307).

6 See for example, Mohanty (1988), Butler (1990 and 1992a), Smart (1990 and 1992).

7 See Dorothy Smith's now classic deconstruction of the concept of 'the everyday' and of 'experience' (1987).

8 See for example Smart (1990). Compare Maureen Cain's development of Sandra Harding's (1986) work on the feminist successor science project (Cain 1990b).

9 For some unexplained reason, Carlen speaks constantly of 'insemination' in her studies of women's imprisonment (e.g. 1983a and 1985).

10 These have been explored elsewhere (e.g. Allen 1988; Carlen 1985 and 1990a). Indeed, the theorisation of 'the criminal woman' – the question of how she is put into discourse, how she is made into an object of knowledge – has been addressed in another book in this series (Worrall 1990).

11   Black women constitute over 20 per cent of the female prison population in the United Kingdom (Rice 1990: 58) and in the United States. In Australia, recent surveys indicate that Aboriginal women are at least fifty times more likely to be imprisoned than white women. Furthermore, the total number of Aboriginal women in Australian prisons has increased over the last few years. In addition, Aboriginal women are massively over-represented in police detention cells. In 1988 almost 50 per cent of all women detained in police cells were Aboriginal women although they constituted less than 1.5 per cent of the female population in Australia (Hogg 1991: 4).

12   Among the exceptions are Rafter (1985a) in the United States and Carlen (1988) in the United Kingdom. For Australian research on the policing and imprisonment of Aboriginal women and girls see note 3.

13   Similarly, Kerry Carrington has insisted that white feminists in Australia need to note research demonstrating the highly disproportionate rates of imprisonment of Aboriginal people. She argues, convincingly, that if feminist readings of delinquency miss the 'differential positioning' of girls in relation to the operation of law, they will overlook the specificity of the over-representation of Aboriginal girls in Australian juvenile penal systems (1990b: 10). Of course, the same could be said for masculinist readings of delinquency.

14   See for example Nava (1984); Hudson (1984); Cain (1990a).

15   At least, they do not acknowledge any explicit theoretical debts in their contribution to Cain's collection of ethnographic studies of the policing of girls in Europe.

16   In a recent Australian reading of 'female deliquency', Kerry Carrington has challenged the view that juvenile justice agencies 'sexualise' girls' behaviours and punish them more harshly than boys. Examining court records for one Australian state, she concludes that girls are 'not necessarily dealt with more harshly than boys and girls are *not* over-represented in statistics for welfare matters in most Australian states' (1990b: 26). Reviewing the statistical evidence indicating that boys are still massively over-represented on criminal charges in juvenile courts, Carrington argues that the crucial issue is 'the *masculinity of criminality*' and not 'the *sexualisation of female delinquency*' (1990b: 15; her emphasis). She also insists that asking why both boys and girls appearing before the courts on welfare matters are treated more harshly than those appearing on criminal charges is an important question which is overlooked in feminist readings of delinquency (1990b: 21). However, a breakdown of welfare cases according to age and a close scrutiny of the 'moral danger' category or its equivalent are required before we can draw firm conclusions which will overturn the established feminist wisdom, which Carrington is bent on challenging, that the sexual behaviour of young women is policed more closely and penalised more frequently than that of boys.

17   Sumner does not explicitly purport to offer a feminist perspective in his contribution to Gelsthorpe and Morris's *Feminist Perspectives in Criminology*, but in his series editor's preface to that book, he insists that the project of progressively reconstructing criminology 'cannot even begin . . . without a recognition of the full implications of feminist work, and without the full participation of feminists' (1990: xii).

18   I am not suggesting that feminists deploying Foucault's ideas were the first to theorise the gaze as a control mechanism. See for example, John Berger's now classic *Ways of Seeing* (1972).

6 TOWARDS A POSTMODERN PENAL POLITICS?

1   See Robert Young's appreciative critique of Spivak's problematisation of the subaltern's voice (1990: 157–75).

2   Foucault's biographer claims that the GIP, Foucault's main concern in the early 1970s, was 'really his movement – his and Daniel Defert's' (Eribon 1991: 229).

3   For a Foucauldian-influenced critique of abolitionism developed in an Australian penal context see Brown and Hogg (1985b and 1992).

4   For an early 'feminist and prison abolitionist approach to violence against women' see Davidson (1985). Rene Van Swaaningen has at least addressed the questions provoked by feminist calls for the criminalisation of violent men, but she does not provide any persuasive reasons for abandoning the use of criminal sanctions against violent men (1989). For a critique of the abolitionist movement's manifest failure to address seriously feminist concerns about non-custodial punishment options for violent men see Schwartz and DeKeseredy (1991). See also Liv Finstad's 'principles for a realist utopia' involving the abolition of custodial sentences for sex offenders (Finstad 1990).

Bibliography

Acker, J. (1988) 'Class, gender and the relations of distribution', *Signs*, 13 (3): 473–97.

Adamson, C. (1983) 'Punishment after slavery: southern state penal systems, 1855–1890', *Social Problems*, 30 (5): 555–69.

—— (1984) 'Towards a marxian penology: captive criminal populations as economic threats and resources', *Social Problems*, 31 (4): 435–58.

Allen, H. (1987) 'Rendering them harmless: the professional portrayal of women charged with serious violent crimes' in P. Carlen and A. Worrall (eds) *Gender, Crime and Justice*, Milton Keynes: Open University Press.

Allen, J. (1988) 'The "masculinity" of criminality and criminology' in M. Findlay and R. Hogg (eds) *Understanding Crime and Criminal Justice*, Sydney: The Law Book Company.

Andrieu-Sanz, R. and Vasquez-Anton, K. (1989) 'Young women prostitutes in Bilbao' in M. Cain (ed.) *Growing up Good*, London: Sage.

Austin, J. and Krisberg, B. (1981) 'Wider, stronger and different nets: the dialectics of criminal justice reform', *Journal of Research in Crime and Delinquency*, 18 (1): 165–96.

Barret-Kriegel, B. (1992) 'Michel Foucault and the police state' in T. J. Armstrong (ed.) *Michel Foucault: Philosopher*, New York: Routledge.

Barrett, M. (1980) *Women's Oppression Today*, London: Verso.

Bartky, S. (1988) 'Foucault, femininity and the modernisation of patriarchal power' in I. Diamond and L. Quinby (eds) *Feminism and Foucault: Reflections on Resistance*, Boston: Northeastern University Press.

Baskin, D. R. and Sommers, I. B. (1990) 'The gender question in research on female criminality', *Social Justice*, 17 (2): 148–56.

Baxi, U. (1974) 'Durkheim and legal evolution: some problems of disproof', *Law and Society Review*, 8: 645–51.

Beier, A. L. (1985) *Masterless Men: The Vagrancy Problem in England, 1560–1640*, London: Methuen.

Berger, J. (1972) *Ways of Seeing*, Harmondsworth: Penguin.

Bernauer, J. W. (1990) *Michel Foucault's Force of Flight: Towards an Ethics for Thought*, London: Humanities Press International.

Bernauer, J. W. and Rasmussen, D. (1988) *The Final Foucault*, Cambridge, Mass.: MIT Press.

Berzins, L. and Cooper, S. (1982) 'The political economy of correctional planning for women: the case of the bankrupt bureaucracy', *Canadian Journal of Criminology*, 24 (4): 399–416.

Blom, M. and van den Berg, T. (1989) 'A typology of the life and work styles of "heroin-prostitutes"' in M. Cain (ed.) *Growing up Good: Policing the Behaviour of Girls in Europe*, London: Sage.

Blumstein, A. and Cohen, J. (1973) 'A theory of the stability of punishment', *Journal of Criminal Law and Criminology*, 64: 317–34.

Blumstein, A., Cohen, J. and Nagin, D. (1976) 'The dynamics of a homeostatic punishment process', *Journal of Criminal Law and Criminology*, 67: 317–34.

Bonger, W. (1916) *Criminality and Economic Conditions*, Boston: Little, Brown & Co.

Bordo, S. (1988) 'Anorexia nervosa: psychopathology and the crystallisation of culture' in I. Diamond and L. Quinby (eds) *Feminism and Foucault: Reflections on Resistance*, Boston: Northeastern University Press.

—— (1989) 'The body and the reproduction of femininity: a feminist appropiation of Foucault' in A. Jagger and S. Bordo (eds) *Gender/Body/Knowledge: Feminist Reconstructions of Being and Knowing*, New Brunswick: Rutgers University Press.

—— (1990) 'Feminism, postmodernism and gender-scepticism' in L. J. Nicholson (ed.) *Femnism/Postmodernism*, New York: Routledge.

Bottoms, A. (1983) 'Neglected features of contemporary penal systems' in D. Garland and P. Young (eds) *The Power to Punish*, London: Heinemann.

Bové, P. (1988) 'Foreword – the Foucault phenomenon: the problematics of style' in G. Deleuze, *Foucault*, Minneapolis: University of Minnesota Press.

Box, S. (1987) *Recession, Crime and Unemployment*, London: Macmillan.

Box, S. and Hale, C. (1982) 'Economic crisis and the rising prisoner population in England and Wales', *Crime and Social Justice*, 17: 20–35.

Braithwaite, J. (1980) 'The political economy of punishment', in K. Buckley and E. L. Wheelwright (eds) *Essays in the Political Economy of Australian Capitalism*, 4, Sydney: Australia and New Zealand Book Co.

Brown, B. (1986) 'Women and the dark figures of criminology', *Economy and Society*, 15 (3): 355–402.

—— (1990) 'Reassessing the critique of biologism' in L. Gelsthorpe and A. Morris (eds) *Feminist Perspectives in Criminology*, Milton Keynes: Open University Press.

Brown, D. (1987) 'Some preconditions for sentencing and penal reform' in G. Wickham (ed.) *Social Theory and Legal Politics*, Sydney: Local Consumption.

Brown, D. (1989) 'Returning to sight: contemporary Australian penality', *Social Justice*, 16 (3): 141–57.

Brown, D. and Hogg, R. (1985a) 'Reforming juvenile justice: issues and prospects', in A. Borowski and J. M. Murray (eds) *Juvenile Justice in Australia*, Sydney: Methuen.

—— (1985b) 'Abolitionism reconsidered: issues and problems', *Australian Journal of Law and Society*, 2 (2): 56–75.

—— (1992) 'Essentialism, radical criminology and left realism', *Australian and New Zealand Journal of Criminology*, 25 (3): 195–230.

Brown, D., Kramer, H. and Quinn, M. (1988) 'Women in prison: Task Force Reform', in M. Findlay and R. Hogg (eds) *Understanding Crime and Criminal Justice*, Sydney: Law Book Company.

Burchell, G., Gordon, C. and Miller, P. (eds) (1991) *The Foucault Effect: Studies in Governmentality*, London: Harvester Wheatsheaf.

Butler, J. (1990) *Gender Trouble: Feminism and the Subversion of Identity*, New York: Routledge.

—— (1992a) 'Contingent foundations: feminism and the question of "postmodernism"' in J. Butler and J. W. Scott (eds) *Feminists Theorise the Political*, New York: Routledge.

—— (1992b) 'Response to Bordo's "feminist scepticism and the maleness of philsophy"', *Hypatia*, 7 (3): 162–5.

Butler, J. and Scott, J. (eds) (1992) *Feminists Theorise the Political*, New York: Routledge.

Byrne, P. J. (1993) *Criminal Law and Colonial Subject: New South Wales, 1810–1830*, Cambridge: Cambridge University Press.

Cain, M. (1986) 'Socio-legal studies and social justice for women', Unpublished paper.

—— (1989) *Growing up Good: Policing the Behaviour of Girls in Europe*, London: Sage.

—— (1990a) 'Towards transgression: new directions in feminist criminology', *International Journal of the Sociology of Law*, 18 (1): 1–18.

—— (1990b) 'Realist philosophy and standpoint epistemologies or feminist criminology as a successor science' in L. Gelsthorpe and A. Morris (eds) *Feminist Perspectives in Criminology*, Milton Keynes: Open University Press.

Cain, M. and Hunt, A. (1979) *Marx and Engels on Law*, London: Academic Press.

Cain, M. and Smart, C. (1990) 'Series editors' preface' in A. Worrall, *Offending Women: Female Lawbreakers and the Criminal Justice System*, London: Routledge.

Carlen, P. (1980) 'Radical criminology, penal politics and the rule of law' in P. Carlen and M. Collison (eds) *Radical Issues in Criminology*, Oxford: Martin Robertson.

—— (1982) 'Review of *The Prison and the Factory*', *Sociological Review*, 30: 685–7.

—— (1983a) *Women's Imprisonment: A Study in Social Control*, London: Routledge.

—— (1983b) 'On rights and powers: some notes on penal politics' in D. Garland and P. Young (eds) *The Power to Punish*, London: Heinemann.

—— (1988) *Women, Crime and Poverty*, Milton Keynes: Open University Press.

—— (1989) 'Women's imprisonment: a strategy for abolition', Occasional Paper, 3, University of Keele, Centre for Criminology.

—— (1990a) 'Women, crime, feminism and realism', *Social Justice*, 17 (4): 106–23.

—— (1990b) *Alternatives to Women's Imprisonment*, Milton Keynes: Open University Press.

Carlen, P. (ed.) (1985) *Criminal Women*, Cambridge: Polity Press.

Carlen, P. and Worrall, A. (eds) (1987) *Gender, Crime and Justice*, Milton Keynes: Open University Press.

Carrington, K. (1990a) 'Aboriginal girls and juvenile justice: what justice? White justice', *Journal for Social Justice Studies*, 3: 1–18.

—— (1990b) 'Feminist readings of female delinquency', *Law in Context*, 8 (2): 5–31.

Chadwick, K. and Little, C. (1987) 'The criminalisation of women', in P. Scraton (ed.) *Law, Order and the Authoritarian State*, London: Open University Press.

Chesney-Lind, M. (1978) 'Chivalry reexamined: women and the criminal justice system', in L. H. Bowker (ed.) *Women, Crime and the Criminal Justice System*, Lexington: Lexington Books.

Chiricos, T. G. and Bales, W. D. (1991) 'Unemployment and punishment: an empirical assessment', *Criminology*, 29 (4): 701–23.

Cipollini, R, Faccioli, F. and Pitch, T. (1989) 'Gypsy girls in an Italian juvenile court' in M. Cain (ed.) *Growing Up Good: Policing the Behaviour of Girls in Europe*, London: Sage.

Cohen, S. (1979) 'The punitive city: notes on the dispersal of social control', *Contemporary Crises*, 3 (4): 339–63.

—— (1983) 'Social-control talk: telling stories about correctional change' in D. Garland and P. Young (eds) *The Power to Punish*, London: Heinemann.

—— (1985) *Visions of Social Control*, Cambridge: Polity Press.

Cohen, S. and Scull, A. (1983) *Social Control and the State*, Oxford: Martin Robertson.

Colvin, M. (1981) 'The contradictions of control: prisons in class society', *The Insurgent Sociologist*, 10 (4): 33–45.

—— (1986) 'Controlling the surplus population: the latent functions of imprisonment and welfare in late U.S. capitalism', in B. D. MacLean (ed.) *The Political Economy of Crime*, Scarborough: Prentice-Hall Canada.

Combahee River Collective (1983) 'A black feminist statement' in C. Moraga and G. Anzaldua (eds) *This Bridge Called My Back: Writings by Radical Women of Colour*, New York: Kitchen Table: Women of Colour Press.

Conley, J. (1980) 'Prisons, production and profit: reconsidering the importance of prison industries', *Journal of Social History*, 14 (2): 257–75.

—— (1982) 'Economics and the social reality of prisons', *Journal of Criminal Justice*, 10: 25–35.

Cotterrell, R. (1977) 'Durkheim on legal development and social solidarity', *British Journal of Law and Society*, 3: 241–52.

Cousins, M. (1980) '"Men's rea": a note on sexual differences, criminology and the law' in P. Carlen and M. Collison (eds) *Radical Issues in Criminology*, Oxford: Martin Robertson.

Cousins, M. and Hussain, A. (1984) *Michel Foucault*, New York: St Martin's Press.

Currie, D. (1986) 'Female criminality: a crisis in feminist theory', in B. D. MacLean (ed.) *The Political Economy of Crime*, Scarborough: Prentice-Hall Canada.

Dahl, T. S. and Snare, A. (1978) 'The coercion of privacy' in C. Smart and B. Smart (eds) *Women, Sexuality and Social Control*, London: Routledge & Kegan Paul.

Daniels, K. (1985) 'Feminism and social history', *Australian Feminist Studies*, 1: 27–40.

Davidson, H. S. (1985) 'Community-control without state-control: issues surrounding a feminist and abolitionist approach to violence against women', *Canadian Criminology Forum*, 7 (2): 93–101.

DeLacy, M. E. (1981) 'Grinding men good? Lancashire's prisons at mid-century' in V. Bailey (ed.) *Policing and Punishment in Nineteenth Century Britain*, London: Croom Helm.

—— (1986) *Prison Reform in Lancashire, 1700–1850*, Stanford: Stanford University Press.

Deleuze, G. (1988) *Foucault*, Minneapolis: University of Minnesota Press.

Dews, P. (1986) 'The *Nouvelle Philosophie* and Foucault' in M. Gane (ed.) *Towards a Critique of Foucault*, London: Routledge & Kegan Paul.

—— (1987) *Logics of Disintegration: Post-structuralist Thought and the Claims of Critical Theory*, London: Verso.

Diamond, I. and Quinby, L. (1988) *Feminism and Foucault: Reflections on Resistance*, Boston: Northeastern Press.

Di Stefano, C. (1990) 'Dilemmas of difference: feminism, modernity and post-modernism' in L. J. Nicholson (ed.) *Feminism/Postmodernism*, New York: Routledge.

Ditton, J. (1983) 'Review', *British Journal of Criminology*, 23 (1): 72–8.

Dobash, R. P., Dobash, R. E. and Gutteridge, S. (1986) *The Imprisonment of Women*, London: Basil Blackwell.

Dominelli, L. (1984) 'Differential justice: domestic labour, community service and female offenders', *Probation Journal*, 31 (3): 100–3.

Donnelly, M. (1986) 'Foucault's genealogy of the human sciences' in M. Gane (ed.) *Towards a Critique of Foucault*, London: Routledge & Kegan Paul.

Donzelot, J. (1979) *The Policing of Families*, London: Hutchinson.

Douglas, R. (1987) 'Is chivalry dead? Gender and sentence in the Victorian magistrates' courts', *The Australian and New Zealand Journal of Criminology*, 23 (3): 343–57.

Downes, D. (1988) *Contrasts in Tolerance: Post-War Penal Policy in the Netherlands*, Oxford: Clarendon Press.

Dreyfus, H. L. and Rabinow, P. (1983) *Michel Foucault: Beyond Structuralism and Hermeneutics*, Chicago: University of Chicago Press.

Durkheim, E. (1964) *The Division of Labour in Society*, New York: Free Press.

—— (1973) 'Two laws of penal evolution', *Economy and Society*, 2: 285–308.

Eaton, M. (1986) *Justice for Women? Family, Court and Social Control*, Milton Keynes: Open University Press.

Edwards, A. R. (1989) 'Sex/Gender, sexism and criminal justice: some theoretical considerations', *International Journal of the Sociology of Law*, 17 (2): 165–84.

Eribon, D. (1991) *Michel Foucault*, Cambridge, Mass.: Harvard University Press.

Ewald, F. (1992) 'A power without an exterior' in T. J. Armstrong (ed.) *Michel Foucault: Philosopher*, New York: Routledge.

Farrington, D. P. and Morris, A. M. (1983) 'Sex, sentencing and reconviction', *British Journal of Criminology*, 23 (3): 229–48.

Faugeron, C. and Houchon, G. (1987) 'Prison and the penal system: from penology to a sociology of penal policies', *International Journal of the Sociology of Law*, 15 (4): 393–422.

Ferrajoli, L. and Zolo, D. (1985) 'Marxism and the criminal question', *Law and Philosophy*, 4: 71–99.

Ferrari-Bravo, G. and Arcidiacono, C. (1989) 'Relations between staff and girls in an Italian juvenile prison' in M. Cain (ed.) *Growing up Good: Policing the Behaviour of Girls in Europe*, London: Sage.

Finch, J. (1984) '"It's great to have someone to talk to": the ethics and politics of interviewing women' in C. Bell and H. Roberts (eds) *Social Researching: Politics, Problems, Practice*, London: Routledge & Kegan Paul.

Fine, B. (1979) 'Struggles against discipline: the theory and politics of Michel Foucault', *Capital and Class*, 9: 75–96.

—— (1980) 'The birth of bourgeois punishment', *Crime and Social Justice*, 13: 19–26.

—— (1986) 'What is social about social control?', *Contemporary Crises*, 10 (4): 321–7.

Fineman, M. and Thomasden, N. S. (eds) (1990) *At the Boundaries of Law: Feminism and Legal Theory*, New York: Routledge.

Finnane, M. (1991) 'After the convicts: towards a history of imprisonment in Australia', *The Australian and New Zealand Journal of Criminology*, 24 (2): 105–17.

Finstad, L. (1990) 'Sexual offenders out of prison: principles for a realistic utopia', *International Journal of the Sociology of Law*, 18 (2): 157–77.

Forsythe, B. (1989) 'National socialists and the English prison commission: the Berlin Penitentiary Congress of 1935', *International Journal of the Sociology of Law*, 17 (2): 131–45.

Foucault, M. (1973) *The Order of Things*, New York: Vintage Books.

—— (1977a) *Discipline and Punish: the Birth of the Prison*, Penguin: London.

—— (1977b) 'What is an author?' in D. F Bouchard (ed.) *Language, Counter-Memory, Practice*, Ithaca: Cornell University Press.

—— (1977c) 'Intellectuals and power' in D. F. Bouchard (ed.) *Language, Counter-Memory, Practice*, Ithaca: Cornell University Press.

—— (1979) *The History of Sexuality*, vol. 1, London: Allen Lane.

—— (1980a) 'Prison Talk' in C. Gordon (ed.) *Michel Foucault: Power/Knowledge, Selected Interviews and Other Writings, 1972–1977*, Brighton: Harvester Press.

—— (1980b) 'Body/Power' in C. Gordon (ed.) *Michel Foucault: Power/Knowledge, Selected Interviews and Other Writings, 1972–1977*, Brighton: Harvester Press.

—— (1980c) 'Truth and Power' in C. Gordon (ed.) *Michel Foucault: Power/Knowledge, Selected Interviews and Other Writings, 1972–1977*, Brighton: Harvester Press.

—— (1980d) 'Two lectures' in C. Gordon (ed.) *Michel Foucault: Power/Knowledge, Selected Interviews and Other Writings, 1972–1977*, Brighton: Harvester.

—— (1980e) 'The history of sexuality' in C. Gordon (ed.) *Michel Foucault: Power/Knowledge, Selected Interviews, 1972–1977*, Brighton: Harvester Press.

—— (1980f) 'La poussière et le nuage' in M. Perrot (ed.) *L'impossible prison*, Paris: Seuil.

—— (1980g) 'Questions on geography' in C. Gordon (ed.) *Michel Foucault: Power/Knowledge, Selected Interviews and Other Writings, 1972–1977*, Brighton: Harvester Press.

—— (1981) 'Questions of method: an interview with Michel Foucault', *Ideology and Consciousness*, 8: 3–14.

—— (1982) *I, Pierre Rivière*, Lincoln: Bison Books.

—— (1983a) 'The subject and power' in H. L. Dreyfus and P. Rabinow (eds) *Michel Foucault: Beyond Structuralism and Hermeneutics*, Chicago: University of Chicago Press.

—— (1983b) 'On the genealogy of ethics: an overview of work in progress' in H. L. Dreyfus and P. Rabinow (eds) *Michel Foucault: Beyond Structuralism and Hermeneutics*, Chicago, University of Chicago Press.

—— (1987) *The Use of Pleasure: The History of Sexuality*, vol. 2, London: Routledge.

—— (1988a) 'On Power' in L. D. Kritzman (ed.) *Michel Foucault: Politics, Philosophy, Culture – Interviews and Other Writings, 1977–1984*, New York: Routledge.

—— (1988b) 'The ethic of care for the self as a practice of freedom' in J. Bernauer and D. Rasmussen (eds) *The Final Foucault*, Cambridge, Mass.: MIT Press.

——(1988c) 'The concern for truth' in L. D. Kritzman (ed.) *Michel Foucault: Politics, Philosophy, Culture*, Cambridge, Mass.: MIT Press.

—— (1989a) 'Clarifications on the question of power' in S. Lotringer (ed.) *Foucault Live: Interviews, 1966–84*, New York: Semiotext(e).

—— (1989b) 'What calls for punishment?' in S. Lotringer (ed.) *Foucault Live: Interviews, 1966–1984*, New York: Semiotexte(e).

Franke, H. (1992) 'The rise and decline of solitary confinement: socio-historical explanations of long-term penal changes', *The British Journal of Criminology*, 32 (2): 125–43.

Fraser, N. (1989) 'Foucault's body language' in N. Fraser, *Unruly Practices: Power, Discourse and Gender in Contemporary Social Theory*, Minneapolis: University of Minnesota Press.

Freedman, E. B. (1981) *Their Sisters' Keepers: Women's Prison Reform in America, 1830–1930*, Ann Arbor: The University of Michigan Press.

Freiberg, A. (1987) 'Reconceptualising sanctions', *Criminology*, 25 (2): 223–55.

Gandal, K. (1986) 'Michel Foucault: intellectual work and politics', *Telos*, 67: 121–34.

Gane, M. (1986) 'The form of Foucault', *Economy and Society*, 15 (1): 110–22.

Gardner, G. (1987) 'The emergence of the New York state prison system: a critique of the Rusche–Kirchheimer model', *Crime and Social Justice*, 29: 88–109.

Garland, D. (1983a) 'Durkheim's theory of punishment: a critique' in D. Garland and P. Young (eds) *The Power to Punish: Contemporary Penality and Social Analysis*, London: Heinemann.

—— (1983b) 'Philosophical argument and ideological effect: an essay review', *Contemporary Crises*, 7 (1): 79–85.

—— (1985) *Punishment and Welfare: A History of Penal Strategies*, Aldershot: Gower.

—— (1986) 'Review essay – Foucault's *Discipline and Punish*: an exposition and critique', *American Bar Foundation Research Journal*, 4: 847–80.

—— (1990a) *Punishment and Modern Society*, Oxford: Clarendon Press.

—— (1990b) 'Frameworks of inquiry in the sociology of punishment', *British Journal of Sociology*, 41 (1): 1–15.

Garland, D. and Young, P. (1983) ' Towards a social analysis of penality' in D. Garland and P. Young (eds) *The Power to Punish*, London: Heinemann.

Garton, S. (1982) 'Bad or mad? Developments in incarceration in NSW, 1880–1920' in Sydney Labour History Group (ed.) *What Rough Beast*, Sydney: Allen & Unwin.

—— (1988) 'The state, labour markets and incarceration' in M. Findlay and R. Hogg (eds) *Understanding Crime and Criminal Justice*, Sydney: Law Book Company.

—— (1991) 'The convict origins debate: historians and the problem of the "criminal class"', *The Australian and New Zealand Journal of Criminology*, 24 (2): 66–82.

Gelfland, E. (1983) *Imagination in Confinement*, Ithaca: Cornell University Press.

Gelsthorpe, L. (1986) 'Towards a sceptical look at sexism', *International Journal of the Sociology of Law*, 14 (2): 125–52.

—— (1987) 'The differential treatment of males and females in the criminal justice system' in G. Horobin (ed.) *Sex, Gender and Care Work*, London: Jessica Kinglsey.

Gelsthorpe, L. and Morris, M. (eds) (1990) *Feminist Perspectives in Criminology*, Milton Keynes: Open University Press.

Genders, E. and Player, E. (1986) 'Women's imprisonment: the effects of youth custody', *British Journal of Criminology*, 26 (4): 357–71.

Genovese, E. F. and Genovese, E. D. (1976) 'The political crisis of social history', *Journal of Social History*, 10 (2): 205–21.

Giallombardo, R. (1966) *Society of Women: A Study of a Women's Prison*, New York: Wiley.

Gordon, C. (ed.) (1980) *Michel Foucault: Power/Knowledge, Selected Interviews and other Writings, 1972–1977*, Brighton: Harvester Press.

Graycar, R. and Morgan, J. (1990) *The Hidden Gender of Law*, Sydney: Federation Press.

Greenberg, D. (1977) 'The dynamics of oscillatory punishment processes', *The Journal of Criminal Law and Criminology*, 68 (4): 643–51.

—— (1980) 'Penal sanctions in Poland: a test of alternative models', *Social Problems*, 28 (2): 194–204.

Greenwood, V. (1981) 'The myths of female crime' in A. Morris (ed.) *Women and Crime: Papers Presented to the Cropwood Round Table Conference*, Cambridge: Cambridge University Press.

Hale, C. (1989) 'Economy, punishment and imprisonment', *Contemporary Crises*, 13 (4): 327–350.

Hall, J. (1939) 'Review of *Punishment and Social Structure*', *Journal of Criminal Law and Criminology*, XXX (6): 971–2.

Hampton, B. (1993) *Prisons and Women*, Sydney: New South Wales University Press.

Harding, C. and Ireland, R. W. (1989) *Punishment, Rhetoric, Rule and Practice*, London: Routledge.

Harding, S. (1986) *The Science Question in Feminism*, Ithaca: Cornell University Press.

Harlow, B. (1986) 'From the women's prison: Third World women's narratives of prison' *Feminist Studies*, 12 (3): 501–24.

Harris, R. and Webb, D. (1987) *Welfare, Power and Juvenile Justice*, London: Tavistock.

Hartsock, N. (1990) 'Foucault on power: a theory for women?' in L. J. Nicholson (ed.) *Feminism/Postmodernism*, New York: Routledge.

Heidensohn, F. (1985) *Women and Crime*, London: Macmillan.

—— (1987) 'Women and crime: questions for criminology' in P. Carlen and A. Worrall (eds) *Gender, Crime and Justice*, Milton Keynes: Open University Press.

Hogg, R. (1980) 'Imprisonment and society under early British capitalism' in T. Platt and P. Takagi (eds) *Punishment and Penal Discipline*, Berkeley: Crime and Social Justice Asssociates.

—— (1991) 'Policing and penality', *Journal for Social Justice Studies*, 4: 1–26.

Horwitz, A. (1977) 'Marxist theories of deviance and teleology: a critique of Spitzer', *Social Problems*, 24 (3): 362–3.

Howe, A. (1986) 'Equal justice for women prisoners: why settle for less?', *Refractory Girl*, 29: 20–3.

—— (1987) '"Social injury revisted": towards a feminist theory of social justice', *International Journal of the Sociology of Law*, 15 (4): 423–38.

—— (1988) 'Aboriginal women in custody: a footnote to the Royal Commission', *Aboriginal Legal Bulletin*, 30: 5–7.

—— (1990a) 'The problem of privatised injuries: feminist strategies for litigation', in M. Fineman (ed.) *At the Boundaries of Law: Feminism and Legal Theory*, New York: Routledge.

—— (1990b) 'Sweet dreams: deinstitutionalising young women' in R. Graycar (ed.) *Dissenting Opinions: Feminist Explorations in Law and Society*, Sydney: Allen & Unwin.

—— (1990c) 'Sentencing women to prison in Victoria: a research and political agenda', *Law in Context*, 8 (2): 32–53.

—— (1991) 'Postmodern penal politics? Further footnotes on women prisoners', *Journal for Social Justice Studies*, 4: 61–72.

Hudson, A. (1990) '"Elusive subjects": researching young women in trouble' in L. Gelsthorpe and A. Morris (eds) *Feminist Perspectives in Criminology*, Milton Keynes: Open University Press.

Hudson, B. (1984) 'Femininity and adolescence' in A. McRobbie and M. Nava (eds) *Gender and Generation*, London: Macmillan.

—— (1987) *Justice Through Punishment: A Critique of the Justice Model of Corrections*, London: Macmillan.

—— (1989) 'Justice or welfare? A comparison of recent developments in the English and French juvenile justice systems' in M. Cain (ed.) *Growing up Good: Policing the Behaviour of Girls in Europe*, London: Sage.

Hughes, R. (1987) *The Fatal Shore*, London: Collins Harvill.

Humphries, D. and Greenberg, D. F. (1981) 'The dialectics of crime control' in D. F. Greenberg (ed.) *Crime and Capitalism: Readings in Marxist Criminology*, Palo Alto, Cal.: Mayfield.

Hutter, B. and Williams, G. (eds) (1981) *Controlling Women: The Normal and the Deviant*, London: Croom Helm.

Ignatieff, M. (1978) *A Just Measure of Pain: The Penitentiary in the Industrial Revolution, 1750–1850*, New York: Pantheon.

—— (1981) 'Review: the prison and the factory', *New Society*, 237–8.

—— (1982) 'Class interests and the penitentiary: a response to Rothman', *Canadian Criminology Forum*, 5.

—— (1983a) 'State, civil society and total institutions: a critique of recent social histories of punishment' in S. Cohen and A. Scull (eds) *Social Control and the State*, Oxford: Martin Robertson.

—— (1983b) 'Total institutions and working classes: a review essay', *History Workshop*, 15: 167–73.

Innes, J. (1987) 'Prisons for the poor: English bridewells, 1555–1800' in F. Synder and D. Hay (eds) *Labour, Law and Crime: An Historical Perspective*, London: Tavistock.

Inverarity, J. and Grattet, R. (1989) 'Institutional responses to unemployment: a comparison of U.S. trends, 1948–85', *Contemporary Crises*, 13 (4): 351–70.

Jacobs. J. B. (1977) 'Macrosociology and imprisonment' in D. F. Greenberg (ed.) *Corrections and Punishment*, London: Sage.

Jankovic, I. (1977) 'Labour market and imprisonment', *Crime and Social Justice*, 8: 17–31.

—— (1983) 'Review of *The Prison and the Factory*', *Contemporary Crises*, 7 (4): 393–6.

Jessop, B. (1980) 'On recent Marxist theories of law, the state and juridico-political ideology', *International Journal of the Sociology of Law*, 8 (4): 339–68.

Jones, K. B. (1988) 'On authority: or, why women are not entitled to speak' in I. Diamond and L. Quinby (eds) *Feminism and Foucault: Reflections on Resistance*, Boston: Northeastern University Press.

Judt, T. (1979) 'A clown in regal purple: social history and the historians', *History Workshop*, 7: 67–94.

Kaplan, E. A. (1983) 'Is the gaze male?' in A. Snitow and C. Stanswell (eds) *Desire: The Politics of Sexuality*, London: Virago.

Kempinen, C. (1983) 'Changes in the sentencing patterns of male and female defendants', *The Prison Journal*, 63 (2): 3–11.

Labrum, B. (1992) 'Looking beyond the asylum: gender and the process of committal in Auckland, 1870–1910', *The New Zealand Journal of History*, 26 (2): 125–45.

Laffargue, B. and Godefroy, T. (1989) 'Economic cycles and punishment: unemployment and imprisonment', *Contemporary Crises*, 13 (4): 371–404.

Lagree, J. and Lew Fai, P. (1989) 'Girls in street gangs in the suburbs of Paris' in M. Cain (ed.) *Growing up Good: Policing the Behaviour of Girls in Europe*, London: Sage.

Langbein, J. H. (1983) 'Albion's fatal flaws', *Past and Present*, 98: 96–120.

Lauretis, T. de (1990) 'Eccentric subjects: feminist theory and historical consciousness', *Feminist Studies*, 16 (1): 115–50.

Lea, J. (1979) 'Discipline and capitalist development' in B. Fine *et al.* (eds) *Capitalism and the Rule of Law*, London: Hutchinson.

Lees, S. (1986) *Losing Out: Sexuality and Adolescent Girls*, London: Hutchinson.

—— (1989) 'Learning to love: sexual reputation, morality and the social control of girls' in M. Cain (ed.) *Growing up Good: Policing the Behaviour of Girls in Europe*, London: Sage.

Lemert, C. and Gillan, G. (1982) *Michel Foucault: Social Theory and Transgression*, New York: Columbia University Press.

Lessan, G. T. (1991) 'Macro-economic determinants of penal policy: estimating the unemployment and inflation influences on imprisonment rate changes in the United States, 1948–1985', *Crime, Law and Social Change*, 16 (3): 177–98.

Linebaugh, P. (1985) '(Marxist) social history and (conservative) legal history: a reply to professor Langbein', *New York University Law Review*, 60 (2): 212–43.

Lowman, J., Menzies, R. J. and Palys, T. S. (eds) (1987) *Transcarceration: Essays in the Sociology of Social Control*, Brookfield, Vt: Gower.

Lukes, S. and Scull, A. (1983) *Durkheim and the Law*, Oxford: Martin Robertson.

Lynch, M. J. (1988) 'The extraction of surplus value, crime and punishment: a preliminary examination', *Contemporary Crises*, 12 (4): 329–44.

McClellan, D. S. (1990) 'Two books on women and imprisonment', *Social Justice*, 17 (2): 141–7.

McMullan J. L. (1987) 'Crime, law and order in early modern England', *British Journal of Criminology*, 27 (3): 252–74.

McRobbie, A. (1978) 'Working class girls and the culture of femininity' in Women's Studies Group (eds) *Women Take Issue: Aspects of Women's Subordination*, London: Hutchinson.

—— (1982) 'Review', *International Journal of the Sociology of Law*, 10 (2): 217–20.

McRobbie, A. and Nava, M. (1984) *Gender and Generation*, London: Macmillan.

Mandel, M. (1982) 'Review of *The Prison and the Factory*', *Journal of Criminal Law and Criminology*, 73 (2): 848–50.

Maquieira, V. (1989) 'Boys, girls and the discourse of identity' in M. Cain (ed.) *Growing up Good: Policing the Behaviour of Girls in Europe*, London: Sage.

Marcus, J. (1989) 'The death of the family: Pierre Riviere, Foucault and gender', *Criticism, Heresy and Interpretation*, 2: 67–82.

Martin, J. P. (1988) 'Review', *British Journal of Criminology*, 28 (3): 404–7.

Marx, K. (1970) *Capital*, 1, London: Lawrence & Wishart.

Matthews, J. (1984) *Good and Mad Women*, Sydney: George Allen & Unwin.

Mayer, J. A. (1983) 'Notes towards a working definition of social control in historical analysis' in S. Cohen and A. Scull (eds) *Social Control and the State*, Oxford, Martin Robertson.

Megill, A. (1985) *Prophets of Extremity: Nietzsche, Heidegger, Foucault, Derrida*, Berkeley: University of California Press.

—— (1987) 'The reception of Foucault by historians', *Journal of the History of Ideas*, XLVIII (1): 117–41.

Melossi, D. (1976) 'The penal question in capital', *Crime and Social Justice*, 6: 26–33.

—— (1978) 'Georg Rusche and Otto Kirchheimer: *Punishment and Social Structure*', *Crime and Social Justice*, 9: 73–85.

—— (1979) 'Institutions of social control and the capitalist orgnaisation of work' in B. Fine *et al.* (eds) *Capitalism and the Rule of Law*, London: Heinemann.

—— (1980) 'Georg Rusche: a biographical essay', *Crime and Social Justice*, 14: 51–63.

—— (1985a) 'Punishment and social action: changing vocabularies of punitive motive within a political business cycle', *Current Perspectives in Social Theory*, 6: 169–97.

—— (1985b) 'Overcoming the crisis in critical criminology: toward a grounded labelling theory', *Criminology*, 23 (2): 193–208.

—— (1989) 'An introduction: fifty years later, *Punishment and Social Structure* in comparative analysis', *Contemporary Crises*, 13 (4): 311–26.

—— (1990) *The State of Social Control*, Oxford: Basil Blackwell.

Melossi, D. and Pavarini, M. (1981) *The Prison and the Factory: Origins of the Penitentiary System*, London: Macmillan.

Merquior, J. G. (1985) *Foucault*, London: Fontana Press.

Miller, N. K. (1986) 'Changing the subject: authorship, writing and the reader' in T. de Lauretis (ed.) *Feminist Studies/Critical Studies*, Bloomington: Indiana University Press.

Minson, J. (1985) *Genealogies of Morals: Nietzsche, Foucault, Donzelot and the Eccentricity of Ethics*, London: Macmillan.

—— (1986) 'Strategies for socialists? Foucault's conception of power' in M. Gane (ed.) *Towards a Critique of Foucault*, London: Routledge & Kegan Paul.

Mohanty, C. (1988) 'Under western eyes: feminist scholarship and colonial discourses', *Feminist Review*, 30: 61–88.

Morris, M. (1988) 'The pirate's fiancée' in M. Morris, *The Pirate's Fiancée: Feminism, Reading, Postmodernism*, London: Verso.

Muñoz Gómez, J. (1988) 'Notes toward a historical understanding of the Columbian penal system', *Crime and Social Justice*, 30: 60–77.

Muraskin, W. A. (1976) 'The social-control theory in American history: a critique', *Journal of Social History*, 9 (4): 559–69.

Nava, M. (1984) 'Youth service provision, social order and the question of girls' in A. McRobbie and M. Nava (eds) *Gender and Generation*, London: Macmillan.

Nelken, D. (1989) 'Discipline and punish: some notes on the margin', *The Howard Journal*, 28 (4): 245–54.

Nicholson, L. (1990) (ed.) *Feminism/Postmodernism*, London: Routledge.

O'Brien, P. (1978) 'Crime and punishment as historical problem', *Journal of Social History*, 11 (4): 508–20.

—— (1982) *The Promise of Punishment: Prisons in Nineteenth Century France*, Princeton: Princeton University Press.

O'Hara, D. T. (1988) 'What was Foucault?' in J. Arac (ed.) *After Foucault: Humanistic Knowledge: Postmodern Challenges*, New Brunswick: Rutgers University Press.

O'Malley, P. (1983) *Law, Capitalism and Democracy*, Sydney: George Allen & Unwin.

Oxley, D. (1991) 'Women transported: gendered images and realities', *The Australian and New Zealand Journal of Criminology*, 24 (2): 83–98.

Palmer, J. and Pearce, F. (1983) 'Legal discourse and state power: Foucault and the juridical relation', *International Journal of the Sociology of Law*, 1 (4): 361–83.

Parisi, N. (1982) 'Are females treated differently?' in N. Rafter and E. A. Stanko (eds) *Judge, Lawyer, Victim, Thief: Women, Gender Roles and Criminal Justice*, Boston: Northeastern University Press.

Parker, D. (1987) 'The administration of justice and its penal consequences' in K. Hazlehurst (ed.) *Ivory Scales: Black Australia and the Law*, Sydney: University of New South Wales Press.

Pashukanis, E. (1978) *Law and Marxism: A General Theory*, London: Ink Links.

Pasquino, P. (1986) 'Michel Foucault (1926–84): the will to knowledge', *Economy and Society*, 15 (1): 97–109.

Patton, P. (1979) 'Of power and prisons' in M. Morris and P. Patton (eds) *Michel Foucault: Power, Truth, Strategy*, Sydney: Feral Publications.

Pearce, F. (1988) 'Review', *International Journal of the Sociology of Law*, 16 (2): 257–74.

Perrot, M. (1978) 'Delinquency and the penitentiary system in nineteenth-century France' in R. Forster and O. Ranum (eds) *Deviants and the Abandoned in French Society*, Baltimore: Johns Hopkins University Press.

Petchesky, R. P. (1981) 'At hard labour: penal confinement and production in nineteenth-century America' in G. F. Greenberg (ed.) *Crime and Capitalism: Readings in Marxist Criminology*, Palo Alto, Cal.: Mayfield.

Philips, D. (1983) '"A just measure of crime, authority, hunters and blue locusts": the "revisionist" social history of crime and the law in Britain, 1780–1850' in S. Cohen and A. Scull (eds) *Social Control and the State*, Oxford: Martin Robertson.

Platt, A. (1969) *The Child Savers: The Invention of Delinquency*, Chicago: University of Chicago Press.

Platt, A. and Takagi, P. (eds) (1980) *Punishment and Penal Discipline*, Berkeley: Crime and Social Justice Associates.

Poster, M. (1984) *Foucault, Marxism and History*, Cambridge, Polity Press.

—— (1989) *Critical Theory and Poststructuralism*, Ithaca: Cornell University Press.

Pratt, J. (1991) 'Punishment, history and empire', *The Australian and New Zealand Journal of Criminology*, 24 (2): 118–38.

Prisoners Action Group (1980) 'Submission to the Royal Commission into NSW Prisons', *Alternative Criminology Journal*, 3 (4).

Quinney, R. (1980) *Class, State and Crime*, New York: Longman.

Radzinowicz, L. and Hood, R. (1986) *History of English Criminal Law and its Administration from 1750: The Emergence of Penal Policy*, London: Stevens.

Rafter, N. (1980) 'Matrons and molls: the study of women's prison history' in J. A. Inciardi and C. E. Faupel (eds) *History and Crime: Implications for Criminal Justice Policy*, Beverly Hills: Sage.

—— (1982) 'Hard times: custodial prisons for women' in N. Rafter and E. Stanko (eds) *Judge, Lawyer, Victim, Thief*, Boston: Northeastern University Press.

—— (1983) 'Chastising the unchaste: social control functions of a women's reformatory, 1894–1931' in S. Cohen and A. Scull (eds) *Social Control and the State*, Oxford: Martin Robertson.

—— (1984) 'Review', *Contemporary Crises*, 8 (4): 388–9.

—— (1985a) *Partial Justice: Women in State Prisons, 1800– 1935*, Boston: Northeastern University Press.

—— (1985b) 'Gender, prisons and prison history', *Social Science History*, 9 (3): 233–47.

—— (1990) *Partial Justice: Women, Prisons and Social Control*, 2nd edition, New Brunswick, Transaction Publishers.

Ratner, R. S. (1986) 'Capital, state and criminal justice' in B. D. MacLean (ed.) *The Political Economy of Crime*, Scarborough: Prentice-Hall Canada.

Raulet, G. (1983) 'Structuralism and post-structuralism: an interview with Michel Foucault', *Telos*, 55: 195–211.

Ray, L. (1988) 'Foucault, critical theory and the decomposition of the historical subject', *Philosophy and Social Criticism*, 14: 69–110.

Rice, M. (1990) 'Challenging orthodoxies in feminist theory: a black feminist critique' in L. Gelsthorpe and A. Morris (eds) *Feminist Perspectives in Criminology*, Milton Keynes: Open University Press.

Riley, D. (1988) *Am I That Name? Feminism and the Category of 'Women'*, London: Macmillan.

Rothman, D. (1971) *The Discovery of the Asylum*, Boston: Little, Brown.

—— (1980) *Conscience and Convenience: The Asylum and its Alternatives in Progressive America*, Boston: Little, Brown.

—— (1983) 'Social control: the uses and abuses of the concept in the history of incarceration' in S. Cohen and A. Scull (eds) *Social Control and the State*, Oxford: Martin Robertson.

Rusche, G. (1978) 'Labour market and penal sanction: thoughts on the sociology of criminal justice', *Crime and Social Justice*, 10: 2–8.

—— (1980) 'Prison revolts or social policy lessons from America', *Crime and Social Justice*, 14: 41–4.

Rusche, G. and Kirchheimer, O. (1968) *Punishment and Social Structure*, New York: Russell & Russell.

Sargent, L. (ed.) (1981) *Women and Revolution: A Discussion of the Unhappy Marriage of Marxism and Feminism*, Boston: South End Press.

Sawicki, J. (1988) 'Feminism and the power of Foucauldian discourse' in J. Arac (ed.) *After Foucault: Humanistic Knowledge, Postmodern Challenges*, New Brunswick: Rutgers University Press.

Schumann, K. F. (1983) 'Comparative research on legal sanctions: problems and proposals', *International Journal of the Sociology of Law*, 11 (3): 267–76.

Schwartz, M. D. and DeKeseredy, W. S. (1991) 'Left realist criminology: strengths, weaknesses and the feminist critique', *Crime, Law and Social Change*, 15 (1): 51–72.

Schwartz, R. D. and Miller, J. C. (1964) 'Legal evolution and societal complexity', *American Journal of Sociology*, 70 (1): 159–69.

Scott, J. W. (1988a) 'Women's history' in J. W. Scott, *Gender and the Politics of History*, New York: Columbia University Press.

—— (1988b) 'Gender: a useful category of historical analysis' in J. W. Scott, *Gender and the Politics of History*, New York: Columbia University Press.

—— (1988c) 'Women in *The Making of the English Working Class*' in J. W. Scott, *Gender and the Politics of History*, New York: Columbia University Press.

—— (1992) '"Experience"' in J. Butler and J. W. Scott (eds) *Feminists Theorise the Political*, New York: Routledge.

Sedgwick, P. (1982) *Psycho Politics*, London: Pluto.

Shank, G. (1980) 'J. Thorsten Sellin's penology' in T. Platt and P. Takagi (eds) *Punishment and Penal Discipline*, Berkeley: Crime and Social Justice Associates.

Sheridan, A. (1980) *Michel Foucault: The Will to Truth*, London: Tavistock.

Simon, J. (1985) 'Review essay – back to the future: Newman on corporal punishment', *American Bar Foundation Research Journal*, 4: 927–41.

Smart, B. (1983a) 'On discipline and regulation: a review of Foucault's Genealogical Analysis' in D. Garland and P. Young (eds) *The Power to Punish*, London: Heinemann.

—— (1983b) *Foucault, Marxism and Critique*, London: Routledge.

—— (1986) 'The politics of truth and the problem of hegemony' in D. Couzens Hoy (ed.) *Foucault: A Critical Reader*, Oxford: Basil Blackwell.

Smart, C. (1976) *Women, Crime and Criminology*, London: Routledge.

—— (1989a) *Feminism and the Power of Law*, London: Routledge.

—— (1989b) 'Review of *Women, Crime and Poverty*' *Journal of Law and Society*, 16 (4): 521–4.

—— (1990) 'Feminist approaches to criminology or postmodern woman meets atavistic man' in L. Gelsthorpe and A. Morris (eds) *Feminist Perspectives in Criminology*, Milton Keynes: Open University Press.

—— (1992) 'The woman of legal discourse', *Social and Legal Studies*, 1 (1): 29–44.

Smart, C. and Smart, B. (1978) *Women, Sexuality and Social Control*, London: Routledge & Kegan Paul.

Smith, A. (1962) *Women in Prison*, London: Stevens.

Smith, D. (1987) *The Everyday World as Problematic: A Feminist Sociology*, Boston: Northeastern University Press.

Snyder, F. and Hay, D. (eds) (1987) *Labour, Law and Crime: An Historical Perspective*, London: Tavistock.

Spierenburg, P. (1984) *The Spectacle of Suffering*, Cambridge: Cambridge University Press.

Spitzer, S. (1975a) 'Punishment and social organisation: a study of Durkheim's theory of penal evolution', *Law and Society Review*, 9 (4): 613–37.

—— (1975b) 'Toward a Marxist theory of deviance', *Social Problems*, 22 (5): 638–51.

—— (1977) 'On the Marxist theory of social control: a reply to Horwitz', *Social Problems*, 24 (3): 364–6.

—— (1979) 'Notes towards a theory of punishment and social change', *Research in Law and Sociology*, 2: 207–29.

—— (1983) 'The rationalisation of crime control in capitalist society' in S. Cohen and A. Scull (eds) *Social Control and the State*, Oxford: Martin Robertson.

—— (1984) 'Review essay – the embeddedness of law: reflections on Lukes and Scull's *Durkheim and the Law*, *American Bar Foundation Research Journal*, 4: 859–68.

—— (1985) 'Review essay', *Criminology*, 23 (3): 575–82.

Spivak, G. (1988) 'Can the subaltern speak?' in C. Nelson and L. Grossberg (eds) *Marxism and the Interpretation of Culture*, London: Macmillan.

—— (1990a) 'The problem of cultural self-representation' in S. Harasym (ed.) *The Post-Colonial Critic: Interviews, Strategies, Dialogues*, New York: Routledge.

—— (1990b) 'Criticism, feminism and the institution' in S. Harasym (ed.) *The Post-Colonial Critic*, New York: Routledge.

—— (1990c) 'Questions of multi-culturalism' in S. Harasym (ed.) *The Post-Colonial Critic*, New York: Routledge.

Stearns, P. (1980) 'Towards a wider vision: trends in social history' in M. Kammen (ed.) *The Past Before Us: Contemporary Historical Writing in the United States*, Ithaca: Cornell University Press.

Stedman Jones, G. (1983) 'Class expression versus social control? A critique of recent trends in the social history of "leisure"' in S. Cohen and A. Scull (eds) *Social Control and the State*, Oxford: Martin Robertson.

Steffensmeier, D. J. (1980) 'Assessing the impact of the women's movement on sex-based differences in the handling of adult criminal defendants', *Crime and Delinquency*, 26 (3): 344–57.

Steinert, H. (1977) 'Against a conspiracy theory of criminal law a propos Hepburn's "social control and legal order"', *Contemporary Crises*, 1: 437–40.

—— (1983) 'The development of "discipline" according to Michel Foucault: discourse analysis versus social history', *Crime and Social Justice*, 20: 83–98.

Sumner, C. (1983) 'Rethinking deviance' in S. Spitzer (ed.) *Research in Law, Deviance and Social Control*, 5, Greenwich: JAI Press.

—— (1990) 'Foucault, gender and the censure of deviance' in L. Gelsthorpe and A. Morris (eds) *Feminist Perspectives in Criminology*, Milton Keynes: Open University Press.

Taylor, I., Walton, P. and Young, J. (1973) *The New Criminology*, London: Routledge & Kegan Paul.

Tomlins, C. (1985) 'Whose law? What order? Historicist interventions in the "war against crime"', *Law in Context*, 3: 130–47.

Tremblay, P. (1986) 'The stability of punishment: a follow-up of Blumstein's hypothesis', *Journal of Quantitative Criminology*, 2: 157–80.

Tyler, D. (1990) 'Going too far? The function of "Foucault" in recent feminist writing', Unpublished paper.

Van Swaaningen, R. (1989) 'Feminism and abolitionism as critiques of criminology', *International Journal of the Sociology of Law*, 17 (3): 287–306.

Wallace, D. (1980) 'The political economy of incarceration trends in late U.S. capitalism: 1971–1977', *Insurgent Sociologist*, 9: 59–65.

Ward, T. (1991) 'Review essay on *Prison under Protest*', *Social Justice*, 18 (3): 225–9.

Weedon, C. (1987) *Feminist Practice and Poststructuralist Theory*, Oxford: Basil Blackwell.

Wiener, M. (1987) 'The march of penal progress?', *The Journal of British Studies*, 26 (1): 83–96.

Wilf, S. (1989) 'Anatomy and punishment in late eighteenth-century New York', *Journal of Social History*, 22 (3): 507–30.

Wilkinson (1983) 'Review of *The Prison and the Factory*' *International Journal of the Sociology of Law*, 11 (4): 437–40.

Wolfgang, M. E. (1990) 'Crime and punishment in Renaissance Florence', *The Journal of Criminal Law and Criminology*, 81 (3): 567–84.

Worrall, A. (1990) *Offending Women: Female Lawbreakers and the Criminal Justice System*, London: Routledge.

Young, A. (1988) '"Wild women": the censure of the suffragette movement', *International Journal of the Sociology of Law*, 16 (3): 279–93.
—— (1990) *Femininity in Dissent*, London: Routledge.
Young, R. (1990) *White Mythologies: Writing History and the West*, London: Routledge.
Zdenkowski, G. and Brown, D. (1982) *The Prison Struggle*, Melbourne: Penguin.
Zedner, L. (1991) *Women, Crime and Custody in Victorian England*, Oxford: Clarendon Press.
Zingraff, M. and Thomson, R. (1984) 'Differential sentencing of Women and Men in the USA', *International Journal of the Sociology of Law*, 12 (4): 401–13.

Name index

Subject index